I0071941

A Medical Guide to Anesthesia

A Medical Guide to Anesthesia

Edited by Norman Tucker

hayle
medical

New York

Hayle Medical,
750 Third Avenue, 9th Floor,
New York, NY 10017, USA

Visit us on the World Wide Web at:
www.haylemedical.com

© Hayle Medical, 2019

This book contains information obtained from authentic and highly regarded sources. Copyright for all individual chapters remain with the respective authors as indicated. All chapters are published with permission under the Creative Commons Attribution License or equivalent. A wide variety of references are listed. Permission and sources are indicated; for detailed attributions, please refer to the permissions page and list of contributors. Reasonable efforts have been made to publish reliable data and information, but the authors, editors and publisher cannot assume any responsibility for the validity of all materials or the consequences of their use.

ISBN: 978-1-63241-536-3

Trademark Notice: Registered trademark of products or corporate names are used only for explanation and identification without intent to infringe.

Cataloging-in-Publication Data

A medical guide to anesthesia / edited by Norman Tucker.
    p. cm.
Includes bibliographical references and index.
ISBN 978-1-63241-536-3
1. Anesthesia. 2. Anesthesiology. I. Tucker, Norman.
RD82 .M44 2019
617.96--dc23

Table of Contents

Preface..IX

Chapter 1 **Accurate Measurement of Intraoperative Blood Loss Improves Prediction of Postoperative Hemoglobin Levels**..1
Robert L Thurer, Jose Muniz Castro, Mazyar Javidroozi, Kimberly Burton and Nicole P Bernal

Chapter 2 **Anesthetic Considerations for Management of Cancer Patients to Decrease Cancer Recurrence**..8
Krzysztof Laudanski, Rose Wei and Linda Korley

Chapter 3 **Assessment of Dental Students' Cardiopulmonary Resuscitation Knowledge and Experience in Turkey**..13
Aysun Caglar Torun

Chapter 4 **Bacteriological Aspects of Late Pneumonia in Ventilated Patient in Intensive Care Units: A Single Center Study in Morocco**..17
Frikh Mohammed, Abdelhay Lemnouer, Nabil Alem, Adil Maleb and Mostafa Elouennass

Chapter 5 **Break Through Inspiration During IPPV is Seen as "Curare Crest" in Sevograph**...............22
Mukesh Tripathi, Sanjay Kumar, Nilay Tripathi and Mamta Pandey

Chapter 6 **Clipping versus Coiling for Intracranial Aneurysms: Recent Trends**.............................26
Catarina Barbosa Petiz and Humberto S Machado

Chapter 7 **Combined Thoracic Epidural with General Anesthesia *vs.* General Anesthesia Alone for Major Abdominal Surgery: Anesthetic Requirements and Stress Response**..36
Alaa M Atia and Khaled A Abdel-Rahman

Chapter 8 **Comparative Study between General and Spinal Anaesthesia in Laparoscopic Appendectomy**..42
Ahmed Medhat Ahmed Mokhtar Mehanna and Atteia Gad Ibrahim

Chapter 9 **Comparative Study between Intravenous Ketamine and Lidocaine Infusion in Controlling of Refractory Trigeminal Neuralgia**...47
Mona Mohamed Mogahed, Atteia Gad Anwar and Rabab Mohamed Mohamed

Chapter 10 **Comparison between General Anesthesia and Epidural Anesthesia in Inguinal Herniorrhaphy Regarding the Incidence of Urinary Retention**...55
Seyed Mohammad Mireskandari, Kasra Karvandian, Yashar Iranpour, Sanaz Shabani, Afshin Jafarzadeh, Shahram Samadi, Jalil Makarem, Negar Eftekhar and Jayran Zebardast

Chapter 11   **Comparison of Different Bupivacaine and Fentanyl Combinations When used with a Single Shut Spinal Block for Labor Analgesia**..**59**
Aslan Bilge, Arıkan Müge, Gedikli Ahmet, Kısa Karakaya Burcu and
Moraloğlu Özlem

Chapter 12   **Comparison of the Effectiveness of Unimodal Opioid Analgesia with Multimodal Analgesia in the Management of Postoperative Pain in Patients Undergoing Surgery under Spinal Anesthesia-Double Blind Study**..**62**
Madhu Mala, Prabha Parthasarathy and Raghavendra Rao

Chapter 13   **Controlled Hypotensive Anesthesia in Children Undergoing Nasal Surgery**............................**69**
Sabry Mohamed Amin, Mohamed Gamal Elmawy and Rabab Mohamed Mohamed

Chapter 14   **Determination of the Effects of Sevoflurane Anesthesia in Different Maturing Stages of the Mouse Hippocampus by Transcriptome Analysis**..**77**
Tomo Hayase, Shunsuke Tachibana and Michiaki Yamakage

Chapter 15   **Dexamethasone as an Additive to Low Volume Interscalene Plexus Blockade: A Randomized Controlled Study**..**83**
Andreas Liedler, Benedikt Sattler, Ingo Zorn, Christian Fohringer,
Sabine Ottenschlager, Herbert Steininger and Christoph Hormann

Chapter 16   **Dexmedetomidine as an Adjuvant to Bupivacaine in Supraclavicular Brachial Plexus Block**..**89**
Rajesh Meena, Sandeep Loha, Arun Raj Pandey, Kavita Meena, Anil Kumar Paswan,
Lalita Chaudhary and Shashi Prakash

Chapter 17   **Dexmedetomidine *vs.* Magnesium Sulphate as an Adjuvant to Rocuronium Bromide, and Local Anaesthetic Mixture in Peribulbar Anaesthesia for Viteroretinal Surgery**..**95**
Mona Mohamed Mogahed, Wessam Mohamed Nassar and Mohamed Ali Abdullah

Chapter 18   **Does the Type of Anesthesia for Caesarean Section Affect the Neonate? A Non-Randomized Observational Study Comparing Spinal versus General Anesthesia**..**103**
Reena Nayar, Jui Lagoo and Chandra Kala

Chapter 19   **Effect of Different Doses of Dexmedetomidine on Stress Response and Emergence Agitation after Laparoscopic Cholecystectomy: Randomized Controlled Double-Blind Study**..**108**
Mohamed F Mostafa, Ragaa Herdan, Mohammed Yahia Farrag Aly and
Azza Abo Elfadle

Chapter 20   **Effect of Heparin Flush in Blood Drawn from Arterial Line on Activated Clotting Time and Thromboelastogram**..**114**
Amit Lehavi, Vitaliy Borissovski, Avishay Zisser and Yeshayahu (Shai) Katz

Chapter 21   **Effects of Types of Anesthesia on Neurobehavioral Response and Apgar Score in Neonates Delivered with Cesarean Section in Dilla University Referral Hospital**............................**117**
Semagn Mekonnen and Kokeb Desta

Chapter 22   **Efficacy and Safety of Dexamethasone as an Adjuvant to Local Anesthetics in Lumbar Plexus Block in Patients Undergoing Arthroscopic Knee Surgeries**............................**125**
Bassant M Abdelhamid, Inas Elshzly, Sahar Badawy and Ayman Yossef

Chapter 23   **Enhanced Recovery after Surgery Pathway: How its Implementation Influenced Digestive Surgery Outcomes?**..132
Carolina Tintim and Humberto S Machado

Chapter 24   **Evaluation of TEE Training for Chinese Anesthesiology Residents using Two Various Simulation Systems**..142
Fei Liu, Fu S Lin, Yong G Peng, Li Liu, Massimiliano Meineri, Hai B Song and Jin Liu

Chapter 25   **Evaluation of USG Guided Transversus Abdominis Plane Block for Post-Operative Analgesia in Total Abdominal Hysterectomy Surgeries**...............................146
Natesh Prabu, Alok Kumar Bharti, Ghanshyam Yadav, Vaibhav Pandey, Yashpal Singh, Anil Paswan, Bikram Kumar Gupta and Dinesh Kumar Singh

Chapter 26   **Fluid Optimization in Liver Surgery**..150
Levantesi Laura, Oggiano Marco, Fiorini Federico, Sessa Flaminio, De Waure Chiara, Congedo Elisabetta and De Cosmo Germano

Chapter 27   **Heart Rate Variability in Children Submitted to Surgery**....................................154
Marta Joao Silva, Raquel Pinheiro, Rute Almeida, Francisco Cunha, Augusto Ribeiro, Ana Paula Rocha and Hercília Guimaraes

Chapter 28   **History and Evolution of Anesthesia Education in United States**...........................164
Mian Ahmad and Rayhan Tariq

Chapter 29   **Optimal Timing for the Initiation of Enteral Feeding in Neonates with Gastroschisis, Depending on Non-Invasive Doppler Ultrasound Evaluation of Hemodynamics in the Bowel Wall Arteries**..173
OV Teplyakova, EA Filippova, YL Podurovskaya, AV Pyregov, VV Zubkov, AA Burov, EI Dorofeeva and MI Pykov

Chapter 30   **Anesthetic and Analgesic Effect of Neostigmine when Added to Lidocaine in Intravenous Regional Anesthesia**..179
Alaa Mohammed Atia and Khaled Abdel-Baqy Abdel-Rahman

Chapter 31   **A Comparative Study of Effect of Propofol, Etomidate and Propofol Plus Etomidate Induction on Hemodynamic Response to Endotracheal Intubation: A RCT**...183
Kavita Meena, Rajesh Meena, Sudhansu Sekhar Nayak, Shashi Prakash and Ajit Kumar

Chapter 32   **A Cross-Sectional Study Evaluating the GuardianCPV™ Supraglottic Airway Device in a Clinical Setting**...189
Michael Hua-Gen Li, Howard Ho-Fung Tang, Celestine Johnny Bouniu and Jun Keat Chan

Chapter 33   **A Comparative Evaluation of General Anesthesia versus Spinal Anesthesia Combined with Paravertebral Block for Renal Surgeries: A Randomized Prospective Study**..196
Ahmed Eldaba and Sabry Mohamed Amin

Permissions

List of Contributors

Index

Preface

It is often said that books are a boon to mankind. They document every progress and pass on the knowledge from one generation to the other. They play a crucial role in our lives. Thus I was both excited and nervous while editing this book. I was pleased by the thought of being able to make a mark but I was also nervous to do it right because the future of students depends upon it. Hence, I took a few months to research further into the discipline, revise my knowledge and also explore some more aspects. Post this process, I begun with the editing of this book.

Anesthesia is a state that is characterized by a temporary loss of sensation and awareness. It facilitates the execution of painful medical procedures that can cause severe distress and pain to the patient. Anesthesia is classified into three categories namely, general anesthesia, sedation and local anesthesia. Drugs that are used in anesthesia include general anesthetics, neuromuscular-blocking drugs, analgesics, sedatives, narcotics and hypnotics. The types and degree of anesthesia vary depending upon the medical procedure to be performed. This book aims to shed light on some of the unexplored aspects of anesthesia and the recent researches in this field. From theories to research to practical applications, case studies related to all contemporary topics of relevance to anesthesia have been included herein. This book is appropriate for students seeking detailed information in this area as well as for experts.

I thank my publisher with all my heart for considering me worthy of this unparalleled opportunity and for showing unwavering faith in my skills. I would also like to thank the editorial team who worked closely with me at every step and contributed immensely towards the successful completion of this book. Last but not the least, I wish to thank my friends and colleagues for their support.

Editor

Accurate Measurement of Intraoperative Blood Loss Improves Prediction of Postoperative Hemoglobin Levels

Robert L Thurer[1*], Jose Muniz Castro[2], Mazyar Javidroozi[3], Kimberly Burton[4] and Nicole P Bernal[4]

[1]*Gauss Surgical Inc., Los Altos, CA, USA*

[2]*Department of General Surgery, Houston Methodist Hospital, Houston, TX, USA*

[3]*Englewood Hospital and Medical Center, Englewood, NJ, USA*

[4]*University of California, Irvine School of Medicine, Irvine, CA, USA*

*Corresponding author:** Robert L Thurer, Gauss Surgical Inc., Los Altos, CA, USA, E-mail: rthurer@gmail.com

Abstract

Background: Restrictive red cell transfusion is preferable to liberal transfusion in most clinical situations. However, intraoperative transfusion decisions are challenging due to uncertainty about the amount and rate of bleeding, the poor correlation of hemoglobin levels with blood loss and the effects of anesthetics on blood volume and physiologic responses. Clinicians frequently use hemoglobin levels to guide transfusion. While these "triggers" assume that the patient is normovolemic, they are often applied in situations confounded by hemodilution or hemoconcentration. We postulated that accurate measurement of surgical blood loss would facilitate prediction of postoperative hemoglobin levels, potentially leading to more accurate intraoperative transfusion decisions.

Methods: Using image-processing algorithms, a novel system accurately measures blood loss by photographing surgical sponges and canisters and calculating their hemoglobin content. A formula to predict postoperative hemoglobin levels was devised and used to calculate postoperative hemoglobin levels in a study group of 167 burn and other wound excision procedures performed on 103 patients using the system. In an historical group (100 similar procedures, 60 patients) clinician estimates of blood loss were used. These predictions were compared with actual values.

Results: The formula using measured blood loss in the study group was a better predictor of the actual postoperative day one hemoglobin value (R^2=0.822) than was the same formula using visually estimated blood loss used in the historical group (R^2=0.615). The mean absolute bias of postoperative day one hemoglobin levels in the study group was significantly lower than the mean bias in the historical group (study=group, mean 0.4, 95% CI 0.2 to 0.5 g/dL; historical group, mean 0.9, 95% CI 0.7 to 1.2 g/dL, p<0.001).

Conclusion: Blood loss measurements using the novel system are a significantly better predictor of hemoglobin values obtained after surgery than traditional blood loss estimates.

Keywords: Hemodilution; Blood loss; Surgical blood transfusion

Introduction

Restrictive red cell transfusion is preferable to liberal transfusion in most clinical situations [1-3]. Published guidelines support the use of predefined restrictive hemoglobin levels to determine the need for transfusion [4,5]. While these guidelines can be useful in normovolemic non-bleeding patients where the hemoglobin level may closely reflect the red cell mass, intraoperative transfusion decisions are more challenging. Changes in blood volume due to anesthetic agents, fluid administration, insensible losses, positioning, temperature and other factors leads to poor correlation between the measured hemoglobin and decreased red cell mass from surgical blood loss [6-8]. Moreover, both the amount and rate of bleeding are difficult to estimate leaving surgeons and anesthesiologists with little meaningful data to help decide whether a red cell transfusion is appropriate [9-11].

Ideally, red cell transfusions would be given only when there is the need to improve oxygen delivery to vital organs and other tissues.

When the patient is normovolemic, the hemoglobin level and arterial oxygen saturation, combined with clinical evaluation, can be used to estimate oxygen delivery and guide transfusion. However, since intraoperative hemoglobin values can be confounded by hemodilution, hemoconcentration or volume redistribution, accurate contemporaneous measurement of surgical blood loss could provide the surgical team with the information they need not only to control bleeding but could also lead to more informed transfusion decisions than those based primarily on the hemoglobin concentration [7].

A recently introduced, FDA-cleared device that measures blood loss on surgical sponges and in suction canisters may provide useful, real-time information to guide surgical and anesthetic care. The performance of the device has been validated in bench-top and clinical settings [12-14]. To demonstrate the utility of this device, we postulated that accurate measurement of operative blood loss would facilitate prediction of postoperative hemoglobin levels following restoration of normovolemia. If this were the case, these contemporaneous measurements could be used in conjunction with knowledge of the patient's clinical condition and preoperative hemoglobin level to guide transfusion decisions during and immediately following surgical procedures.

Materials and Methods

The protocol was approved by the IRB (HS#: 2015-2418) at the University of California, Irvine School of Medicine. As a retrospective chart review, the requirement for written informed consent for this study was waived by the IRB. Procedures in adult patients with a baseline weight ≥ 50 kg having burn and other wound excisions before (January 2014 to November 2014; n=100 procedures, 60 patients; historical group) and after (November, 2014 to January, 2016; n=167 procedures, 103 patients; study group) the introduction of the blood loss measurement system were analyzed retrospectively. Since the hemoglobin levels related to a procedure could affect levels during subsequent procedures on the same patient, subsequent surgeries taking place less than five days from the previous intervention were excluded. The five day period was chosen since the investigator's typical policy was to wait until a patient had hemodynamically and physiologically recovered from one surgical intervention before proceeding with a subsequent excision. It is likely that the five day period coupled with hemodynamic stability prior to each procedure would minimize the effect one procedure might have on a subsequent one.

The novel FDA-cleared mobile application (Triton System™, Gauss Surgical, Inc., Los Altos, CA) on a tablet computer (iPad) was used to measure surgical blood loss. Using the enabled tablet camera, the application captures images of surgical sponges and employs image analysis algorithms (Feature Extraction Technology™) and cloud-based machine learning to accurately estimate hemoglobin mass on the surgical laparotomy sponges in real time (Figure 1). The technology can also measure the hemoglobin content of fluid collected in surgical suction canisters. The accuracy of the method is not affected by the admixture of irrigation or other fluids or the ambient lighting condition [13].

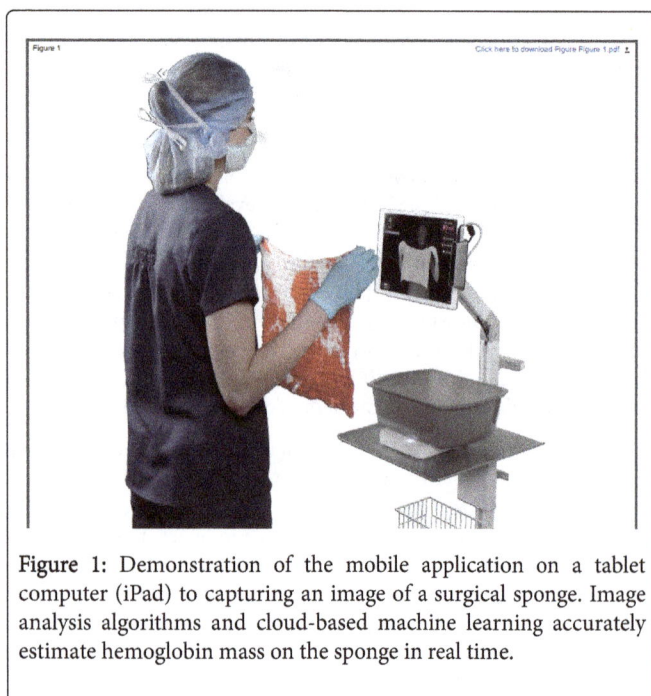

Figure 1: Demonstration of the mobile application on a tablet computer (iPad) to capturing an image of a surgical sponge. Image analysis algorithms and cloud-based machine learning accurately estimate hemoglobin mass on the sponge in real time.

In the historical group (system not used) a visual estimation of blood loss was determined by consensus between the attending surgeon and anesthesiologist. Estimates were typically based on the size of the excised area and observed bleeding. In the study group, all surgical sponges were collected during the procedure and scanned with the system to capture images of the sponges. This resulted in a measured amount of hemoglobin loss per sponge that was converted to a volumetric measure using the patient's pre-procedure hemoglobin value. The operating team attempted to capture all blood loss using surgical sponges. Surgical suction was not used for these procedures so scanning of and estimation of the blood collected in surgical suction canisters was not performed.

Data extracted from the patient's medical records included date of surgery, patient age (years), total body surface area (BSA) (meters^2), total size of burn or wound (% BSA), size of wound excised (cm^2), visually estimated blood loss (in the historical group) (ml) and hemoglobin concentrations (g/dl) preoperatively, immediately following surgery and on postoperative days one, two and three when available. All packed red cell (PRBC) and component transfusions (units) given from the day of surgery through postoperative day two were documented. Measurements of blood loss (ml) on surgical sponges was recorded when the system was used.

A simplified formula to predict postoperative hemoglobin levels was devised and used to calculate hemoglobin levels on postoperative days one, two and three following each surgical procedure for which the patient's baseline weight, preoperative hemoglobin and transfusion data were obtained. These predictions were compared with the actual values when available.

The formula assumed a blood volume of 70 ml/kg body weight [15]. It was also assumed that each transfused unit raised the hemoglobin level by 1 g/dl [16]. Using these assumptions, the predicted postoperative hemoglobin (g/dl) (PPOHgb) is calculated as follows:

PPOHgb (g/dl)=Preop Hgb (g/dl)-((EBL (ml)/(70 × weight (kg))) × Preop Hgb (g/dl))+1 × transfused units

Preop Hgb is the preoperative hemoglobin (g/dl) and EBL is the estimated blood loss (ml), which was obtained from the visual estimate recorded in the chart in the historical group, and the system's measured blood loss in the study group. In this formula, the hemoglobin loss is calculated as a fraction of the blood volume lost multiplied by the preoperative hemoglobin. The number of transfused units given prior to the measurement of the particular postoperative hemoglobin value is included.

Statistical analysis

Data are provided as mean (95% confidence intervals) and frequency (%). Univariate comparisons were performed using chi square, Fisher's exact, Student t-test, or Mann-Whitney U-test as appropriate. The main study endpoint was the bias between the predicted and actual post-operative Day 1 hemoglobin level. Association between the actual and predicted postoperative hemoglobin values were evaluated using scatter plots and further analyzed using linear regression models to obtain the unstandardized and standardized correlation coefficients with corresponding confidence intervals. Further subgroup analyzes were performed depending on whether any red cell transfusions were received or not at any time during the day of surgery. Agreement between the predicted and actual postoperative hemoglobin values was also characterized using the Bland-Altman method by calculating the bias (predicted minus actual values) and limits of agreement (bias ± 1.96 × standard deviation) with corresponding confidence intervals as previously described [17]. A p value of 0.05 or less was considered to be statistically significant. Based on the preliminary studies, it was expected that the absolute bias of postoperative day 1 hemoglobin would be half a standard deviation smaller than the historical group. To detect such a difference using t-test with alpha of 0.05 and power of 90%, 85 subjects were needed per group. This sample size was further adjusted to 99 per group by dividing it by 0.864 according to the Pitman Asymptomatic Relative Efficiency (ARE) method to make it independent of underlying distribution. This number was considered as the minimum sample size needed and additional eligible subject were added if records were available. All analyses were performed using SPSS (SPSS Inc., Chicago, IL).

Results

Characteristics of the historic and study cohorts are provided in Table 1.

	Historic Group (N=100)	Study Group (N=167)	P Value
Age at time of surgery (years)	50.2 (46.4 to 53.9)	46.8 (44.0 to 49.5)	0.148
Weight at admission (Kg)	82.2 (77.5 to 86.8)	85.8 (82.1 to 89.4)	0.231
Case type:			
Burn excision	57 (57.0%)	103 (61.7%)	0.449
Other wound excision	43 (43.0%)	64 (38.3%)	0.449
Total burn/wound surface area (% of total body surface area)	12.6 (8.6 to 16.6)	13.8 (10.1 to 17.4)	0.666
Total area excised:			
Area (cm^2)	923 (608 to 1238)	782 (643 to 921)	0.418
% of total body surface area	4.8 (3.1 to 6.4)	4.0 (3.2 to 4.7)	0.379
Estimated blood loss (mL)	215 (157 to 273)	351 (286 to 417)	0.002
Hemoglobin levels (g/dL):			
Preoperative	10.4 (9.9 to 10.8) N=100	10.5 (10.1 to 10.9) N=167	0.564
Postoperative same day	9.5 (8.7 to 10.2) N=26	9.8 (9.4 to 10.3) N=62	0.35
Postoperative Day 1 (N=100 & 167)	9.6 (9.2 to 10.0) N=100	10.0 (9.6 to 10.3) N=167	0.204
Postoperative Day 2	8.9 (8.4 to 9.3) N=48	9.1 (8.7 to 9.4) N=78	0.482
Postoperative Day 3	9.4 (8.9 to 9.9) N=61	9.2 (8.8 to 9.6) N=74	0.454
Patients transfused red blood cells			
Preoperative same day	4 (4.0%)	6 (3.6%)	1
Intraoperative	22 (22.0%)	39 (23.4%)	0.799
Postoperative same day	3 (3.0%)	1 (0.6%)	0.149
Postoperative Day 1	9 (9.0%)	6 (3.6%)	0.063
Postoperative Day 2	6 (6.0%)	7 (4.2%)	0.563
Any postoperative	18 (18.0%)	14 (8.4%)	0.0199
Any perioperative	33 (33.0%)	51 (30.5%)	0.675

Table 1: Characteristics of historic and study groups. Ranges are 95% confidence intervals.

The formula using measured blood loss in the study group (n=167) was a better predictor of the actual postoperative day one hemoglobin value (R^2=0.822) than was the same formula using visually estimated blood loss used in the historical group (n=100) (R^2=0.615). Additionally, the mean absolute bias of postoperative Day 1 hemoglobin level in the study group was statistically significantly lower than the mean bias of the historical group (mean 0.4, 95% CI 0.2 to 0.5 g/dL in Study and 0.9, 95% CI 0.7 to 1.2 g/dL in Historical group, p<0.001). Cases that had red cell transfusion at any time during the day of surgery (historical group=27, study group=43) and those cases that did not have red cell transfusion on the day of surgery (historical group=73, study group=124) were also analyzed separately. For each of these subgroups, the measured blood loss in the study group was similarly more predictive of actual values (Table 2). This is graphically demonstrated for the transfused subgroup (Figures 2 and 3).

	Historical Group	Study Group	P Value
All Procedures	**N=100**	**N=167**	
PPOHgb bias (g/dl)	0.9 (0.7 to 1.2)	0.4 (0.2 to 0.5)	<0.001
Lower limit of agreement (g/dl)	-1.6 (-2.1 to -1.2)	-1.5 (-1.8 to -1.3)	
Upper limit of agreement (g/dl)	3.5 (3.0 to 3.9)	2.2 (2.0 to 2.5)	
Correlation, R	0.784 (0.695 to 0.849)	0.906 (0.875 to 0.929)	
Procedures with Operative Day Transfusion	**N=27**	**N=43**	
PPOHgb Bias (g/dl)	1.6 (1.0 to 2.2)	0.5 (0.2 to 0.7)	0.001
Lower limit of agreement (g/dl)	-1.3 (-2.3 to -0.3)	-1.1 (-1.5 to -0.7)	
Upper limit of agreement (g/dl)	4.5 (3.5 to 5.5)	2.0 (1.6 to 2.4)	
Correlation, R	0.559 (0.228 to 0.774)	0.734 (0.557 to 0.847)	
Procedures without operative day transfusion	**N=73**	**N=124**	
PPOHgb Bias (g/dl)	0.7 (0.4 to 0.9)	0.3 (0.1 to 0.5)	0.027
Lower limit of agreement (g/dl)	-1.6 (-2.0 to -1.1)	-1.6 (-2.0 to -1.3)	

Upper limit of agreement (g/dl)	2.9 (2.4 to 3.4)	2.3 (2.0 to 2.6)	
Correlation, R	0.844 (0.762 to 0.899)	0.906 (0.869 to 0.933)	

Table 2: Prediction of hemoglobin level on post-operative day 1. Ranges are 95% confidence intervals.

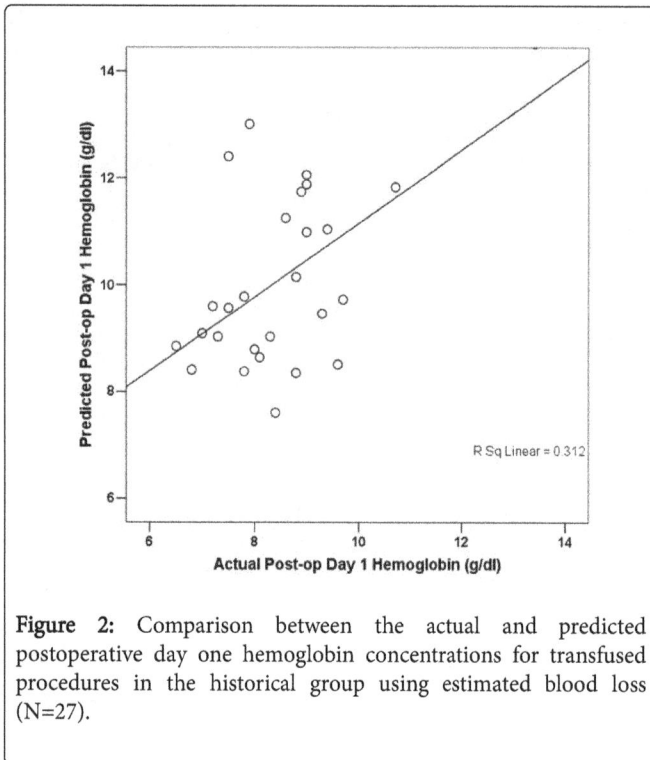

Figure 2: Comparison between the actual and predicted postoperative day one hemoglobin concentrations for transfused procedures in the historical group using estimated blood loss (N=27).

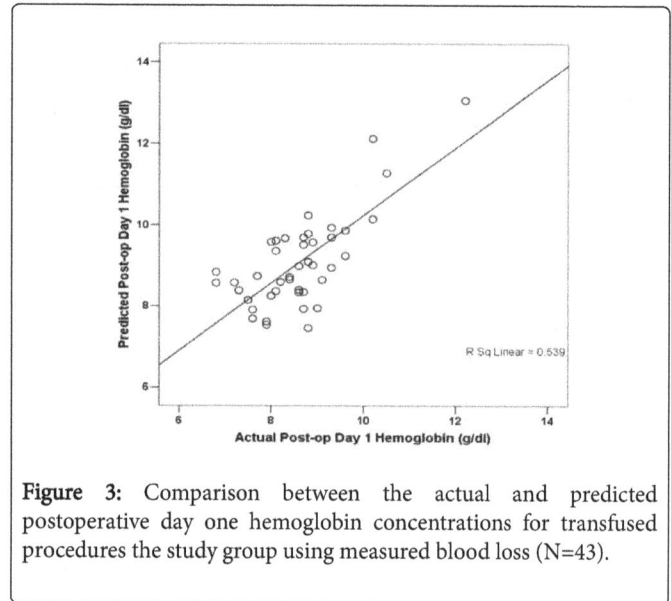

Figure 3: Comparison between the actual and predicted postoperative day one hemoglobin concentrations for transfused procedures the study group using measured blood loss (N=43).

	Historical Group	Study Group	P Value
All Procedures	**N=48**	**N=78**	
PPOHgb Bias (g/dl)	1.5 (1.1 to 1.9)	0.6 (0.3 to 0.9)	<0.001
Lower limit of agreement (g/dl)	-1.2 (-1.9 to -0.5)	-2.0 (-2.5 to -1.5)	
Upper limit of agreement (g/dl)	4.3 (3.6 to 5.0)	3.2 (2.7 to 3.7)	
Correlation, R	0.619 (0.407 to 0.768)	0.686 (0.547 to 0.788)	
Procedures with transfusion prior to POD 2	**N=27**	**N=32**	
PPOHgb Bias (g/dl)	2.0 (1.4 to 2.6)	1.1 (0.6 to 1.7)	0.038
Lower limit of agreement (g/dl)	-1.1 (-2.2 to 0.0)	-1.6 (-2.5 to -0.7)	
Upper limit of agreement (g/dl)	5.1 (4.0 to 6.2)	3.9 (3.0 to 4.8)	
Correlation, R	0.314 (-0.074 to 0.62)	0.608 (0.330 to 0.789)	
Procedures without transfusion prior to POD 2	**N=21**	**N=46**	
PPOHgb Bias (g/dl)	0.9 (0.5 to 1.3)	0.2 (-0.1 to 0.6)	0.017
Lower limit of agreement (g/dl)	-0.7 (-1.3 to 0.0)	-2.0 (-2.6 to -1.4)	
Upper limit of agreement (g/dl)	2.5 (1.9 to 3.1)	2.5 (1.9 to 3.0)	
Correlation, R	0.907 (0.782 to 0.962)	0.785 (0.641 to 0.875)	

Table 3: Prediction of hemoglobin level on post-operative day 2. Ranges are 95% confidence intervals.

	Historical Group	Study Group	P Value

Postoperative day two hemoglobin values were available for 48 procedures in the historical group (31 transfused either on the day of surgery or on the first postoperative day) and 78 procedures in the study group (46 transfused). For the entire group and for subgroup of cases according to transfusion up to day 1, the bias of predictions using measured blood loss versus the actual hemoglobin was smaller in the study group compared with the historical group. However, the correlation between the predicted and actual day 2 hemoglobin was stronger in transfused subset of cases in study group and untransfused subset cases in historical group (Table 3).

Postoperative day three hemoglobin values were available for 61 patients in the historical group (27 transfused) and 74 patients in the study group (35 transfused). For the transfused subgroups and the groups as a whole, the measured blood loss in the study group was a better predictor of actual postoperative day three hemoglobin values (indicated by smaller bias) than the traditionally estimated blood loss, but the difference in bias was not significant in the subgroup of cases without transfusion (Table 4).

All procedures	N=61	N=74	0.028
PPOHgb Bias (g/dl)	1.2 (0.8 to 1.7)	0.6 (0.3 to 0.9)	
Lower limit of agreement (g/dl)	-2.2 (-3.0 to -1.4)	-2.0 (-2.5 to -1.5)	
Upper limit of agreement (g/dl)	4.7 (3.9 to 5.5)	3.3 (2.7 to 3.8)	
Correlation, R	0.519 (0.308 to 0.681)	0.729 (0.601 to 0.820)	
Procedures with transfusion prior to POD 3	N=27	N=35	
PPOHgb Bias (g/dl)	2.2 (1.4 to 2.9)	1.1 (0.6 to 1.6)	0.016
Lower limit of agreement (g/dl)	-1.6 (-2.9 to -0.3)	-1.9 (-2.8 to -1.0)	
Upper limit of agreement (g/dl)	6.0 (4.6 to 7.3)	4.1 (3.2 to 5.0)	
Correlation, R	0.174 (-0.220 to 0.519)	0.436 (0.121 to 0.671)	
Procedures without transfusion prior to POD 3	N=34	N=39	
PPOHgb Bias (g/dl)	0.5 (0.1 to 0.9)	0.2 (-0.1 to 0.5)	0.28
Lower limit of agreement (g/dl)	-1.9 (-2.7 to -1.2)	-1.8 (-2.4 to -1.2)	
Upper limit of agreement (g/dl)	2.9 (2.2 to 3.7)	2.2 (1.6 to 2.8)	
Correlation, R	0.800 (0.634 to 0.895)	0.872 (0.768 to 0.931)	

Table 4: Prediction of hemoglobin level on post-operative day 3. Ranges are 95% confidence intervals.

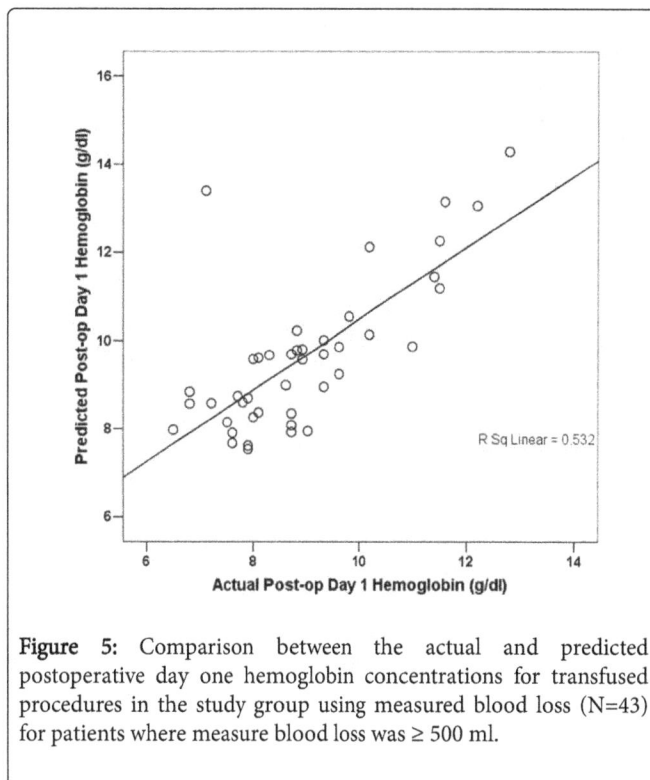

Figure 4: Comparison between the actual and predicted postoperative day one hemoglobin concentrations for transfused procedures in the Historical Group using estimated blood loss (N=15) for patients where estimated blood loss was ≥ 500 ml.

Interestingly, of the 167 procedures in the study group, 43 (25.7%) had a measured blood loss of 500 ml or greater. In the historical group the estimated blood loss equaled or exceeded 500 ml in only 15 of the 100 cases (15%). In these higher blood loss cases, the predicted postoperative day one hemoglobin value using the measured blood loss in the study group was more closely correlated with the actual value (R=0.729) than was the same prediction using the estimated blood loss in the historical group (R=0.421) (Figures 4 and 5).

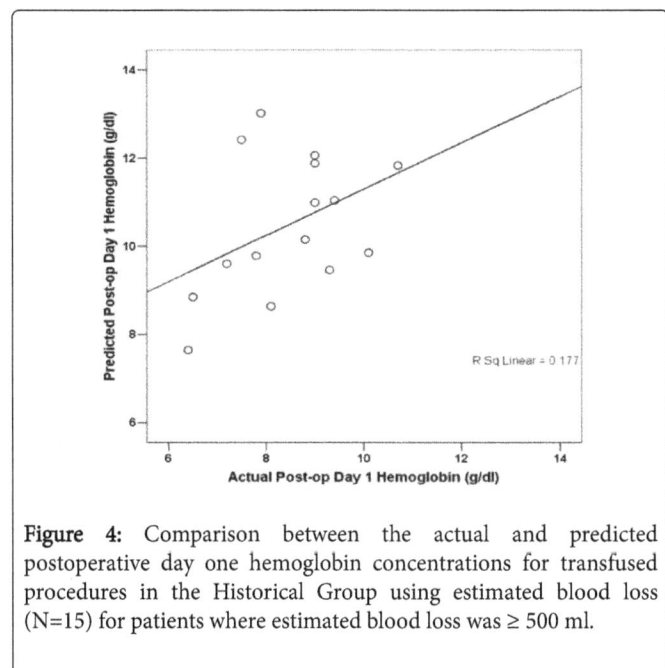

Figure 5: Comparison between the actual and predicted postoperative day one hemoglobin concentrations for transfused procedures in the study group using measured blood loss (N=43) for patients where measure blood loss was ≥ 500 ml.

Discussion

Transfusion of allogeneic red cells is a costly medical procedure with potentially serious adverse consequences [18,19]. Restrictive red cell transfusion policies are recommended since they help avoid unneeded transfusions, conserve the limited blood resource and save money while resulting in similar or better outcomes than more liberal policies [1-5]. However, the inability to accurately determine the extent of blood loss makes it difficult to appropriately manage surgical bleeding. Moreover, transfusion decision-making during and immediately following surgery is problematic not only because of the difficulty in accurately assessing blood loss, but also because of the potential for sudden substantial bleeding and the inaccuracy of the hemoglobin level in reflecting red cell mass. On one hand, evidence-based practice clearly favors limiting transfusions while, conversely, transfusion avoidance can result in inadequate oxygen delivery to vital organs and resultant morbidity and mortality. While visual estimates of surgical blood loss can theoretically be used to keep track of red cell mass, these determinations are known to be inaccurate [10].

Accurate, contemporaneous measurement of surgical bleeding could potentially alleviate these problems by providing surgeons and anesthesiologists with real-time data that, when combined with relevant clinical information, could improve transfusion decisions and overall surgical and anesthetic management. Other methods of obtaining this information including training in visual estimation and gravimetric methods that involve weighing of surgical sponges have been investigated, but are inadequate [20,21]. While the system used in this study is accurate, the clinical relevance of the measurements obtained have not been previously evaluated.

This study demonstrates that the blood loss measurements from the novel system are a much better predictor of hemoglobin values obtained in the first three days after surgery than are traditional blood loss estimates. This confirms the relative inaccuracy of hemoglobin values in the setting of fluctuating blood volume and supports the contention that measured blood loss is more accurate than hemoglobin values in guiding transfusion therapy for patients during and immediately following surgery.

During standard clinical care, many clinicians practice transfusion avoidance intraoperatively and then transfuse postoperatively based on predetermined, evidence-based hemoglobin values. This strategy is problematic since it may lead to under or over transfusion during the most critical periods of surgical instability. Furthermore, most patients are in positive fluid balance postoperatively and experience an initial downward "hemoglobin drift" followed by recovery as this fluid is mobilized. These variations can result in hemoglobin changes of greater than 2 g/dl that occur over several days despite a stable red cell mass, making reliance on hemoglobin values alone a poor strategy [7]. Ideally, clinicians would estimate preoperative red cell mass based on the patient's weight and preoperative hemoglobin level and determine the amount of tolerable blood loss taking into account the clinical situation. Accurate measurement of surgical blood loss would then allow for indicated transfusion at the most appropriate time.

Another consideration is the cost of a transfusion episode [22]. The increased need for nursing resources associated with transfusions given outside of the operating room or recovery area, make those transfusions more costly. Therefore, if a transfusion is indicated, it is best given during or immediately following surgery for both clinical and economic reasons.

This study may be of limited value since it was done in only in procedures involving burn or other wound excisions. These patients were selected since they often have substantial blood loss and the surgical blood loss is readily captured on surgical sponges. The applicability of the system to other patient populations needs further study. Another limitation is that the study was not randomized and retrospectively compared historical data to a novel intervention. However, this approach helped to eliminate any confounding of the visual estimations that could have occurred if the device was introduced using a prospective randomized study design (provider "learning curve"). Furthermore, there were no patients treated between the end of the historical group and the introduction of the system, and the participating clinicians made no other changes in their clinical care. While further studies are needed, the novel device studied accurately measures blood loss and can potentially provide useful, real-time information to guide surgical and anesthetic care.

Acknowledgment

None.

Disclosures

Robert L. Thurer and Mazyar Javidrozzi are paid consultants to Gauss Surgical Inc. and they participated in study design, data analysis and manuscript preparation. No financial support was provided to the University of California Irvine School of Medicine or to the other investigators.

Funding

Gauss Surgical, Inc., Los Altos, CA provided assistance with study design, data analysis and manuscript preparation. The company provided no other support. There were no other funding sources.

References

1. Hebert PC, Wells G, Blajchman MA, Marshall J, Martin C, et al. (1999) A multicenter, randomized, controlled clinical trial of transfusion requirements in critical care. N Engl J Med 340: 409-417.

2. Carson JL, Terrin ML, Noveck H, Sanders DW, Chaitman BR, et al. (2011) Liberal or restrictive transfusion in high-risk patients after hip surgery. N Engl J Med 365: 2453-2462.

3. Villanueva C, Colomo A, Bosch A, Concepción M, Hernandez-Gea V, et al. (2003) Transfusion strategies for acute upper gastrointestinal bleeding. N Engl J Med 368: 11-21.

4. American Society of Anesthesiologists Task Force on Perioperative Blood Management (2015) Practice guidelines for perioperative blood management: an updated report by. Anesthesiology 122: 241-275.

5. Carson JL, Guyatt G, Heddle NM, Grossman BJ, Cohn CS, et al. (2016) Clinical practice guidelines from the AABB: red blood cell transfusion thresholds and storage. JAMA 316: 2025-2035.

6. Valeri CR, Dennis RC, Ragno G, Macgregor H, Menzoian JO, et al. (2016) Limitations of the hematocrit level to assess the need for red blood cell transfusion in hypovolemic anemic patients. Transfusion. 46: 365-371.

7. Grant MC, Whitman GJ, Savage WJ, Ness PM, Frank SM (2014) Clinical predictors of postoperative hemoglobin drift. Transfusion 54: 1460-1468.

8. Berkow L, Rotolo S, Mirski E (2011) Continuous noninvasive hemoglobin monitoring during complex spine surgery. Anesth Analg 113: 1396-1402.

9. Meiser A, Casagranda O, Skipka G, Laubenthal H (2001) Quantification of blood loss. How precise is visual estimation and what does its accuracy depend on? Anaesthesist 50: 13-20.

10. Rothermel LD, Lipman JM (2016) Estimation of blood loss is inaccurate and unreliable. Surgery 160: 946-953.

11. Guinn NR, Broomer BW, White W, Richardson W, Hill SE (2013) Comparison of visually estimated blood loss with direct hemoglobin measurement in multilevel spine surgery. Transfusion 53: 2790-2794.

12. Holmes AA, Konig G, Ting V, Philip B, Puzio T, et al. (2014) Clinical evaluation of a novel system for monitoring surgical hemoglobin loss. Anesth Analg 119: 588-594.

13. Konig G, Holmes AA, Garcia R, Mendoza JM, Javidroozi M, et al. (2014) In vitro evaluation of a novel system for monitoring surgical hemoglobin loss. Anesth Analg 119: 595-600.

14. Sharareh B, Woolwine S, Satish S, Abraham P, Schwarzkopf R (2015) Real time intraoperative monitoring of blood loss with a novel tablet application. Open Orthop J 9: 422-426.

15. http://ether.stanford.edu/calc_mabl.html.

16. Thurer RL, Katz RS, Parce P, Precopio T, Popovsky MA (2010) By how much does a single unit transfusion increase the recipient's hemoglobin? Transfusion 50: 135A.

17. Bland JM, Altman DG (1986) Statistical methods for assessing agreement between two methods of clinical measurement. Lancet 1: 307-310.

18. Murphy GJ, Reeves BC, Rogers CA, Rizvi SI, Culliford L, et al. (2007) Increased mortality, postoperative morbidity, and cost after red blood cell transfusion in patients having cardiac surgery. Circulation 27: 2544-2552.

19. Hofmann A, Ozawa S, Farrugia A, Farmer SL, Shander A (2013) Economic considerations on transfusion medicine and patient blood management. Best Pract Res Clin Anaesthesiol 27: 59-68.

20. Toledo P, Eosakul ST, Goetz K, Wong CA, Grobman WA (2013) Decay in blood loss estimation skills after web-based didactic training. Simul Healthc 7: 18-21.

21. Johar RS, Smith RP (1993) Assessing Gravimetric Estimation of Intraoperative Blood Loss. J Gynecol Surg 9: 151-154.

22. Participants of the Cost of Blood Consensus Conference (2015) The cost of blood: multidisciplinary consensus conference for a standard methodology. Transfus Med Rev 19: 66-78.

23. Stefano G, Kream RM, Mantione KJ, Sheehan M, Cadet P, et al. (2008) Endogenous morphine/nitric oxide-coupled regulation of cellular physiology and gene expression: implications for cancer biology. Semin Cancer Biol 18: 199-210.

24. Cadet P, Rasmussen M, Zhu W, Tonnesen E, Mantione KJ, et al. (2004) Endogenous morphinergic signaling and tumor growth. Front Biosci 9: 3176-3186.

25. Tegeder I, Grosch S, Schmidtko A, Haussler A, Schmidt H, et al. (2003) G protein-independent G1 cell cycle block and apoptosis with morphine in adenocarcinoma cells: involvement of p53 phosphorylation. Cancer Res 63: 1846-1852.

26. Tsujikawa H, Shoda T, Mizota T, Fukuda K (2009) Morphine induces DNA damage and P53 activation in CD3+ T cells. Biochim Biophys Acta 1790: 793-799.

2

Anesthetic Considerations for Management of Cancer Patients to Decrease Cancer Recurrence

Krzysztof Laudanski*, Rose Wei and Linda Korley

Hospital of University of Pennsylvania, Philadelphia, USA

***Corresponding author:** Krzysztof Laudanski, Assistant Professor of Anesthesiology and Critical Care, Hospital of University of Pennsylvania, 3400 Spruce Street, Philadelphia, PA 19104, USA, E-mail: klaudanski@gmail.com

Abstract

Alongside the known direct, short-term effects of anesthesia in general, there is emerging evidence of an immunomodulatory effect with specific anesthetics that may decrease patient's defences against malignant neoplastic growths. This effect is especially important in the setting of surgical management of neoplasms, which is often the best option for long-term survival in patients with solid neoplasm. Many studies have speculated on the best anesthetic technique to reduce the neoplasm recurrence and promote patient survival, however, we often neglect the sympathetic stress response to neoplasia and how anesthetics modulate this effect. In this review, we study the evidence as it pertains to anesthetic techniques and pain control, particularly general vs. regional anesthesia, and opioid analgesia. At this time there is not enough evidence to support that regional anesthesia has a more favorable outcome than general anesthesia, or that opioids should not be used in neoplasm-related pain management because of their potential pro-metastatic properties secondary to opioid-induced immunosuppression. Instead, the debate over anesthetic use should be centered on adequate pain control since overwhelming evidence have shown that pain-related stress reaction mediated via β-adrenergic activation, promotes neoplastic propagation and metastasis, hence decreasing survival rates.

Keywords: Cancer; Anesthetics

Introduction

The use of anesthetics is commonplace in the perioperative setting for sedation, amnesia, analgesia, and immobilization. Alongside the known direct effects of anesthesia in general, there is emerging evidence of an immunomodulatory effect with specific anesthetics that may decrease host defenses against neoplastic growth. Analyzing the effect of the anesthesia on tumor growth, its propensity to metastasize, and its recurrence is an interesting idea that brings about new implications to a seemingly straight forward, routine anesthesia delivery. However, to study this potential long-term effect of anesthesia is complicated and difficult in methodology. Cancer recurrence is multifactorial, and the incidence of recurrence can vary substantially based upon the type of cancer, stage and grade at diagnosis, biologic characteristics of the tumor, initial treatment modalities, and host immune function. The ability of the immune system to restrict, and possible to eradicate neoplastic growth is especially significant in the setting of surgical management, which is often the best option for long-term survival in patients with solid tumors. Surgical resection, however, can inherently promote cancer metastasis or recurrence by the inadvertent release of tumor cells and humoral factors into the circulation and the normal surgical stress response may lead to metabolic and neuroendocrine changes that further inhibit host defenses against the implantation of circulating tumor cells [1,2]. Preservation of host immune function in the perioperative and intraoperative setting can lead to better patient outcomes and the minimization of risks, analogous to pre-operative optimization of any surgical patient. However, modulation of immune function has been shown to be influenced by anesthetic technique. This was demonstrated in *in vivo* and *in vitro*, in both manual models and with the utilization of the human species but the vast majority of the studies focused on modulation of the short-term immunological responses by anesthetic techniques or compounds. However, it is unclear how these results translate into long-term outcome. The study of patient outcomes with different anesthetic techniques can be challenging, yet it may be essential to cause a change of practice in the surgical management of oncology patients. Here, we review most recent studies and attempt to chart a potential way in which anesthesia can modulate immune response in the long-term time frame via modulation of the sympathetic system. First, we will examine the effects of regional versus general anesthesia on the growth and recurrence of neoplasms.

The Effect of General Anesthesia on Cancer Recurrence

Wigmore et al. published a study in 2015 comparing mortality rates over 3 years after elective surgery in a comprehensive cancer center. In a retrospective analysis, they compared mortality after cancer surgery in more than 7,000 patients given volatile general anesthesia (INHA) or total intravenous anesthesia (TIVA) [3]. Patients in the TIVA group received sedation with propofol and remifentanil, while patients in the volatile anesthetic group received either sevoflurane or isoflurane, along with an adjunct opioid at the anesthesiologist's discretion. Variables included patient's age at the time of procedure, severity of malignancy, tumor site and group, intraoperative transfusion of blood products, severity of surgery, sex, height and weight, and the use of epidural analgesia, as these are all potentially confounding. The study by Wigmore et al. cannot estimate the effect of opioids since most the enrolled individuals received opioids. Such an effect would be difficult to estimate since medical provider had freedom to use to use different opioids in one arm versus remifentanil in another arm of the study. Perhaps the most significant limitation of the study is the uneven distribution of patients with more favorable prognosis and lack of the tumor staging data. The patients who were expected to have better prognosis, such as breast cancer patients, had a lower proportion in the inhaled volatile anesthetic group [3].

Interestingly, results showed that the mortality was approximately 50% greater with volatile than with IV anesthesia, with an adjusted hazard ratio of 1.46 (1.29 to 1.66), no matter their ASA score, surgical severity, or whether the patient had metastasis at the time of the procedure [3]. The study, as with many studies of this nature, showed an association but not causation between the type of anesthetic delivered and survival rates. There is a need for further large and prospective studies to investigate this association, as well as the expansion of laboratory and animal studies to explore the possible biological mechanism. This study in particular, suggests the differential effect of volatile anesthetics versus TIVA on tumor progression, and potential implications of their effect on the immune system in the perioperative period [3].

Inherited limitations of the study by Wigmore et al. are difficult to overcome in a rigorous fashion. However, his observations are well aligned with studies from more than four decades ago, when the association between volatile anesthetics and neoplasm progression was first observed. Lundy et al. proposed that the combination of halothane, surgery and immunosuppression increased pulmonary metastases in mice inoculated with tumor cells [4]. Shapiro et al. found that lung tumor progression was accelerated in mouse models when exposed to halothane and nitrous oxide [5]. There are no human studies on the isolated effect of volatile anesthetics on tumor spread and metastasis. Nevertheless, since inhaled anesthetics have direct and indirect effects on different aspects of the immune response, it is reasonable to assert that they are important actors in postoperative immunosuppression and residual malignant cell migration and invasion.

Interestingly, recent evidence shows oxidative DNA damage induced by isoflurane in elective surgery suggesting that inhalation anesthesia could potentially trigger tumor growth. Coincidently, Musak et al. showed that healthcare personnel exposed to volatile anesthetics exhibit higher frequency of chromosomal damage [6]. These findings imply direct carcinogenic effects of inhaled anesthetic agents, making the issue of perioperative tumor progression an even more complex matter.

The Effect of Regional Anesthesia on Cancer Recurrence

In a retrospective study using patient's medical records, Exadaktylos et al. compared recurrence rates in breast cancer patients undergoing mastectomy and axillary clearance/ simple complete mastectomy [7]. One group received a combined general and paravertebral anesthetic while the general anesthesia group received GA and patient controlled analgesia with morphine. Recurrence or metastasis was documented in 3 of 50 patients (6%) in the paravertebral group and in 19 of 79 patients (24%) in the general anesthesia group throughout the follow-up period. A Kaplan-Meier analysis was used to adjust for the varied duration of follow-up for each patient. The study showed that the paravertebral group had longer time to recurrence (P=0.013) Furthermore, in a multivariable analysis adjusting for histologic grade and axillary node involvement, recurrence risk proved significantly less in the paravertebral group [7]. Despite showing interesting and provocative result selection bias and a small sample size are severe limitation of this study. Biki et al. addressed the issue of the effect of

epidural anesthesia/analgesia on cancer recurrence after radical prostatectomy [8]. This retrospective review showed that the epidural plus general anesthesia group had a 57% (95 CI, 17-78%) lower risk of recurrence compared with the general anesthesia plus opioid group. However, the results of study can be difficult to translate considering incomplete information provided by authors in regards to clinical protocol [8]. There is no mention of the quantitative postoperative opioid requirement. It is unclear how many individuals patients dropped off the study, or was not qualified in the first place weakening the validity of this study. Though the evidence provided by Biki et al. is not enough to change practice; nonetheless, it remains as an important study as it encouraged other authors to design prospective studies to clarify the cause-effect relationship between anesthetic technique and cancer recurrence.

Unfortunately, recent literature review do not support uniformly the idea that regional anesthesia is superior to general anesthesia [9]. Wuethrich et al. published a retrospective study of 148 patients with prostate cancer, concluding that general anesthesia combined with epidural analgesia did not reduce the risk of cancer progression or improve survival after radical prostatectomy after 14 years of observation [10]. The main strength of this study was the prolonged follow-up time of 14 years. Conclusions are limited since no power or error estimations were done. Also, as in any retrospective study, selection bias cannot be excluded. Finally, the general anesthesia group included ketorolac in the analgesic regimen. It has been shown that ketorolac, by its action on the enzyme cyclooxygenase-2, may suppress neoplasm relapse [11]. It is possible that this effect could have influenced the results. In a similar study, Tsui et al. performed a secondary analysis on 99 patients undergoing radical prostatectomy, who had participated in a previous randomized controlled trial evaluating pain control, blood loss, and transfusion. They found no difference between epidural and control groups in terms of disease free survival after a follow-up time of 4.5 years [12]. Among the 99 patients, 22 were lost to follow-up. Biochemical markers of neoplastic recurrence was detected in 31% of epidural patients compared to 40% of general anesthesia patients, with a hazard ratio of 1.3 slightly favoring general anesthesia, but with a 95% confidence interval of 0.6-2.7. Despite randomization, the fact that the study was originally designed for different endpoints renders the study conclusion of the study somewhat limited [12]. Again, the authors call for design of larger prospective trials.

Regional has widely been studied as an alternate and arguably safer anesthetic technique in cancer patients. This is based on the concept of regional anesthesia decreasing or preventing the surgical stress response [13]. Such a stress is perceived as inducing immuno-inhibition or immuno-suppression thus theoretically can contribute to progression of the neoplasm. Regional anesthesia also decreases the need for perioperative opioids, which are believed to have a pro-tumoral effect [14,15]. In addition, studies on bupivacaine suggest that it has direct anti-neoplastic properties via activation of both intrinsic and extrinsic apoptotic pathways in ovarian cancer and the intrinsic pathway in prostate cancer [16]. Still, confounding evidence must be taken into account. Although regional anesthesia can be perceived more favorable than general anesthesia based other studies, there is a predilection in selecting patients for regional anesthesia secondary to their frailty or perceiving patient with widespread disease as better suited for general anesthesia [17]. This significantly biased the results. In fact, once confounders are controlled, studies by Cakmakkaya et al. showed no evidence of improved tumor recurrence and evidence by Cata et al. showed no evidence of prolonged cancer survivall [7,18].

Mechanism Favoring Type of Anesthesia and Cancer Recurrence

Long-term effect of opioids on neoplasm progression

Post-operatively, opioids are a common choice for pain management in cancer patients. Although the immunosuppressive effect of opioids has been widely documented, some reports argue that opioids' immunomodulatory effects may be beneficial in the context of malignancy [16-18]. The effects of opioids on neoplasia progression likely depend on the extent of their analgesic action, counterbalancing their immunomodulatory effect by decreasing acute pain and attenuating the stress response. Here, we review the confounding evidence for opioid effect on malignancy, which should illustrate the urgency of further studies in humans, comparing patient outcomes with and without opioid use for cancer pain. Intentionally, we will not focus on the direct effects of opioids on immunosuppression since this subject has been reviewed many times [19,20].

Opioids effect on neoplasm survival: Morphine has been the most widely studied opioid with regards to cancer recurrence. It has been found that peripheral opioid receptors help modulate cell proliferation and apoptosis [21,22]. In vitro studies have shown the pro-apoptotic action of morphine on cancer cells by different mechanisms including inhibition of NF-κB via nitric oxide [23,24] whereas other studies have shown inhibition of apoptotic processes via p53, a key factor in programmed cell death [25-27]. These findings are somewhat conflicting with data showing an inhibitory effect of morphine tumor cell proliferation in vitro [28-31].

Opioids for acute pain: Treatment of postoperative pain with opioids has been shown to reduce cancer recurrence, despite their potential prometastatic effect [32]. Recognizably, it is difficult to ascertain the independent effect of acute postoperative pain on tumor progression, as it overlaps with the bimodal effect of opioids. It is likely that the stimulating effect of opioids on tumor cells is only evident in the absence of acute pain [19]. Unfortunately there is a lack of studies evaluating the impact of chronic pain on cancer recurrence due to the obvious limitation of such studies.

Other perioperative considerations

These are outlined in order to acknowledge other ways anesthesiologists can modify neoplasia progression. Although beyond the scope of this review, we hope to use this data to map out comprehensive anesthetic planning to improve outcomes in cancer patients.

Blood transfusion: Theoretically, transfusion-associated immunomodulation (TRIM) is the driving force behind allogeneic blood transfusion related tumor recurrence. This is related to the widely studied immunosuppressive effects of allogeneic blood and the modulation of WBCs in allogenic vs. autologous transfusions [33]. A study investigating patients undergoing resection of gastric cancer randomized patients to allogeneic or autologous transfusion. IFNγ, T-helper cell, and T-helper/cytotoxic T-cell ratio were reduced in both groups after operation but the suppression was most profound in the allogeneic transfusion group. Five days after the operation, levels had returned to baseline for patients receiving autologous transfusions but remained suppressed in the allogeneic group [34]. Studies on this effect are controversial and remain inconclusive, as current literature does not clearly correlate TRIM with cancer recurrence [33,34].

Perioperative use of β-blockers: It became almost a common practice to use of β-blockers in patients undergoing anesthesia due to the cardiovascular-related issues [35]. However, some studies investigated the effect of pharmacological β-blockade on neoplastic growth. Two studies have shown less distant metastases in patients with prostate and lung cancer [35,36]. In the breast cancer subgroup, evidence strongly suggests a favorable benefit in the use of B-blockers for the reduction of long-term cancer recurrence in particular [37,38]. This was attributed to the attenuation of the natural stress response with β-blockade, resulting in diminished interleukin release during the initial phase of neoplastic seeding. These studies, however, are all retrospective in nature. Stronger blinded randomized trials combined with therapeutic intervention offer better evidence to prompt a change in practice.

The most popular proposed mechanism in which the adrenergic pathway affects tumor progression is via the stress responses, which is correlated with release of adrenergic hormones linked to NK cell suppression, enhanced tumor retention, and perioperative immunosuppression [39,40]. Human studies have shown that patients with depressed NK cell function have higher cancer incidence and metastatic disease after excisional surgery suggesting that this acute, or short-term suppression, can be translated into long-term effect [39,41-43]. Consequently, diminishing the adrenergic pathway, particularly via B-adrenergic inhibition, has been shown to block progression of stress-induced tumors [44,45]. These findings have to be separated from the effect of B-adrenergic agonists itself, which has also been shown to stimulate malignant cell proliferation.

Recently, a paper by Chang et al. 2015 highlighted the importance of chronic stress as a physiological regulator of neural-tumor interactions, and how that microenvironment drives the progression of pancreatic cancer, particularly through B-adrenergic receptor signalling. He has demonstrated that stress on mice, in terms of repeated restraints, changes in cage composition, sound stress, resulted in systemic increase in epinephrine and adrenal gland enlargement as well as pancreatic tumor volume [46]. In fact, majority of pancreatic cancer cell lines and its stromal cells in its vicinity, including macrophages, endothelial cells, and fibroblasts express β-adrenergic receptors. They have even demonstrated that isoproterenol, a non-selective β-adrenergic receptor agonist, increased pancreatic cancer cell proliferation in vitro! More importantly, it increased Panc-1 type pancreatic tumor cells' basement membrane invasion in a dose-dependent manner, and these effects were blocked with propranolol, a B-blocker. When exposed to norepinephrine, tumor's expression of matrix metalloproteinases (MMPs), an enzyme that degrades the extracellular matrix, is upregulated. Similar to the upregulation of MMPs as a tumor grows in grade. Inhibiting β-adrenergic signaling to pancreatic cancer cells induced apoptosis by suppressing the Ras/Akt/NFκB signaling pathway [47,48]. Similar findings were also reported in studies of hemangioma, neuroblastoma, melanoma and gastric cancer [49-52]. Chang et al. go as far as to support the use of β-blockers as a possible novel therapeutic intervention, but that claim must be utilized with caution, as recent studies by Wang et al. stated that B2 adrenergic stimulation with norepinephrine has actually attenuated invasion of certain types of breast CA's migration [53]. Thus despite overwhelming evidence that B-adrenergic stress responses is pro-cancerous, there is still need to quantify the exact types of cancers that are amenable to this type of therapy.

Hypothermia: Current literature suggests that hypothermia stimulates a stress response and glucocorticoid release augmenting immunosuppressive effects. Thus, hypothermia could be mechanistically linked to neoplastic recurrence in a similar fashion as the use of β-blockers. Although further studies in humans are needed, animal studies show that a temperature of 30.8°C suppresses NK cell activity and also suppresses resistance to neoplastic metastasis [54]. Similarly, mild hypothermia has been shown to exacerbate immunosuppression in abdominal surgeries of non-cancer patients [55]. Further studies of could elucidate whether a change in intraoperative body temperature management would provide better patient outcomes after surgical resection of the neoplasm.

How Optimal Management of Anesthesia can Impact Patient Recovery from Neoplasm

How we should modify our anesthetic plan to improve outcomes for cancer patients will continue to be a difficult debate. This debate also touches on the issue of future of our profession in both clinical importance and academic development. As indicated above, multiple studies have attempted to answer this question by looking at specific anesthetics or anesthetic procedure types and their immunomodulatory outcomes. In hopes to answer how we should modify anesthetic plan to diminish cancer recurrence or propagation, one thing is clear- a proper balance has to be established. As written above, not only does the anesthetic type matter, but also the mode in which these anesthetic are implemented, for example whether via general or regional, should be considered in how it translates to cancer outcome. Unfortunately, most studies have been retrospective trials, and these studies are subject to some confounders. Although regional anesthesia seems to be better than general anesthesia as implicated before, cancer patients who were designated to receive general rather than regional anesthesia may have more tumors that needed to be excised, which correlates to the extent of cancer metastasis and so higher cancer severity and poorer outcomes already.

In conclusion, there is still not enough evidence to make a definitive anesthetic plan for cancerous patients to diminish cancer recurrence or propagation. However, some broad statements can be drawn- first, opioids should be avoided except in acute pain, and if an opioid is utilized morphine rather than fentanyl is preferred. Obviously the type of surgery and the length of anesthetic requirements are still going to largely dictate the type of anesthetic use, prospective studies with these variables held constant while comparing morphine versus fentanyl use would be helpful. Second, there is still no significant difference in regional versus general anesthetic modalities found in prospective studies, even though overwhelming retrospective studies have shown otherwise. At this time, the type of anesthetic modality a cancer patient receives should depend on which modality or even modalities will offer the best pain control during and after surgery. And the stresses of pain causing catecholamine release and subsequent cancer progression via the B-adrenergic pathway is much more validated.

References

1. Baum M, Demicheli R, Hrushesky W, Retsky M (2005) Does surgery unfavourably perturb the "natural history" of early breast cancer by accelerating the appearance of distant metastases? Cancer 41: 508-515.

2. Ben-Eliyahu S (2003) The promotion of tumor metastasis by surgery and stress: immunological basis and implications for psychoneuroimmunology. Brain Behav Immun 1: S27-36.

3. Wigmore TJ, Mohammed K, Jhanji S (2016) Long-term Survival for Patients Undergoing Volatile versus IV Anesthesia for Cancer Surgery: A Retrospective Analysis. Anesthesiology 124: 69-79.

4. Lundy J, Lovett EJ 3rd, Hamilton S, Conran P (1978) Halothane, surgery, immunosuppression and artificial pulmonary metastases. Cancer 41: 827-830.

5. Shapiro J, Jersky J, Katzav S, Feldman M, Segal S (1981) Anesthetic drugs accelerate the progression of postoperative metastases of mouse tumors. J Clin Invest 68: 678-685.

6. Musak L, Smerhovsky Z, Halasova E, Osina O, Letkova L, et al. (2013) Chromosomal damage among medical staff occupationally exposed to volatile anesthetics, antineoplastic drugs, and formaldehyde. Scan J Work Env. Health 39: 618-630.

7. Exadaktylos AK, Buggy DJ, Moriarty DC, Mascha E, Sessler DI (2006) Can anesthetic technique for primary breast cancer surgery affect recurrence or metastasis? Anesthesiology 105: 660-664.

8. Biki B, Mascha E, Moriarty DC, Fitzpatrick JM, Sessler DI, et al. (2008) Anesthetic technique for radical prostatectomy surgery affects cancer recurrence: a retrospective analysis. Anesthesiology. Anesthesiology 109; 180-187.

9. Daley MD, Norman PH (2009) Retrospective but not rigorous. Anesthesiology 111: 203.

10. Wuethrich P, Thalmann G, Studer U, Burkhard F (2013) Epidural Analgesia during Open Radical Prostatectomy Does Not Improve Long-Term Cancer-Related Outcome: A Retrospective Study in Patients with Advanced Prostate Cancer. PLoS One 8: e72873.

11. Retsky M, Rogers R, Demicheli R, Hrushesky WJ, Gukas I, et al. (2012) NSAID analgesic ketorolac used perioperatively may suppress early breast cancer relapse: particular relevance to triple negative subgroup. Breast Cancer Res Treat 134: 881-888.

12. Tsui BC, Rashiq S, Schopflocher D, Murtha A, Broemling S, et al. (2010) Epidural anesthesia and cancer recurrence rates after radical prostatectomy. Can J Anaesth 57: 107-112.

13. Yamaguchi K, Takagi Y, Aoki S, Futamura M, Saji S (2000) Significant detection of circulating cancer cells in the blood by reverse transcriptase-polymerase chain reaction during colorectal cancer resection. Ann Surg 232: 58-65.

14. Sessler DI (2010) Regional anesthesia and prostate cancer recurrence. Can J Anaesth 57: 99-102.

15. Page G (2005) Acute pain and immune impairment. Pain Clin Updat 13: 1-4.

16. Xuan W, Zhao H, Hankin J, Chen L, Yao S, et al. (2016) Local anesthetic bupivacaine induced ovarian and prostate cancer apoptotic cell death and underlying mechanisms in vitro. Sci Rep 6: 26277.

17. Cakmakkaya OS, Kolodzie K, Apfel CC, Pace NL (2014) Anaesthetic techniques for risk of malignant tumour recurrence. Cochrane Database Syst Rev : CD008877.

18. Cata J, Hernandez M, Lewis V, Kurz A (2014) Can regional anesthesia and analgesia prolong cancer survival after orthopaedic oncologic surgery? Clin Orthop Relat Res 472: 1434-1441.

19. Page GG, Ben-Eliyahu S, Liebeskind JC (1994) The role of LGL/NK cells in surgery-induced promotion of metastasis and its attenuation by morphine. Brain Behav Immun 8: 241-250.

20. Beilin B, Martin FC, Shavit Y, Gale RP, Liebeskind JC (1989) Suppression of natural killer cell activity by high-dose narcotic anesthesia in rats. Brain Behav Immun 3: 129-137.

21. McLaughlin PJ, Zagon IS (2012) The opioid growth factor-opioid growth factor receptor axis: homeostatic regulator of cell proliferation and its implications for health and disease. Biochem Pharmacol 84: 746-755.

22. Spirkoski J, Melo FR, Grujic M, Calounova G, Lundequist A, et al. (2012) Mast cell apoptosis induced by siramesine, a sigma-2 receptor agonist. Biochem Pharmacol 84: 1671-1680.

23. Stefano G, Kream RM, Mantione KJ, Sheehan M, Cadet P, et al. (2008) Endogenous morphine/nitric oxide-coupled regulation of cellular physiology and gene expression: implications for cancer biology. Semin Cancer Biol 18: 199-210.

24. Cadet P, Rasmussen M, Zhu W, Tonnesen E, Mantione KJ, et al. (2004) Endogenous morphinergic signaling and tumor growth. Front Biosci 9: 3176-3186.

25. Tegeder I, Grosch S, Schmidtko A, Haussler A, Schmidt H, et al. (2003) G protein-independent G1 cell cycle block and apoptosis with morphine in adenocarcinoma cells: involvement of p53 phosphorylation. Cancer Res 63: 1846-1852.

26. Tsujikawa H, Shoda T, Mizota T, Fukuda K (2009) Morphine induces DNA damage and P53 activation in CD3+ T cells. Biochim Biophys Acta 1790: 793-799.

27. Yin D, Woodruff M, Zhang Y, Whaley S, Miao J, et al. (2006) Morphine promotes Jurkat cell apoptosis through pro-apoptotic FADD/P53 and anti-apoptotic PI3K/Akt/NF-kappaB pathways. J Neuroimmunol 174: 101-107.

28. Qin Y, Chen J, Li L, Liao CJ, Liang YB, et al. (2012) Exogenous morphine inhibits human gastric cancer MGC- 803 cell growth by cell cycle arrest and apoptosis induction. Asian Pac J Cancer Prev 13: 1377-1382.

29. Gach K, Wyrebska A, Fichna J, Janecka A (2011) The role of morphine in regulation of cancer cell growth. Naunyn Schmiedebergs Arch Pharmacol 384: 221-230.

30. Chen YL, Law PY, Loh HH (2008) The other side of the opioid story: modulation of cell growth and survival signaling. Curr Med Chem 15: 772-778.

31. Yeager MP, Colacchio TA (1991) Effect of morphine on growth of metastatic colon cancer in vivo. Arch Surg 126: 454-456.

32. Page GG, Ben-Eliyahu S, Yirmiya R, Liebeskind JC (1993) Morphine attenuates surgery-induced enhancement of metastatic colonization in rats. Pain 54: 21-28.

33. Weber RS, Jabbour N, Martin RC 2nd (2008) Anemia and transfusions in patients undergoing surgery for cancer. Ann Surg Oncol 15: 34-45.

34. Blajchman M (1999) Transfusion-associated immunomodulation and universal white cell reduction: are we putting the cart before the horse? Transfusion (Paris) 39: 665-670.

35. Grytli HH, Fagerland MW, Fosså SD, Taskén KA, Håheim LL (2013) Use of Î²-blockers is associated with prostate cancer-specific survival in prostate cancer patients on androgen deprivation therapy. Prostate 73: 250-260.

36. Wang HM, Liao ZX, Komaki R, Welsh JW, O'Reilly MS, et al. (2013) Improved survival outcomes with the incidental use of beta-blockers among patients with non-small-cell lung cancer treated with definitive radiation therapy. Ann Oncol 24: 1312-1319.

37. Barron TI, Connolly RM, Sharp L, Bennett K, Visvanathan K (2011) Beta blockers and breast cancer mortality: a population- based study. J Clin Oncol 29: 2635-2644.

38. Melhem-Bertrandt A, Chavez-Macgregor M, Lei X, Brown EN, Lee RT, et al. (2011) Beta-blocker use is associated with improved relapse-free survival in patients with triple-negative breast cancer. J Clin Oncol 29: 2645-2652.

39. Andersen BL, Farrar WB, Golden-Kreutz D, Kutz LA, MacCallum R, et al. (1998) Stress and immune responses after surgical treatment for regional breast cancer. J Natl Cancer Inst 90: 30-36.

40. Stefanski V, Ben-Eliyahu S (1996) Social confrontation and tumor metastasis in rats: defeat and beta-adrenergic mechanisms. Physiol Behav 60: 277-282.

41. Orange JS (2006) Human natural killer cell deficiencies. Curr Opin Allergy Clin Immunol 6: 399-409.

42. Liljefors M, Nilsson B, Hjelm Skog AL, Ragnhammar P, Mellstedt H, et al. (2003) Natural killer (NK) cell function is a strong prognostic factor in colorectal carcinoma patients treated with the monoclonal antibody 17-1A. Int J Cancer 105: 717-723.

43. Kondo E, Koda K, Takiguchi N, Oda K, Seike K, et al. (2003) Preoperative natural killer cell activity as a prognostic factor for distant metastasis following surgery for colon cancer. Dig Surg 20: 445-451.

44. Palm D, Lang K, Niggemann B, Drell TL 4th, Masur K, et al. (2006) The norepinephrine-driven metastasis development of PC-3 human prostate cancer cells in BALB/c nude mice is inhibited by beta-blockers. Int J Cancer 118: 2744-2749.

45. Cole SW, Sood AK (2012) Molecular pathways: beta-adrenergic signaling in cancer. Clin Cancer Res 18: 1201-1206.

46. Chang A, Kim-Fuchs C, Le CP, Hollande F, et al. (2015) Neural Regulation of Pancreatic Cancer: A Novel Target for Intervention. Cancers (Basel) 7: 1292-1312.

47. Zhang D, Ma Q, Shen S, Hu H (2009)) Inhibition of pancreatic cancer cell proliferation by propranolol occurs through apoptosis induction: The study of beta-adrenoceptor antagonist's anticancer effect in pancreatic cancer cell. Pancreas 38: 94-100.

48. Zhang D, Ma Q, Wang Z, Zhang M, Guo K, et al. (2011) β2-adrenoceptor blockage induces G1/S phase arrest and apoptosis in pancreatic cancer cells via Ras/Akt/NFκB pathway. Mol Cancer 10: 146.

49. Ji Y, Li K, Xiao X, Zheng S, Xu T, et al. (2012) Effects of propranolol on the proliferation and apoptosis of hemangioma-derived endothelial cells. J Pediatr Surg 47: 2216-2223.

50. Wolter JK, Wolter NE, Blanch A, Partridge T, Cheng L, et al. (2014) Anti-tumor activity of the beta-adrenergic receptor antagonist propranolol in neuroblastoma. Oncotarget 5: 161-172.

51. Wrobel LJ, Le Gal FA1 (2015) Inhibition of human melanoma growth by a non-cardioselective Î²-blocker. J Invest Dermatol 135: 525-531.

52. Liao X, Che X, Zhao W, Zhang D, Bi T, et al. (2010) The beta-adrenoceptor antagonist, propranolol, induces human gastric cancer cell apoptosis and cell cycle arrest via inhibiting nuclear factor kappa-b signaling. Oncol Rep 24: 1669-1676.

53. Wang T, Li Y, Lu HL, Meng QW, Cai L, et al. (2015) β-Adrenergic Receptors : New Target in Breast Cancer. Asian Pac J Cancer Prev 16: 8031-8039.

54. Ben-Eliyahu S, Shakhar G, Rosenne E, Levinson Y, Beilin B (1999) Hypothermia in barbiturate-anesthetized rats suppresses natural killer cell activity and compromises resistance to tumor metastasis: a role for adrenergic mechanisms. Anesthesiology 91: 732-740.

55. Beilin B, Shavit Y, Razumovsky J, Wolloch Y, Zeidel A, et al. (1998) Effects of mild perioperative hypothermia on cellular immune responses. Anesthesiology 89: 1133-1140.

3

Assessment of Dental Students' Cardiopulmonary Resuscitation Knowledge and Experience in Turkey

Aysun Caglar Torun*

Department of Oral and Maxillofacail Surgery, Faculty of Dentistry, Ondokuz Mayis University, Samsun, Turkey

*Corresponding author: Aysun Caglar Torun, Assistant Professor, Department of Oral and Maxillofacail Surgery, Faculty of Dentistry, Ondokuz Mayis University, Samsun, Turkey, E-mail: aysunct@hotmail.com

Abstract

Background: This questionnaire-based study aimed to evaluate the CPR knowledge and experiences of Turkish trainee dentists and research assistants at the Faculty of Dentistry of Ondokuz Mayis University in Turkey.

Methods: All the dentists completed a 23-item questionnaire about basic and advanced life support. The survey questions focused on the CPR knowledge and experiences of the dentists.

Results: During their undergraduate education, 68.7% (n=68) of the trainee dentists and 60.5% (n=23) of the research assistants stated they had received CPR training (p=0.010 and p=0.016, respectively). In postgraduate education, 7.9% (n=3) of the research assistants said they had received CPR training (p=0.028). With regard to performing orotracheal intubation on a model, 31.3% (n=3) of the interns and 68.4% (n=26) of the research assistants had never performed this procedure (p=0.009 and p=0.006). There was a significant difference in the number of interns versus that of research assistant who had performed orotracheal intubation on a model (p=0.009). The interns gave correct answers to 5 (0-10) of the questions, and the research assistants correctly answered 6 (0-10) of the questions, on average (p=0.034).

Conclusion: An inability to manage medical emergencies properly can lead to legal complications and sometimes have tragic consequences. To ensure that dentists are able to manage medical emergencies in daily practice and enhance patient safety, training on CPR skills should be increased and made mandatory in all undergraduate and postgraduate dental courses.

Keywords: Dentistry; Cardiopulmonary resuscitation; Experience

Introduction

The need for emergency interventions is common in dentistry. Vasovagal syncope, orthostatic hypotension, and hypoglycemia, side effects due to local anesthetics, are the most commonly encountered emergencies [1-3]. In these and similar emergencies, cardiopulmonary resuscitation (CPR) may be required to ensure the continuity of the patient's respiration and circulation. The physician's knowledge and experience of CPR can save a patient's life. In Turkey and other countries, dentists receive training on CPR during their studies and after graduation. However, due to inadequate training and the failure of dentists to refresh their knowledge via education programs, many dentist practitioners may be unable to perform CPR correctly.

This questionnaire-based study aimed to evaluate the CPR knowledge and experiences of Turkish trainee dentists and research assistants at the Faculty of Dentistry of Ondokuz Mayis University in Turkey.

Materials and Methods

This was a cross-sectional study approved by the ethics committee of Ondokuz Mayis University in Turkey. Turkish trainee dentists at Faculty of Dentistry of Ondokuz Mayis University and research assistants with at least 1 year of experience were included in the study. All the dentists completed a 23-item questionnaire about basic and advanced life support, and all the participants signed a consent form. The survey questions focused on the CPR knowledge and experiences of the dentists. The first seven questions asked about the CPR training and experience of the participants. They were questioned about their departments, whether they had received CPR training during and after undergraduate education, their orotracheal intubation experience on a model or patient, their experience of using a defibrillator, and the annual average number of CPR procedures they had performed. Questions 8–13 were multiple-choice questions on CPR related to the compression/ventilation ratio, application and location of chest compression, epinephrine dose and implementation of the precordial thump. The final 10 questions asked the participants to rate their knowledge of various aspects of CPR using a 5-point Likert scale.

Statistical analysis

The data were analyzed using IBM SPSS V21 (Chicago, USA). The Kolmogorov–Smirnov test was performed to determine the normality of the data. The Mann-Whitney U test and Kruskal-Wallis test were used in the analysis of quantitative data that was not normally distributed. A Chi-square test was used in the comparison of qualitative data. The results are presented as frequencies, percentages, and median (min-max). The significance level was taken as $p<0.05$.

Results

Ninety-nine trainee dentists and 38 research assistants participated in the study. Of the research assistants who participated in the study, 23.6% (n=9) were training in pediatric dentistry, 21.0% (n=8) in oral and maxillofacial surgery, 18.5% (n=7) in oral and maxillofacial radiology, 7.9% (n=3) in restorative dental treatment, 13.3% (n=5) in prosthesis, and 15.7% (n=6) in orthodontics (Table 1).

During their undergraduate education, 68.7% (n=68) of the trainee dentists and 60.5% (n=23) of the research assistants stated they had received CPR training (p=0.010 and p=0.016, respectively) (Table 2).

In postgraduate education, 7.9% (n=3) of the research assistants said they had received CPR training (p=0.028). With regard to the average annual number of CPR procedures that the participants had performed, the majority of dentists stated they had never performed CPR (Table 3).

With regard to performing orotracheal intubation on patients, 68.7% (n=68) of the trainee dentists and 89.5% (n=34) of the research assistants said they had never performed this intervention (p=0.200 and p=0.81, respectively).

Departments		n (%)
Trainee dentist		99 (70.7%)
Research assistants		38 (29.3%)
	Paedodontics	9 (23.6%)
	OMFS	8 (21.0%)
	Oral Diagnosis	7 (18.5%)
	RDT	3 (7.9%)
	Prosthodontics	5 (13.3%)
	Orthodontics	6 (15.7%)
OMFS: Oral and MaxilloFacial Surgery; RDT; Restorative Dental Treatment.		

Table 1: Departments of participants.

	Yes	No	p-value	Yes	No	p-value
	% (n)[1]	%(n)[1]		% (n)[2]	%(n)[2]	
Trainee dentist	68.7%(68)	31.1%)(31)	0.327	-	-	-
Research assistant	60.5%(23)	39.5%(15)	0.343	7.9%(3)	92.1%(35)	0.028
[1]Receiving CPR training during undergraduate education, [2]Receiving CPR training after undergraduate education.						

Table 2: Participants CPR training rates.

	0/year	1/year	2/year	3/year	4/year	p-value
	% (n)	% (n)	% (n)	% (n)	% (n)	
Trainee dentist	67.7% (67)	20.2% (20)	8.1% (8)	1.0% (1)	3.0% (3)	0.01
Research assistant	65.8% (25)	13.2% (5)	2.6% (1)	0.0% (0)	18.4% (7)	0.016

Table 3: Average annual CPR number of participants.

There was no significant difference between the number of trainee dentists and research assistants who had performed orotracheal intubation on patients (p=0.200). With regard to performing orotracheal intubation on a model, 31.3% (n=3) of the interns and 68.4% (n=26) of the research assistants had never performed this procedure (p=0.009 and p=0.006, respectively). There was a significant difference in the number of interns versus that of research assistant who had performed orotracheal intubation on a model (p=0.009). In terms of defibrillator usage, 96% (n=95) of the interns and 97.4% (n=37) of the research assistants had never used a defibrillator (p=0.000 and p=0.192, respectively).

There was no significant difference in the numbers of interns who had used a defibrillator versus the numbers of research assistants who had done so (p=0.054) Table 4. In the analysis of the participants' answers to the 16 questions about CPR, the interns gave correct answers to 5 (0-10) of the questions, and the research assistants correctly answered 6 (0-10) of the questions, on average (p=0.034) (Table 5).

	Never Performed	It was not effective	It was effective	I cannot rate myself	p-value
	% (n)	% (n)	% (n)	% (n)	
Oratrakeal intubation on patients					
Trainee dentist	68.7%(68)	16.2%(16)	8.1%(8)	7.1%(7)	0.2
Research assistant	89.5%(34)	5.3%(2)	0.0%(0)	5.3%(2)	0.081
p-value	0.2				
Orotracheal intubation on model					
Trainee dentist	31.3%(31)	38.4%(38)	23.2%(23)	7.1%(7)	0.009

Research assistant	68.4%(26)	21.1%(8)	7.9%(3)	2.6%(1)	0.006
p-value	0.009				
	Defibrillator usege				
Trainee dentist	96%(95)	3.0%(3)	0.0%(0)	1.0%(1)	0
Research assistant	97.4%(37)	2.0%(1)	0.0%(0)	0.0%(0)	0.192
p-value	0.054				

Table 4: Participants orotracheal intubation execution and defibrillator usage rates.

	Median (Min-Max)	p-value
Trainee dentist	5(0-10)	0.034
Research Assistant	6(0-10)	
	Median (Min-Max)	0.115
Yes[1]	6(0-10)	
No[1]	5(0-9)	
	Median (Min-Max)	0.694
Yes[2]	5(3-7)	
No[2]	5(0-10)	
	Median (Min-Max)	0.713
Never Performed[3]	5(0-10)	
I did but it was not effective[3]	6(2-9)	
I did effectively[3]	6(2-10)	
I can't fully rate myself[3]	6(4-10)	
	Median (Min-Max)	0.059
Never Performed[4]	6(0-8)	
I did but it was not effective[4]	5(0-10)	
I did effectively[4]	6(2-10)	
I can't fully rate myself[4]	4.5(1-6)	
	Median (Min-Max)	0.764
Never Performed[5]	5(0-10)	
I did but it was not effective[5]	7(0-10)	
I did effectively[5]	6(5-7)	
I can't fully rate myself[5]	6(5-8)	

[1]Have you received CPR training during undergraduate education?, [2]Have you received CPR training in postgraduate education?, [3]Have you performed orotracheal intubation on patients?, [4]Have you performed orotracheal intubation on model?, [5]Have you used defibrillator on a patient?

Table 5: Comparison of the effects different variables on correctly answering the questionnaire.

As shown in Table 5, the comparison of the average numbers of correct answers of the participants who had/had not received CPR training during undergraduate education, had/had not performed orotracheal intubation, and had/had not used a defibrillator revealed no significant difference (p=0.115, p=0.713, and p=0.764, respectively). Five dentists answered none of the questions correctly, and none of the dentists answered all the questions correctly.

Discussion

This study examined the CPR knowledge and experiences of dental interns and research assistants at the Faculty of Dentistry of Ondokuz Mayis University in Turkey. According to the findings of this study, the majority of the participants had never performed orotracheal intubation on a patient and they had never encountered a situation that required the use of CPR. These results showed that dentists have little experience of CPR during their dentistry education. The results may be explained by the fact that most students are involved only in minor surgeries and operations on patients that do not affect patients' vital functions. A study conducted in Brazil also reported that dentists rarely encountered life-threatening complications in clinical practice and that syncope, orthostatic hypotension, and moderate allergic reactions were the most common complications [4,5]. A study conducted in Australia found similar results, with only one of seven dentists encountering an event that required resuscitation [1]. Another study reported that the rate of life-threatening complications, such as foreign object aspiration, asthma attacks, and cardiac problems, was 5.5-11% in dentistry [3]. Therefore, in dental clinical practice, life-threatening complications seem to be very uncommon. Nevertheless, dentists should be prepared for emergency management when such complications occur.

In cases of emergency management, the dentist must be familiar with the complete CPR algorithm used to ensure the sustainability of the respiratory and circulatory systems. To ensure familiarity with current CPR methods, the dentist should also take part in education programs at regular intervals. In a study of dental interns and postgraduate students, Narayan et al. in India found that the percentage of dentists with good knowledge of CPR was quite low [6]. They stated that training on CPR in the dental curriculum should be increased [6]. Similarly, a study in Iran reported that dentists had little knowledge and experience of CPR and suggested that training could address this lack of knowledge [7]. The same study reported that ongoing CPR training was a necessity for dentists. In the present study, although the experiences and CPR-related training of the dental research assistants and interns were similar, on average, the research assistants answered more questions correctly (6 of 16) than did the interns (5 of 16). There was no significant difference in various factors (e.g., previously receiving CPR training, practicing orotracheal intubation, and using a defibrillator) that could have affected the level of correct answers of the dentists who participated in the survey. The results of this study demonstrate that dentistry students in Turkey have insufficient knowledge and experience of CPR, in common with findings in many other countries [8-11].

CPR training during dentistry courses varies by country in terms of time allotted to training and necessity. In the United Kingdom, 93.9% of dentistry students receive CPR training during undergraduate education, and 98.9% receive such training during postgraduate education [4]. In Iran, since 2013, on a weekly basis, dental students receive 26 h of training (a combination of theory and practice) [12]. CPR training is compulsory in 95% of dentistry schools in the United

States (U.S.) [13]. In the U.S., many states request a CPR certificate from the dentist after graduation for state board dental registration [14]. In contrast, in Turkey, a first aid and emergency management course is an elective option in the 4th year of undergraduate education. This course covers basic life support and involves practice using a model. However, as this is an elective course, not all dental students undertake this type of training. In addition, CPR is included in the curriculum of general anesthesia in the 4th year of training. After undergraduate education, dentists in Turkey are not required to take part in compulsory training on CPR. Furthermore, after graduation, for those who continue to practice dentistry in the clinic, CPR certification is not mandatory. However, all dental practices are required to possess equipment, such as an ambu bag, adrenaline, and dopamine, to deal with potential emergencies. According to the present study, only 68.7% of dental interns and 60.5% of research assistants received CPR training during their undergraduate education.

An inability to manage medical emergencies properly can lead to legal complications and sometimes have tragic consequences. To ensure that dentists are able to manage medical emergencies in daily practice and enhance patient safety, training on CPR skills should be increased and made mandatory in all undergraduate and postgraduate dental courses.

Funding

No funding declared.

References

1. Chapman PJ (1997) Medical emergencies in dental practice and choice of emergency drugs and equipment: a survey of Australian dentists. Aust Dent J 42: 103-108.

2. Jevon P (2012) Updated guidance on medical emergencies and resuscitation in the dental practice. Br Dent J 212: 41-43.

3. Alhamad M, Alnahwi T, Alshayeb H, Alzayer A, Aldawood O, et al. (2015) Medical emergencies encountered in dental clinics: A study from the Eastern Province of Saudi Arabia. J Family Community Med 22: 175-179.

4. Atherton GJ, Pemberton MN, Thornhill MH (2000) Medical emergencies: the experience of staff of a UK dental teaching hospital. Br Dent J 188: 320-324.

5. Arsati F, Montalli VA, Flório FM, Ramacciato JC, da Cunha FL, et al. (2010) Brazilian dentists' attitudes about medical emergencie during dental treatment. J Dent Educ 74: 661-666.

6. Narayan DP, Biradar SV, Reddy MT, Bk S (2015) Assessment of knowledge and attitude about basic life support among dental interns and postgraduate students in Bangalore city, India. World J Emerg Med 6: 118-122.

7. Jamalpour MR, Asadi HK, Zarei K (2015) Basic life support knowledge and skills of Iranian general dental practitioners to perform cardiopulmonary resuscitation. Niger Med J 56: 148-152.

8. Boddu S, Prathigudupu RS, Somuri AV, Lingamaneni KP, Rao P, et al. (2012) Evaluation of knowledge and experience among oral and maxillofacial surgeons about cardiopulmonary resuscitation. J Contemp Dent Pract 13: 878-881.

9. Sopka S, Biermann H, Druener S, Skorning M, Knops A, et al. (2012) Practical skills training influences knowledge and attitude of dental students towards emergency medical care. Eur J Dent Educ 16: 179-186.

10. Jodalli PS, Ankola AV (2012) Evaluation of knowledge, experience and perceptions about medical emergencies amongst dental graduates (Interns) of Belgaum City, India. J Clin Exp Dent 4: e14-e18.

11. Müller MP, Hänsel M, Stehr SN, Weber S, Koch T (2008) A state-wide survey of medical emergency management in dental practices: incidence of emergencies and training experience. Emerg Med J 25: 296-300.

12. Iranian curriculum of dentistry, approved at 2007. p.86: Persian.

13. Clark MS, Wall BE, Tholström TC, Christensen EH, Payne BC ((2006) A twenty-year follow-up survey of medical emergency education in U.S. dental schools. J Dent Educ 70: 1316-1319.

14. Peskin RM, Siegelman LI (1995) Emergency cardiac care. Moral, legal, and ethical considerations. Dent Clin North Am 39: 677-688.

4

Bacteriological Aspects of Late Pneumonia in Ventilated Patients in Intensive Care Units: A Single Center Study in Morocco

Frikh Mohammed[1,2*], **Abdelhay Lemnouer**[1,2], **Nabil Alem**[1], **Adil Maleb**[3] and **Mostafa Elouennass**[1,2]

[1]*Department of Bacteriology, Faculty of Medicine and Pharmacy, Military Hospital of Instruction Mohammed V, University Mohammed V, Rabat, Morocco*

[2]*Group of Research and Study for Antibiotic Resistance and Bacterial Infections, University Mohammed V Rabat, Morocco*

[3]*Faculty of Medicine Oujda, University Mohammed First, Morocco*

*****Corresponding author:** Frikh Mohammed, Department of Bacteriology, Military Hospital of Instruction Mohammed V, University Mohammed V, Avenue des FAR, Hay Riad, 10100, Rabat, Morocco, E-mail: frikmed@yahoo.fr

Abstract

Background: The resistance to antimicrobial among patients with late Ventilator-associated pneumonia (VAP) has become increasingly more common in many ICUs in Morocco. There are scarce studies assessing VAP importance in Morocco.

The aim of this study is to determine the bacterial ecology and resistance profile of late VAP in intensive care units in an academic hospital of Rabat.

Methods: A total of 215 sputum samples were collected from endotracheal aspirate in patients with diagnosis of late VAP during the study period, defined from April 1st 2012 to April 2013. The bacteriology interpretations was done following the Referential of Medical Microbiology (REMIC 2010) and were quantitatively cultured with a cut-off of ≥ 10 UFC/ml for endotracheal aspiration samples.

Results: Overall, the Gram-negative bacilli (GNB) represent 81.42% of isolates, while Gram-positive was less represented with a rate of 18.56%. Non-lactose fermenting GNB made up the half of pathogens with the rate of 55.23% and the prevalence of Enteric GNB reaches 26.19%. *Pseudomonas aeruginosa* is the most isolates with the rate of 28.57%, followed by *Acinetobacter baumannii* (24.76%), *Staphylococcus aureus* (9.5%) and *Klebsiella pneumonia* (8.09%). A high level of multi-drug resistance pathogens was found with a rate of 39.52%. They included *Pseudomonas aeruginosa* (14.28%), *Acinetobacter baumannii* (19.04%) and *Klebsiella pneumonia* (5.71%) whereas all *S. aureus* were methicillin-sensitive.

Conclusion: The local bacterial pathogens isolates displayed high levels of antibiotic resistance. Enteric GNB naturally resistant to Polymyxin E and *Corynebacterium* species are likely to be emerging pathogens. This study significantly highlights the need to take into account these potentially drug-resistant isolates when making empiric antibiotic treatment.

Keywords: Ventilator-associated pneumonia (VAP); Antimicrobial resistance; Nosocomial infections

Background

Ventilator-associated pneumonia (VAP) is a very common type of infection in intensive care unit (ICU) patients [1]. Late onset VAP is defined as VAP developing ≥ 5 days of mechanical ventilation. It is caused by multidrug-resistant (MDR) pathogens, and is associated with increased morbidity and mortality [2,3].

VAP could be considered a form of aspiration (gravity) pneumonia in intubated patients. Indeed, pooled secretions present in the subglottic area above inflated endotracheal tube cuff may be aspirated into the lower airways [4]. The international nosocomial infection control consortium (INICC) data suggests a VAP incidence as high as 13.6/1000 mechanical ventilation (MV) days [1]. In developing countries, the rates of VAP infections varied from 10 to 41.7/1000 MV-days, and were generally higher than NHSN benchmark rates [5].

In Morocco, the incidence of VAP in a tertiary medical ICU of Rabat was 43.2 per 1,000 ventilator-days [6] and the prevalence was found to be 71.4 % to 93% [7,8].

VAP are associated with mortality rates ranging between 20% and 70% that can be even more important when VAP are caused by multiple drug-resistant pathogens or when the first antibiotic is inadequate [9-11]. It is also linked with extended ICU and hospital stay, delay in recovery, and augmented health care expenses [12-14].

Many studies investigated the risk factors for VAP infections and found that the male sex, elderly age, higher APACHE II scores, prolonged antibiotic usage, immunosupression, reintubation, etc... are the most common ones [15].

Because of the grave consequences of VAP, its prevention has gained the attention of policy makers for developing patients' safety plans [9,16].

The Institute for Healthcare Improvement (IHI) [17,18] has promoted VAP prevention and safety of patients on mechanical ventilation by implementing a set of interventions known as the 'ventilator bundle' [19]. This bundle includes four components: (1) elevation of the head of the bed to between 30 and 45 degrees, (2) daily interruption of sedation and daily assessment of readiness to extubate, (3) peptic ulcer disease prophylaxis, and (4) deep vein thrombosis prophylaxis. Others reports added to these approaches: staff education programs and implementation of hand hygiene [5] and showed that the VAP rate can be reduced significantly by applying theses preventive measures [20-23].

The VAP causative agents varies according to the population of patients in the ICU, the durations of hospital and ICU stays, and the specific diagnostic method(s) used [5,24-28]. *Pseudomonas aeruginosa, Acinetobacter baumannii, Enterobacteriaceae* producing extended-spectrum beta-lactamase (ESBL) and methicillin-resistant *Staphylococcus aureus* (MRSA) are the species most frequently isolated [24,29,30]. In developping countries, Gram-negative bacilli were responsible for the majority of VAP episodes (41-92%) followed by Gram-positive cocci (6-58%) [31-35].

In Morocco, most studies reported the ecology of VAP including both early and late ones (the latter representing 55 to 66% of cases). Bacteriological profile in these studies was dominated by BGN (48,3-68,3%), *Staphylococcus* (21,2-5,5%) and *Enterobacteriaceae* (10,7-15%) with predominance of multidrug resistance especially for BGN [36,37].

The aim of this study is to describe the bacterial ecology and resistance profile of late VAP in a tertiary ICU in Morocco in order to adapt the empirical antibiotic therapy of late VAP and to prevent the emergence of MDRB.

Methods

This retrospective and descriptive study was conducted between April 2012 and April 2013 at the bacteriology laboratory of Mohammed V Military Instruction Hospital in Rabat. This hospital contains 700 beds capacity with a medical and a surgical care unit of 12 beds each. We included all pulmonary origin samples of intensive care units hospitalized patients who developed later VAP (occurring five days after ventilation [2,3]. VAP was defined according to CDC criteria [3]: a new and persistent infiltration present for more than 48 hours on a chest radiograph, plus two or more of the following: 1) fever of more than 38°C or less than 36°C; 2) leukocytosis of more than 10,000 or leucopenia of less than 5,000 cells/mL; 3) purulent tracheobronchial secretion; and 4) gas exchange degradation. Positive microbiological culture confirmation was also required [38].

Samples were collected by endotracheal aspiration (EA), bronchial aspiration (BA) and protected distal samples or broncho-alveolar washing. They were treated and interpreted according to REMIC recommendations [39], with a quantitative culture threshold of AET ≥ 10^5 CFU/ml. The antibiotic sensitivity tests were performed and interpreted according to CA SFM [40]. Multidrug resistant bacteria included meticillino resistant *Staphylococcus aureus* (MRSA), *Enterobacteriaceae* producing extended-spectrum beta-lactamases (ESBLs) and/or hyper-produced cephalosporinases (HCP) and/or carbapenemase (Carb), non-fermenting negative gram bacilli resistant to third generation cephalosporins or imipenem [29,41]. The microbiological data extraction was performed using the expert system module (OSIRIS® software Biorad, French).

Results

During the study period, we collected 215 significant culture samples with 210 isolates; 112 (53.33%) from the medical intensive care unit and 98 (46.66%) from the surgical one. The Gram negative bacilli represented 81.42% of isolates while Gram positive cocci and Gram positive bacilli are less represented with a rate of 11.42% and 7.14% respectively. Non-lactose fermenting Gram negative bacilli made up the half of pathogens with 55.23% and the frequency of enteric bacilli was 26.19% of all isolates (Table 1).

Famille	Espece	Nombre N	Percentage (%)
BGN non Fermentant 116 (55.23%)	Pseudomonas aeruginosa	60	28.57
	Acinetobacter baumannii	52	24.76
	stenotrphomonas maltophilia	3	1.42
	Achromobacter Xylosoxydans	1	0.47
Enterobacteries 55 (26.19%)	Klebsiella pneumonia	17	8.09
	Proteus spp	11	5.23
	Serrratia sp	11	5.23
	Enterobactor sp	7	3.33
	E. Coli	5	2.38
	Providencia sp	4	1.9
Coccia gram positif 24 (11.42%)	Staphylococcus aureus	20	9.52
	Staphylococcus pneumoniae	2	0.95
	Staphylococcus CN	1	0.47
	Enterococcus faecalis	1	0.47
Bacilles a gram positif 15 (7.14%)	Corynebacterium striatum	8	3.8
	Corynebacterium sp	7	3.33

Table 1: Distribution of bacteria species isolated (n=210).

Bacteria	Our study n=210	Erden et al. n=327	Kollef et al. n=499	Chastre et al. n=2490
P. Aeruginosa	28.60%	23.20%	21.20%	24.40%
A.baumanii	24.70%	37.00%	3.00%	7.90%
K.pneumoniae	8.10%	1.20%	8.40%	-
S.aureus	9.50%	27.80%	42.50%	20.40%
Corynebacterium	7.14%	-	22.90%	-

Table 2: Frequency of principal's species based on studies.

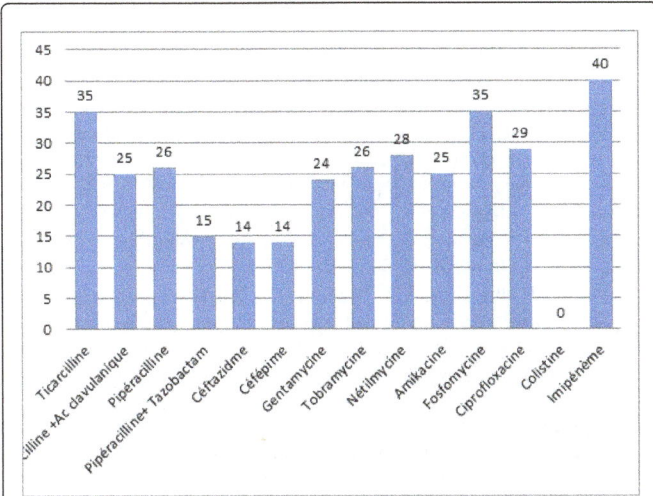

Figure 1: Resistance rates (R+I)* of *P. aeruginosa* isolates (n=60).

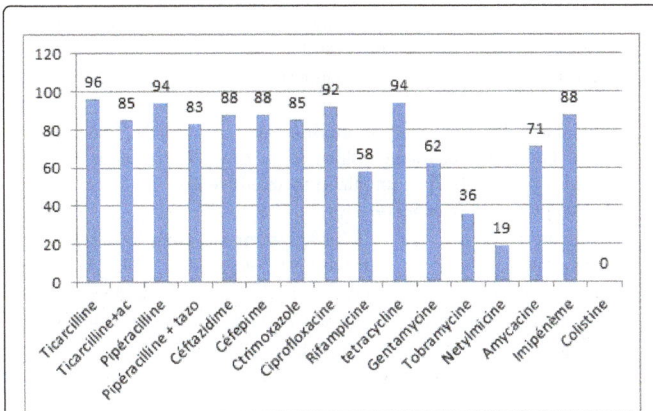

Figure 2: Resistance rates (R+I) of *A. baumannii* isolates (n=52).

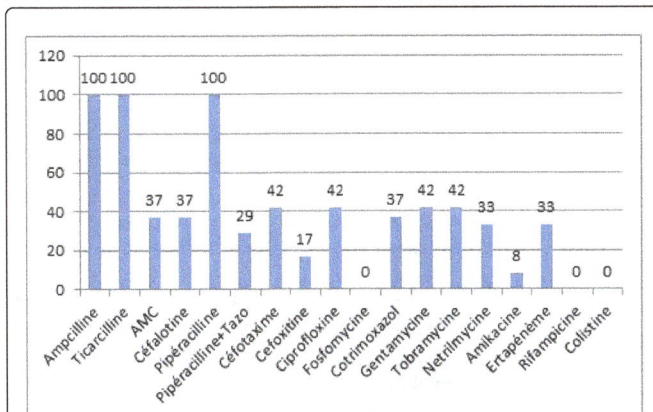

Figure 3: Resistance rates (R+I) of *K. pneumonia* isolates (n=17).

Pseudomonas aeruginosa were the most isolates with the rate of 28.57%, followed by *Acinetobacter Baumannii* (24.76%), *Staphylococcus aureus* (9.52%) and *Klebsiella pneumonia* with the rate

of 8.09% (Table 2). The *corynebacteria* represented 7.14% of all isolates with a resistance rate of 7.10%.

Antimicrobial susceptibility profiles of *Acinetobacter baumannii*, *Pseudomonas aeruginosa* and *Klebsiella pneumoniae* showed a high level of multidrug resistance up to 39.52% (Table 3) especially for *Acinetobacter baumannii*, *Pseudomonas aeruginosa* (Figures 1-3). They included imipenem-resistant *Pseudomonas aeruginosa* strains (14.28%), *Acinetobacter baumannii* carbapenem-resistant strains (19.04%) and ESBL and carbapenem-resistant *Klebsiella pneumonia* strains (5.71%). All *S. aureus* isolates were sensitive to methicillin and glycopeptides.

Species	ESBL(n)	OEC(n)	Carb(n)	Imper(n)	%MDR
P.aeruginosa (n=60)	0	4	3	23	14.28
A. baumannii (n=52)	0	1	40	0	19.52
K. pneumoniae (n=17)	6	0	6	0	5.71

MDR: Bacteria multiple drug resistance, ESBL: Extended-Spectrum Beta-lactamase,

OEC: overexpressed cephalosporinase, Carb: carbapenemase. Imper: impermeability.

Table 3: Betalactams Resistance profile of the main bacteria isolated.

Other species isolated were represented by *Proteus*, *Providencia* and *Serratia* that all accounted for 12.36% of all isolates and *Corynebacteria* with a rate of 7.14%.

Discussion

In our study, the late VAP bacterial epidemiology is dominated by Gram-negative bacilli with 81.42%. The Gram-negative, non-fermenting bacteria accounted for 67.83% and the enterobacteria for 32.16%. This dominance could be explained by the VAP physiopathology; lung contamination being due in one hand by modified endogenous flora of oropharynx and gastric fluid, mainly represented by enteric Gram-negative bacteria and *Pseudomonas aeruginosa* [42-44] and in the second hand, by exogenous flora from respiratory instruments or aerosols [3,42-45].

Pseudomonas aeruginosa, *Acinetobacter baumannii*, *Klebsiella pneumoniae* and *Staphylococcus aureus* are the predominating species. They are usually isolated in nosocomial infections, particularly in intensive care units [46]. However, the frequency of these species is very variable depending on regions, the structure and intensive care unit types [24,42,46,47].

The overall MDRB rate of late VAP in our study is very high (39.52%), but it is still inferior to that of other series namely in Greece [48] and in Brazil with a rates of 50% and 59% respectively [29]. The MDRB are represented first by Carbapenemase-producing *A. baumannii* isolates with the rate of 76.92% that remained only sensitive to polymyxin E, tobramycin and netilmicin (Figure 2). The imipenem *P. aeruginosa* resistance rate is 38.33% in our study with impermeability more prevailing than carbapenemases (Figure 1).

This resistance profile lead in most of case, to using polymixine E (colistine) as the only efficient drug given by parenteral route and by aerosol to the MDRB infections especially *Acinetobacter* and *Enterobacteriaceae* producing carbapenemases [49-52]. Therefore, we recorded an increase incidence of bacterial species that are naturally resistant to polymyxin E (Proteus, Providencia, Serratia and *Corynebacteria* especially, multi-resistant one: *Corynebacterium striatum*). These results are in line with their reported increasing responsibility for VAP [46] and are a risk factor for inducing resistance to colistin in particular in case of its inadequate and inappropriate use as confirmed by other authors [49,50]. This resistance, non-noted in our region, appeared at the beginning of the century and is due to a modification of the lipid A of the bacterial plasma membrane and the presence of an efflux [53,54].

S. aureus accounted for only 9.52% of the isolates in our work, in contrast to other studies where it occupies the first place in Kollef et al. study [55] and the second place after *A. baumannii* in Erdem et al. one [56]. This low *S. aureus* rate is probably multifactorial including low nasal carriage in our context [57].

The frequency by species of ESBL *Klebsiella pneumoniae* isolates and carbapenemase *Klebsiella pneumoniae* isolates (35.29%) was higher than that found by some authors [29,41,58]. The emergence of these MDRB are attributable to multiple proven risk factors that include stay duration more than 5 days, recent antibiotic use, previous hospitalization, the frequency of these bacteria in intensive care units [46], and the empirical broad-spectrum antibiotics [29].

Conclusion

The late VAP is caused in most of cases, by BGN especially non-fermenting ones followed by Enterobacteria and in third rank gram positive bacteria. These species are most often multidrug resistant bacteria. This ecology indicates prescription of second line antimicrobial drug and especially colistine for *Acinetobacter baumannii* and *P. Aeruginosa* which expose to the emergence of naturally resistant species to this drug and some gram-positive bacteria. Hence, we recommend urgent implementation of efficient preventive actions, of note VAP bundles that had been proven to reduce the incidence of VAP.

Acknowledgement

The authors would like to thank technicians and all participants of bacteriological unit in the study for their cooperation during data collection by providing and/or facilitating collection of valuable information.

Authors Contributions

FM, LA, EM conceived of the Study conception and design: AN, MA participated in Data acquisition. FM, LA, MA performed analysis and interpretation of data. FM, LA: participated in drafting the manuscript. FM, EM had been involved in Critical revision of the manuscript for important intellectual content. AN performed statistical analysis. FM, LA, AN, MA and EM have given final approval of this version to be published.

References

1. Rosenthal VD, Maki DG, Jamulitrat S, Medeiros EA, Todi SK, et al. (2010) International Nosocomial Infection Control Consortium (INICC) report, data summary for 2003-2008, issued June 2009. Am J Infect Control 38: 95-104.

2. American Thoracic Society, Infectious Diseases Society of America (2005) Guidelines for the management of adults with hospital-acquired, ventilator associated, and healthcare-associated pneumonia. Am J Respir Crit Care Med 171: 388-416.

3. Niederman MS, Craven DE (2005) Guidelines for the management of adults with hospital-acquired, ventilator-associated, and healthcare-associated pneumonia. Am J Respir Crit Care Med 171: 388-416.

4. Vijai MN, Ravi PR, Setlur R, Vardhan H (2016) Efficacy of intermittent sub-glottic suctioning in prevention of ventilator-associated pneumonia-A preliminary study of 100 patients. Indian J Anaesth 60: 319-324.

5. Arabi Y, Al-Shirawi N, Memish Z, Anzueto A (2008) Ventilator-associated pneumonia in adults in developing countries: A systematic review. Int J Infect Dis 12: 505-512.

6. Madani N, Rosenthal VD, Dendane T, Abidi K, Zeggwagh AA, et al. (2009) Health-care associated infections rates, length of stay, and bacterial resistance in an intensive care unit of Morocco: Findings of the International Nosocomial Infection Control Consortium (INICC). Int Arch Med 2: 29.

7. Lahsoune M, Boutayeb H, Zerouali K, Belabbes H, El mdaghri N (2007) Prévalence et état de sensibilité aux antibiotiques d'A. baumanii dans un CHU marocain. Méd Mal Infect 37: 828-831.

8. Razine R, Azzouzi A, Barkat A, Khoudri I, Hassouni F, et al. (2012) Prevalence of hospital-acquired infections in the university medical center of Rabat, Morocco. Int Arch Med 5: 26.

9. Muscedere J, Dodek P, Keenan S, Fowler R, Cook D, et al. (2008) Comprehensive evidence-based clinical practice guidelinesfor ventilator associated pneumonia: diagnosis and treatment. J Crit Care 23: 138-147.

10. Chastre J, Fagon JY (2003) Ventilator-associated pneumonia. Am J Respir Crit Care Med 165: 867-903.

11. Berenholtz SM, Pharm JC, Thompson DA, Nadham DM, Lubomski LH, et al. (2011) Collaborative cohort study of an intervention to reduce ventilator-associated pneumonia in theintensive care unit. Infect Control Hosp Epidemiol 32: 305-314.

12. Andrews T, Steen C (2013) A review of oral preventative strategies to reduce ventilator-associated pneumonia. Nurs Crit Care 18: 116-122.

13. Bouza E, Burillo A (2009) Advances in the prevention and management of ventilator-associated pneumonia. Curr Opin Infect Dis 22: 345-351.

14. Vincent JL, Sakar Y, Sprung CL, Ranier VM, Reinhart K, et al. (2006) Sepsis in European intensive care units: results of SOAP study. Crit Care Med 34: 344-353.

15. Chawla R (2008) Epidemiology, etiology, and diagnosis of hospital-acquired pneumonia and ventilator-associated pneumonia in Asian countries. Am J Infect Control 36: S93-S100.

16. Arabi Y, Haddad S, Hawes R, Moore T, Pillay M, et al. (2007) Changing sedation practices in the intensive care unit: protocol implementation, multifaceted multidisciplinary approach and teamwork. Middle East J Anesthesiol 19: 429-447.

17. http://www.ihi.org/IHI/Programs/Campaign/100kLivesCampaignSuccessStories.htm

18. http://www.ihi.org/IHI/Programs/Campaign/Campaign.htm?TabId=1

19. Resar R, Pronovost P, Haraden C, Simmonds T, Rainey T, et al. (2005) Using a bundle approach to improve ventilator care processes and reduce ventilator-associated pneumonia. Jt Comm J Qual Patient Saf 31: 243-248.

20. Al-Tawfiq JA, Abed MS (2010) Decreasing ventilator-associated pneumonia in adult intensive care units using the Institute for Healthcare Improvement bundle. Am J Infect Control 38: 552-556.

21. Unahalekhaka A, Jamulitrat S, Chongsuvivatwong V, Ovretveit J (2007) Using a collaborative to reduce ventilator-associated pneumonia in Thailand. Jt Comm J Qual Patient Saf 33: 387-394.

22. Bonello RS, Fletcher CE, Becker WK, Clutter KL, Arjes SL, et al. (2008) An intensive care unit quality improvement collaborative in nine Department of Veterans Affairs hospitals: reducing ventilator-associated pneumonia and catheter-related bloodstream infection rates. Jt Comm J Qual Patient Saf 34: 639-645.

23. Hawe CS, Ellis KS, Cairns CJ, Longmate A (2009) Reduction of ventilator

associated pneumonia: active versus passive guideline implementation. Intensive Care Med 35: 1180-1186.

24. Legras A, Malvy D, Quinioux Al, Villiers D, Bouachour G, et al. (1998) Nosocomial infections: prospective surveiy of incidence in five french intensive care units. Intensive Care Med 24: 1040-1046.

25. Woske HJ, Röding T, Schulz I, Lode H (2001) Ventilator -associated pneumonia in a surgical intensive care unit: epidemiology, etiology and comparison of three bronchoscopic methods for microbiological specimen sampling. Crit Care 5: 167-173.

26. Bouza E, Perez A, Munoz P, Jesus Perez M, Rincon C, et al. (2003) Ventilator-associated pneumonia after heart surgey: a prospective analysis and the value of surveillance. Crit Care Med 31: 1964-1970.

27. Urli T, Perone G, Acquarolo A, Zappa S, Antonini B, et al. (2002) Surveillance of infections acquierd in intensive care: usefulness in clinical practice. J Hosp Infect 52: 130-135.

28. Resende M M, Monteiro S G, Callegari B, Figueiredo P M S, Monteiro C R A V, et al. (2013) Epidemiology and outcomes of ventilator-associated pneumonia in northern Brazil: an analytical descriptive prospective cohort study. BMC Infect Dis 13: 119.

29. Camargo LF, De Marco FV, Barbas CS, Hoelz C, Bueno MA, et al. (2004) Ventilator associated pneumonia: comparison between quantitative and qualitative cultures of tracheal aspirates. Crit Care 8: R422-R430.

30. Kanafani ZA, Kara L, Hayek S, Kanj SS (2003) Ventilator-associated pneumonia at a tertiary-care center in a developing country: incidence, microbiology, and susceptibility patterns of isolated microorganisms. Infect Control Hosp Epidemiol 24: 864-869.

31. Thongpiyapoom S, Narong MN, Suwalak N, Jamulitrat S, Intaraksa P, et al. (2004) Device-associated infections and patterns of antimicrobial resistance in a medical-surgical intensive care unit in a university hospital in Thailand. J Med Assoc Thai 87: 819-824.

32. Ertugrul BM, Yildirim A, Ay P, Oncu S, Cagatay A, et al. (2006) Ventilator-associated pneumonia in surgical emergency intensive care unit. Saudi Med J 27: 52-57.

33. Luna CM, Aruj P, Niederman MS, Garzon J, Violi D, et al. (2006) Appropriateness and delay to initiate therapy in ventilatorassociated pneumonia. Eur Respir J 27: 158-164.

34. Wu CL, Yang D,Wang NY, Kuo HT, Chen PZ (2002) Quantitative culture of endotracheal aspirates in the diagnosis of ventilator-associated pneumonia in patientswith treatment failure. Chest 122: 662-668.

35. Amor M, Talha Y, Maazouzi W (2014) Facteurs de risque de pneumopathie acquise sous ventilation mécanique (PAVM) chez les patients cérébrolésés. Réanimation 24: S118-S122.

36. Shimi A, Touzani S, Elbakouri N, Bechri B, Derkaoui A, et al. (2015) Pneumopathie nosocomiales en réanimation de CHU Hassan II de Fès. Pan African Medical Journal 22: 285.

37. Kollef MH, Silver P, Murphy DM, Trovillion E (1995) The effect of late-onset ventilator-associated pneumonia in determining patient mortality. Chest 108: 1655–1662.

38. Repository of medical microbiology (Remic) (2010) Microbiological diagnosis of bronchopulmonary infections, 4th edition 2010 Chapter 13: 93-98.

39. Soussy JC (2014) Antibiogram committee of the French society of Microbiology.

40. Depuydt PO, Vandijck DM, Bekaert MA, Decruyenaere JM, Blot SI, et al. (2008) Determinants and impact of multidrug antibiotic resistance in pathogens causing ventilator-associated-pneumonia. Crit Care 12: R142.

41. Joseph N M (2010) Ventiltor-associated pneumoniae: A review. Euro j of int med 21: 360-368.

42. Niederman MS, Craven DE (2005) Guidelines for the management of adults with hospital-acquired, ventilator-associated, and healthcare-associated pneumonia. Am J Respir Crit Care Med 171: 388-416.

43. Safdar N, Crnich CJ, Maki DG (2005) The pathogenesis of ventilator-associated pneumonia: its relevance to developing effective strategies for prevention. Respir Care 50: 725-739.

44. Ewig S, Torres A, El-Ebiary M, (1999) Bacterial colonization patterns in mechanically ventilated patients with traumatic and medical head injury. Incidence, risk factors, and association with ventilator associated pneumonia. Am J Respir Crit Care Med 159: 188-98.

45. Torres A, El-Ebiary M, Soler N, Monton C, Fabregas N, et al. (1996) Stomach as a source of colonization of the respiratory tract during mechanical ventilation: association with ventilator-associated pneumonia. Eur Respir J 9: 1729-1735.

46. Park DR (2005) The microbiology of ventilator-associated pneumonia. Respir Care 50: 742-763.

47. Niederman MS (2001) Cost effectiveness in treating ventilator-associated pneumonia. Am J Respir Crit Care 5: 243-244.

48. Wertheim H, Kinh Van Nguyen, Gabriel Levy Hara, Hellen Gelband, Ramanan Laxminarayan, et al. (2013) Global survey of polymixin use: a call for international guidelines. J of Global Antimicrobial Resistance 1: 131-134.

49. Salomon J (2011) Pansusceptible Proteus mirabilis septicemia in a patient multicolonized by pan-resistant bacteria. Med mal infect 41: 262-263.

50. Hayakawa K, Marchaim D, Divine G W, Pogue J M., Kumar S, et al. (2012) Growing prevalence of Providencia stuartii associated with the increased usage of colistin at a tertiary health care center International. J Infect Dis 16: 646-648.

51. Hays C, Benouda A, Poirel L, Elouennass M, Nordmann P et al. (2012) Nosocomial occurrence of OXA-48-producing enterobacterial isolates in a Moroccan hospitalInt. J Antimicrob Agents 39: 545-547.

52. Rios FG, Luna CM, Maskin B, Saenz Valiente A, (2007) Ventilator-associated pneumonia due to colistin susceptible-only microorganisms. Eur Respir J 30: 307-313.

53. Mezghani Maalej S, Rekik Meziou M, Mahjoubi F, Hammami A (2012) Epidemiological study of Enterobacteriaceae resistance to colistin in Sfax. Méd Mal Inf 42: 256–263.

54. Kontopoulou K, Protonotariou E, Vasilakos K, Kriti M, Koteli A, et al. (2010) Hospital outbreak caused by Klebsiella pneumoniae producing KPC-2 beta-lactamase resistant to colistin. J Hosp Infect. 76: 70-73.

55. Kollef MH, Morrow LE, Niederman MS, Leeper KV, Anzueto A, et al. (2006) Clinical characteristic and treatment pterns among patients with ventilator-associated pneumonia. Chest 129: 1210-1218.

56. Erdem I, Ozgultekin A, Inan AS, Dincer E, Turan G, et al. (2008) Incidence, etiology, and antibiotic resistance patterns of gram-negative microorganisms isolated from patients with ventilator-associated pneumonia in a medical-surgical intensive care unit of a teaching hospital in istanbul, Turkey (2004-2006). Jpn J Infect Dis 61: 339-342.

57. Oztoprak N, Cevik MA, Akinci E, Korkmaz M, Erbay A, et al. (2006) Risk factors for ICU-acquired methicillin-resistant Staphylococcus aureus infections. Am J Infect Control 34: 1-5.

58. Guimares MM, Rocco JR (2006) Prevalence of ventilator-associated pneumonia in a university hospital and prognosis for the patients affected. J Bras Pneumol 32: 339-346.

5

Break Through Inspiration During IPPV is Seen as "Curare Crest" in Sevograph

Mukesh Tripathi[1,2*]**, Sanjay Kumar**[2]**, Nilay Tripathi**[3] **and Mamta Pandey**[4]

[1]*Department of Anesthesiology, All India Institute of Medical Sciences, Rishikesh, India*

[2]*Department of Anesthesiology, Sanjay Gandhi Postgraduate Institute of Medical Sciences, Lucknow, India*

[3]*Internist, Department of Medicine, King George's Medical University, Lucknow, India*

[4]*Department of Emergency Medicine, Sanjay Gandhi Postgraduate Institute of Medical Sciences, Lucknow, India*

[*]**Corresponding author:** Mukesh Tripathi, Professor and Head, Department of Anesthesiology, Type V-B/20, Campus SGPGIMS, Lucknow-226014, India, E-mail: mukesh_tripathi@yahoo.com

Abstract

Background: The break through spontaneous effort in anaesthetized and ventilated patients is seen as 'curare-cleft' during expiratory plateau phase of the capnography. At the open position of the sevoflurane vaporizer, the sevograph displays a mirror image graph to the capnograph. We studied the sevograph changes corresponding to 'curare-cleft' in capnography.

Methods: We have observed that during break through spontaneous breaths the sevograph complemented 'curare-crest' corresponding to 'curare-cleft' in six patients. In second part of study 25 consenting adult patients coming for surgery were given general anaesthesia using fentanyl, propofol and suxamethonium. After tracheal intubation, controlled ventilation was started under sevoflurane anaesthesia. We allowed the onset of spontaneous effort and observed for the onset time to 'curare-cleft' in capnograph, 'curare-crest' in sevograph, visible negative deflection of the needle in airway pressure gauge till negative airway pressure of 5 cm H_2O. The onset time for the both changes were statistically analysed for agreement analysis using Blend and Altman test.

Results: 'Curare-crest' in sevograph was visible at the same breath in majority (76%) of instances along with that of 'curare-cleft' in capnograph. Both appeared in respective graphs significantly earlier than the negative deflection of airway gauge needle by 5 cm H_2O and disappeared after vecuronium. Onset time for both 'curare-cleft' in capnograph and 'curare-crest' in sevograph had significant (p<0.01) correlation (R=0.97) too.

Conclusions: The authors feel that both changes 'curare-crest' in sevograph complemented 'curare-cleft' in capnograph and can be equivocally used as warning signal for lighter planes of anesthesia or diminishing effect of muscle relaxant.

Keywords: Sevography; Capnography; Curare crest; Curare cleft; Monitoring

Introduction

In patient under controlled ventilation during general anesthesia, if patients get break through spontaneous inspiratory efforts, a cleft is seen in the expiratory plateau phase of capnograph. These are popularly referred as 'curare-cleft' and represent diaphragmatic contraction [1]. These defects are associated with diaphragmatic contraction when no response is elicited at the adductor pollicis under muscle relaxant effect [1].

Modern anesthesia monitors give simultaneous graphic display of multiple vital parameters. Anesthesia gas monitoring graphs have also been included along with the digital values of the inspiratory and expiratory levels. Sevograph displays a mirror image graph to capnograph during inspiratory and expiratory phases during positive pressure ventilation (Figure 1).

The mirror image pattern is also reflected as a downslope in expiratory phase in sevograph during bronchospasm vis-a-vis upslope in capnography [2]. Therefore we got interested to look for the changes in sevograph in the event of 'curare-cleft' seen during break through breaths under controlled ventilation. After extensive scientific search when we did not find any report, we wish to report our observations of the 'curare-crest' seen on the expiratory sevograph.

Materials and Methods

A female aged 45 yr was posted for emergency laparotomy. Written informed consent was taken and we monitored electrocardiography, non-invasive arterial blood pressure, central venous pressure, capnography and sevography using anesthesia work station (Dragger Fabius GS premium, Dragger Medical AG and Co KG 23542, Lubeck, Germany).

We performed rapid sequence induction of general anesthesia by giving intravenous injection of fentanyl (100 mcg), thiopental (250 mg) and suxamethonium (100 mg). After cessation of the fasciculation we intubated trachea. Anesthesia was maintained with sevoflurane at 2% along with N_2O and O_2 (50:50). Just below the capnograph a mirror image sevograph was seen on monitor (Figure 1).

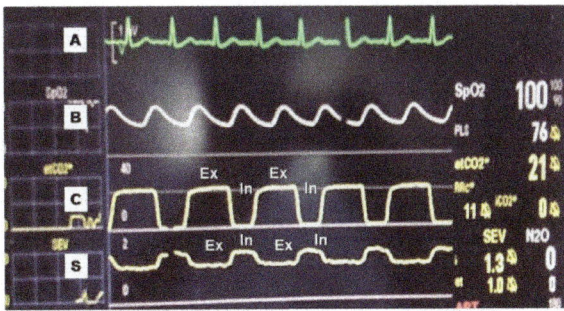

Figure 1: The Multi-channel monitoring screen displaying various wave-forms; A) Electrocardiogram; B) Plethysmograph of pulse oximetry; C) Capnograph; S) Sevograph. The sevograph displayed mirror image of inspiratory (Ins) and expiratory (Ex) phases during positive pressure ventilation during open position of sevoflurane vaporizer characteristically showing 'i-sevo' levels higher than 'et-sevo' levels.

After 10 min patient started breathing and break through breaths were reflected as 'curare-cleft' during expiratory phase in the capnograph. Interestingly we also noticed a corresponding 'curare-crest' in sevograph at same point in expiratory phase of respiratory cycle replicating the mirror image pattern to the capnograph (Figure 2A). After intravenous vecuronium bromide (7 mg) both changes in expiratory phase disappeared to restore plateau character in both graphs (Figure 2B). In next five consecutive anesthetised patients for surgery, we again confirmed similar changes of curare-cleft in capnograph vis-a-vis curare-crest in sevograph during break through breaths. The two changes appeared in on position of the sevoflurane vaporizer.

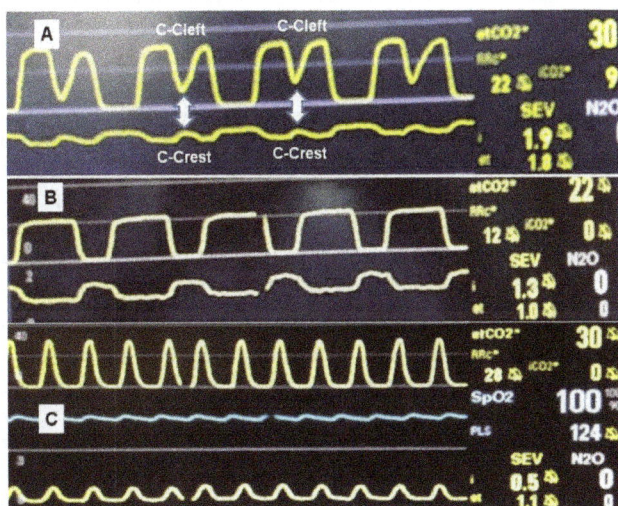

Figure 2: A) Mirror image capnograph and sevograph; B) Curare-cleft' in capnograph corresponds a 'curare-crest' in sevograph (white arrow); C) Sevograph becomes similar to capnograph as vaporizer is switched off.

Based on these results, second part of the simple observational study was conducted on the randomly selected 25 adult (28 yr to 55 yr), ASA grade I, patients of both gender (female=10 and male=15) coming for surgery under general anesthesia. A written informed consent was obtained from all patients after explaining the study protocol. Ethical approval for conducting routine anesthesia protocol for the observations during allowed breathing under anesthesia was taken from the Institute Ethics Committee.

We induced general anesthesia by fentanyl (1 µg/kg), propofol (1 to 1.5 mg/kg) and suxamethonium (1 mg/kg) to facilitate laryngoscopy and intubation. We ventilated lungs on positive pressure ventilation of tidal volume (10 ml/kg) and respiratory rate (12/min) at switched-on sevoflurane vaporizer at 3% during study period. We allowed the patient till we observed the 'curare-cleft', 'curare-crest' negative deflection of breathing pressure gauge needle and the generation of negative airway pressure of 5 cm H_2O. We noted onset time from the induction of anesthesia for the respective changes as above. At the end of study vecuronium (0.1 mg/kg) was given to continue general anesthesia for surgery.

All data were entered in SPSS-16.0 (Statistical Package Social Sciences, Chicago, US) and MS-Excel (Microsoft Office inc., US) for the statistical analysis. The Paired students'-t test was applied to compare mean values. To find out the agreement between 'curare-cleft' and 'curare-crest' the regression analysis was performed between the onset times of the two changes. The Blend and Altman graph was prepared using Excel software.

Results

We observed that in all six occasions, the inspiratory sevoflurane (i-sevo) levels (2.4 ± 0.9 %) were persistently higher than the expiratory sevoflurane (et-sevo) levels (1.7 ± 1.1%) during open position of the vaporizer. Interestingly when we switched off the sevoflurane vaporizer, the sevograph displayed the respiratory phases same as of capnograph (Figure 2C). The i-sevo (1.3 ± 0.5 %) levels at this pattern were also lesser than the et-sevo (0.7 ± 0.8 %) levels during IPPV (Figure 2C). Similar findings were noted on all the occasion in both the graphic display.

The second part of study included 25 observations on 25 adult patients weighing (55 ± 18.5 kg) and height (158 ± 12 cm) (Table 1). The onset time of curare-cleft (394 ± 43.1 sec) was insignificantly ($p>0.05$) earlier than the onset 'curare-crest' (400 ± 46.3 sec). However the onset times of the two parameters were significantly ($p<0.01$) earlier than the onset time (445 ± 40.9 sec) of visible negative deflection of the needle of the airway pressure gauge and the onset time (467 ± 40.4 sec) of the negative airway pressure by 5 cm H_2O during break through breaths (Table 1). We also found that in majority (19/25; 76%) patients, the curare-cleft in capnograph and 'curare-crest' in sevograph was visible in same breath on monitor. The 'curare-cleft' and 'curare-crest' disappeared after vecuronium injection in all patients.

A significant ($p<0.01$) correlation existed between the onset times of the curare-cleft and the 'curare-crest' (R^2-0.94) (Table 2). The Bland and Altman plot of 25 paired samples again depicted significant ($p<0.01$) correlation with slope 0.085 (Figure 3).

	Curare cleft	Curare crest	Negative needle deflection	Negative airway pressure (5 cm H_2O)
Number of observation (n)	25	25	25	25
Onset time (sec) (mean ± SD)	394 ± 43.1	400 ± 46.3	445 ± 40.9[*]	467 ± 40.4[*]
Median onset time (sec)	390	390	430	466
Range (min-max)	340-480	340-480	380-520	400-550
[*]-Statistically significant (p<0.01) difference from other onset times				

Table 1: Showing the observations of the study.

		Onset time to curare-cleft (s)	Onset time to curare-crest (s)
Pearson Correlation	Onset time to curare-cleft (s)	1	0.972
	Onset time to curare-crest (s)	0.972	1
Sig. (1-tailed)	Onset time to curare-cleft (s)	.	0
	Onset time to curare-crest (s)	0	.
Correlation coefficients	R=0.972	R^2=0.94	P<0.001

Table 2: Showing observations of the correlation analysis between onsets of 'curare-cleft' with 'curare-crest'.

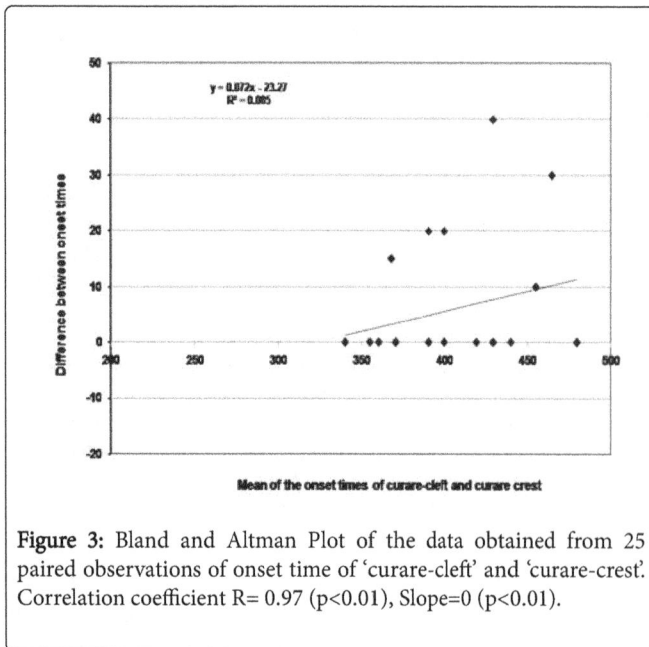

Figure 3: Bland and Altman Plot of the data obtained from 25 paired observations of onset time of 'curare-cleft' and 'curare-crest'. Correlation coefficient R= 0.97 (p<0.01), Slope=0 (p<0.01).

Discussion

These observations confirm that the mirror image configuration of sevograph is seen during 'open-position' of its vaporizer under controlled ventilation in general anesthesia. The 'curare-cleft' in capnograph on break-through breath was also complemented as 'curare-crest' during expiratory phase of ventilation on sevograph. Both the changes 'curare-cleft' and 'curare-crest appeared in majority of patients at the same breath of ventilation. The onset time of the two changes were significantly earlier than the diaphragmatic contractions forceful enough to cause negative deflection of the airway pressure measuring needle or generating negative airway pressure of 5 cm H_2O. There was significant correlation between the onset times of the 'curare-cleft' and 'curare-crest' during allowed break-through breaths and both disappeared after the injection of vecuronium.

The 'curare-cleft' in capnograph was associated with the diaphragm activity [1]. It results from the in-drawing of the gases from the inspiratory limb of the breathing circuit containing lower levels of the carbon dioxide. Since these inspiratory gases contain higher levels of sevoflurane during 'open-position' of the vaporizer, contrary to capnograph this sudden in-drawing of the gases from inspiratory limb was displayed as "curare-crest" on the sevograph at the identical point of the expiratory plateau phase (Figure 2).

Although 'curare-cleft' have been correlated with the diaphragm activity in the paralyzed and ventilated patients and disappears after repeat dose of muscle relaxant, it has failed to measure degree of muscle relaxation of the peripherally monitored muscles (adductor pollicis) [3]. We too found that 'curare-cleft' and 'curare-crest' appeared simultaneously in the expiratory phase of ventilated patients significantly earlier than the diaphragmatic contractions to generate visible negative deflection of the needle of the airway pressure monitoring gauze or generate a negative airway pressure of 5 cm H_2O. The related mechanism has been correlated with rapid kinetics of the muscle relaxant in the diaphragm than the adductor pollicis [4,5].

Anesthesiologists are interested to detect the break through breaths of the patients when the muscle relaxants affect vanes off. If remained unnoticed such efforts are fraught with the problems of the jerky movement, swallowing, gagging movement, tight abdomen and even hemodynamic changes. Recently 'curare-cleft' have also been described during non-specific conditions related to breathing circuit [6,7] unilateral capnothorax [8] and even without respiratory effort in children [9]. We have found that the two changes correlated very closely and appeared simultaneously as well as significantly earlier than the contractions of the diaphragm intense enough to cause negative reflection of the airway pressure gauge. Thus these changes seen on monitor warn significantly earlier to take measures to correct light anesthesia [10] or perhaps inadequate analgesia in the patient.

The 'curare-crest' has the limitation that this change on sevograph is only visible when the vaporizer is in open position and the sevograph shows similar configuration as of capnograph as soon as the vaporizer is put off [2].

Authors feel that the 'curare-crest' in sevograph is new pattern, which closely follows the 'curare-cleft' of caphograph to detect diaphragmatic activity during positive pressure ventilation and can be a good adjunct to detect early diaphragmatic contractions during general anesthesia under controlled ventilation.

Funding

No external funding and no competing interests declared or Funded by the grant.

Author's Contribution

Mukesh Tripathi: Conception and study design, conduct of case, acquisition of data, photographs, primary drafting of article and editing, approver of final draft.

Sanjay Kumar: Conduct of cases, data acquisition, data interpretation, literature search, editing of article, approver of final draft.

Nilay Tripathi: Data acquisition, computation and interpretation, photograph editing literature search, Manuscript writing and editing and approver of final draft.

Mamta Pandey: Study design, data interpretation, statistical analysis, literature search, editing of article and approver of final draft.

References

1. Bissinger U, Lenz G (1993) Capnographic detection of diaphragm movements ("curare cleft") during complete vecuronium neuromuscular block of the adductor pollicis muscle. Anesth Analg 77: 1303-1304.
2. Kumar S, Tripathi M (2013) Down slope on sevoflurane graph in expiratory phase evidence on monitor to diagnose subtle bronchospasm. Br J Anaesth.
3. Bissinger U, Lenz G, Reiter A, Albrecht T, Schorer R (1993) Monitoring neuromuscular function: capnography versus relaxometry. Anaesthesiol Intensivemed Notfallmed Schmerzther 28: 359-362.
4. Donati F, Meistelman D, Plaud B (1990) Vecuronium neuromuscular blockade at the diaphragm, the orbicularis oculi, and the adductor pollicis muscles. Anesthesiology 73: 870-875.
5. Lebrault C, Chauvin M, Guirimand F, Duvaldestin P (1989) Relative potency of vecuronium on the diaphragm and the adductor pollicis. Br J Anaesth 63: 389-392.
6. Hensler T, Chamee MS (1990) Anesthesia machine malfunction simulating spontaneous respiratory effort. J Clin Monit 6: 128-131.
7. Tripathi M, Tripathi M (1998) A partial disconnection at the main stream CO2 transducer mimics "curare-cleft" capnograph. Anesthesiology 88: 1117-1119.
8. Singh M, Chaudhary K, Uppal R (2014) Jain S. Beware of "curare cleft" like changes during unilateral capnothorax. J Clin Monit Comput 28: 315-318.
9. Seefelder C (2012) The 'curare cleft' is not the first sign of respiratory effort. Paediatr Anaesth 22: 415-416.
10. http://www.multileadmedics.com/www.multileadmedics.com/Capnography_files/Slap%20the%20Cap%20handout%202012_revised.pdf.

6

Clipping versus Coiling for Intracranial Aneurysms: Recent Trends

Catarina Barbosa Petiz[1] and Humberto S Machado[1,2,3*]

[1]Instituto Ciências Biomédicas Abel Salazar, Universidade do Porto, Porto, Portugal

[2]Serviço de Anestesiologia, Centro Hospitlar Universitário do Porto, Porto, Portugal

[3]Centro de Investigação Clínica em Anestesiologia, Centro Hospitalar Universitário do Porto, Porto, Portugal

*Corresponding author: Humberto S Machado, Serviço de Anestesiologia, Centro Hospitlar Universitário do Porto, Porto, Portugal, E-mail: hjs.machado@gmail.com

Abstract

Background: Cerebral aneurysms are relevant conditions, and the best therapeutic approach in a patient with Ruptured and Unruptured Intracranial Aneurysm has been debated in the last decades. Coil Embolization therapy has increasingly gained popularity over Surgical Clipping.

Objectives: The aim of this analysis was to review the surgical and endovascular strategies for intracranial aneurysms, and to find out if one intervention is more suitable than other.

Methods: A literature review was carried out identifying studies published from 2002-2017 through Pubmed using the keywords listed below. 75 articles were selected to write this review.

Results: The International Subarachnoid Aneurysm Trial contributed to a change in practice of Intracranial Aneurysms. Endovascular Coiling reduced in 7,4% the proportion of patients who died or became dependent, even if the incidence of late rebleeding was higher at 1 year compared to Neurosurgery (2,9% *vs.* 0,9%). At 18 years the excess risk of rebleeding has not resulted in a significant worse outcome. Endovascular treatment is usually suitable for anterior and posterior circulating aneurysms. Middle cerebral aneurysms are generally treated through clipping. Asymptomatic Unruptured Intracranial Aneurysms smaller than 7 mm usually benefit from simple observation. Despite its benign natural history the number of Unruptured Intracranial Aneurysms treated has increased overtime. Higher mortality is associated with Neurosurgery compared to Endovascular strategy. Anaesthesia applied in surgical clipping is similar to the one applied in endovascular. The most common approaches are general anaesthesia and conscious sedation.

Conclusions: There is strong evidence to indicate that Endovascular Coil embolization is associated with better outcomes compared to Neurosurgical Clipping in patients amenable to either strategy. Despite the major technical advances in imaging and endovascular treatment of intracranial aneurysms, surgical clipping is still the most efficient treatment for medial cerebral artery aneurysms.

Keywords: Endovascular coiling; Neurosurgical clipping; Unruptured intracranial aneurysms; Ruptured intracranial aneurysm; Subarachnoid haemorrhage; ISAT

Abbreviations: AHA: American Heart Association; ASA: American Stroke Association; BAEPs: Brainstem Auditory Evoked Potentials; CI: Confidence Interval; CT: Computed Tomography; CTA: CT Angiography; DCI: Delayed Cerebral Ischemia ; EC: Endovascular Coiling; FDA: US Food and Drug Administration; IA: Intracranial Aneurysm; ISAT: The International Subarachnoid Aneurysm Trial; ISUIA: International Study of Unruptured intracranial Aneurysms Investigators; MRA: Magnetic Resonance Angiography; NC: Neurosurgery Clipping; NIS: Nationwide Inpatient Survey; OR: Odds Ratio; RIAs: Ruptured Intracranial Aneurysms; SAH: Subarachnoid haemorrhage; SSEPs: Cortical Somatosensory Evoked Potentials; TEAM: Trial on Endovascular Management of Unruptured Intracranial Aneurysms; UCAS: Unruptured Cerebral Aneurysms Study; UIAs: Unruptured Intracranial Aneurysms; USA: United States of Ameri

Introduction

Prevalence of Intracranial Aneurysms (IA) varies among populations due to multiple factors. Rupture of IAs is associated with high grades of morbidity and mortality. Therefore it is important to establish an early diagnosis and proceed with an adequate management in order to improve the outcomes of the patients [1].

Prevalence

Unruptured Intracranial Aneurysms (UIAs) are relatively common, found in approximately 3,2% of the general population. Still, the large majority will never rupture [2]. Most aneurysms are asymptomatic, but approximately 300,000 per year in the United States of America suffer a rupture, usually bleeding into the subarachnoid space [3]. Haemorrhagic risk of UIAs is inferior to the risk associated with rerupture of a Ruptured Intracranial Aneurysm (RIA) (1% *vs.* 30-50% within the first year) [4].

Subarachnoid haemorrhage (SAH) has a grim prognosis and is associated with high morbidity and mortality, and only 1/3 of patients that suffer from SAH have a good outcome [3]. However, mortality rates from SAH appear to have declined in the past 25 years [5]. Mortality rates vary from 8% to 67% across published epidemiological studies [6].

Risk factors

There is a female preponderance for aneurysms (2:1), and the prevalence increases with age, with a typical age of onset >50 years [7-9]. Known Hereditary Syndromes, such as Ehlers Danlos syndrome and pseudoxhantoma have been associated with the development of IAs. Also, patients suffering from Autosomal Dominant Polycystic Kidney Disease develop IA in 10-15%. Even in the absence of a hereditary disorder, 7-20% of patients with a cerebral aneurysm will report a family history of this diagnosis [3].

Some acquired risk factors include hypertension, smoking, alcohol abuse, estrogen deficiency, hypercholesterolemia and carotid artery stenosis [10].

Congenital weakness, degenerative alterations associated with hemodynamic stress contribute to the loss of integrity of the artery wall and therefore predispose to the aneurysm development [11].

Diagnosis

Since symptomatic UIAs are unusual, they are usually found incidentally or on screening. There is little data on the best diagnosis strategy. Magnetic Resonance Angiography (MRA) and CT Angiography (CTA) are able to detect aneurysms 5mm or larger [12]. Digital Subtraction Angiography (DSA) has shown great sensitivity in detection of aneurysms smaller than 3mm, and constitutes the gold standard for aneurysm diagnosis. Moreover, it is the most sensitive imaging for follow-up in treated aneurysms [2].

Noncontrast Head Computed Tomography (CT) is the gold standard for diagnosis of SAH, and its sensitivity is close to 100% in the first 3 days after the occurrence. Lumbar puncture is needed if there is a strong suspicion of SAH based on clinical presentation despite a normal CT [13,14].

Risk of aneurysm rupture

Predicting the natural history of an UIA is important to determine the appropriate management. [15,16]. Behavioural risk factors such as hypertension, smoking, alcohol abuse, sympaticomymetic drugs have been associated with an increased risk of IA rupture. A history of previous SAH, familial aneurysms and certain genetic syndromes mentioned above favour SAH [1].

Aneurysm rupture is related to its rate of growth. Natural history was found to vary according to the size, location and shape of the aneurysm. Patient's characteristics such as age and country of origin may also influence the risk of rupture.

SAH complications

The rupture of an IA is a neurological emergency. Rebleeding is a common complication within the first 24 hours after the occurrence [17].

After the aneurysm obliteration, cerebral vasospasm and decreased cerebral perfusion may occur, representing important causes of poor outcome. Vasospasm (narrowing) occurs in multiple levels among cerebral arteries and it is common 7 to 10 days after aneurysm rupture, often resolving spontaneously [1]. Delayed cerebral ischemia (DCI) occurs in about 1/3 to 1/4 of patients. Poor clinical condition at admission and a high amount of blood on the initial CT scan increase the risk of DCI [18].

Acute hydrocephalus occurs in 15-87% of patients with SAH, and is usually managed by external ventricular drainage or lumbar drainage [19]. Seizure-like episodes occur in a high percentage of individuals with SAH. Aneurysm in the middle cerebral artery, presence of a thick SAH clot, intracerebral haematoma, rebleeding, poor neurological grade and history of hypertension predispose to the occurrence of seizures [1].

Treatment

Treatment of IAs may require Neurosurgical Clipping (NC) or Endovascular Coiling (EC). For a long time, NC has been the primary modality of treatment, but in the last 3 decades EC has evolved and became widely used [20]. The International Subarachnoid Aneurysm Trial (ISAT) published in 2002 strongly influenced the change in practice of both RIAs (the focus of the ISAT trial) and UIAs [8].

Endovascular coiling

Coil variations include bare platinum, polymer coated (Matrix) and hydrophilic gel coated (HydroCoil) coils. No clear advantage in preventing recurrence was demonstrated by coating platinum coils [21].

Detachable Guglielmi Coil, a detachable platinum coil device, was first introduced in the USA clinical practice in 1990 and in 1992 in Europe [22,23]. Guglielmi detachable coils were approved by the US Food and Drug Administration (FDA) in 2003 to treat all brain aneurysms [24]. The detachable coil can be considered an "endovascular controllable occlusive soft coil". After detachment, the coil may be repositioned or exchanged so as to obtain better results. The best results are seen in smaller aneurysms with narrow necks [22].

Stent-assisted coiling has been used to treat wide-neck aneurysms. To avoid stent-associated thromboembolic events, antiplatelet therapy during the procedure is required and can complicate SAH. Complete obliteration of the aneurysm is recommended, and to improve the obliteration rate of coiling a high-porosity stent has been suggested [25].

Matrix is a platinum coil modified with polyglycolic acid braid and has been developed to achieve more durable aneurysm occlusion [26]. The hydrogel-coated coil was designed to improve the aneurysm packing, since this embolic treatment targets the aneurysm dead space [27].

In comparison to clipping, coiling has the advantage of requiring a shorter time of procedure, and reduction of surgical complications such as infection. However, there is a frequent necessity of reintervention due to a less permanent effect of treatment [28]. Intraprocedure aneurysm rupture during endovascular treatment presents a major challenge.

Neurosurgical clipping

The first brain aneurysm clipping took place in 1937, and for many decades has been the exclusive treatment for IAs. It is an entirely extravascular procedure, sparing the endovascular space. The craniotomy, brain retraction, arachnoid dissection and aneurysm manipulation involved in surgery may be rendered as an invasive strategy [29]. Open surgery may be required as a support to the endovascular approach in case of prolapse of a coil through the wall of the aneurysmal sac and intraoperative vasospasm [30].

Methods

A literature review was carried out based on a PubMed research with the following instructions: Title/abstract: ("unruptured intracranial aneurysm" OR "ruptured intracranial aneurysm" OR "intracranial aneurysm" OR "subarachnoid haemorrhage") AND ("neurosurgery clipping" OR "endovascular coil") AND "ISAT". Publications written exclusively in English from 2002 to 2017 were considered. The custom range began in 2002, since it was a decisive year in the intracranial aneurysm treatment story.

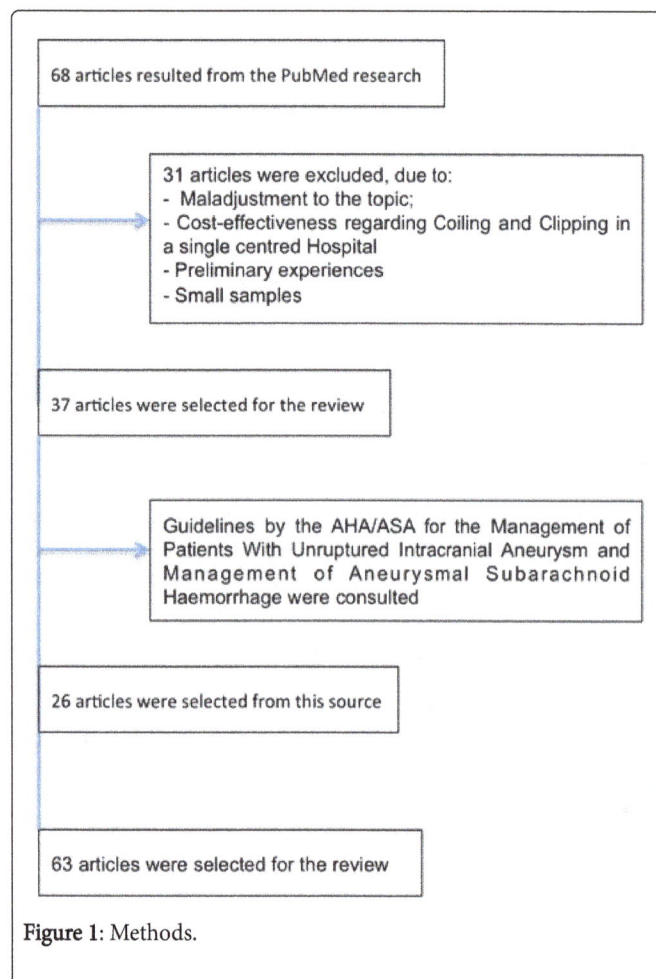

Figure 1: Methods.

From the 68 articles found in the research, 37 were selected for the review taking into consideration the content of the title and abstract. The excluded articles regarded papers that did not adjust to the topics reviewed in this review, publications related to cost-effectiveness of Endovascular Coiling and Neurosurgical Clipping in a single centred Hospital, preliminary experiences of specific techniques and studies regarding small samples.

References from relevant articles and Guidelines presented by the American Heart Association/American Stroke Association (AHA/ASA) for the Management of Patients With Unruptured Intracranial

Aneurysm and Management of Aneurysmal Subarachnoid Haemorrhage were also consulted, in order to better debate the subject. This source added 26 studies to the previous from PubMed, engaging a total of 63 references (Figure 1).

Results

Ruptured intracranial aneurysms

American Heart Association presented in 2012 guidelines for the management of Aneurysmal Subarachnoid Haemorrhage based on literature and recommendations from 2006 to 2010. [1] Medical measures and Surgical or Endovascular treatment are required to achieve the best outcomes in patients who suffered SAH.

Surgical and endovascular methods

ISAT: ISAT was the only multicentre, randomized, and controlled clinical trial that compared outcomes of surgical and endovascular repair across 42 neurosurgical centres, mainly in Europe and in the UK. Patients were randomly assigned to NC (n=1070) or EC (n=1073). To be eligible for the trial aneurysms had to be suitable for surgery and endovascular therapy. Most of the enrolled patients had good clinical grade and the aneurysms were localised in the anterior circulation. Patients older than 70 years old were not randomized [31].

The study concluded that patients who underwent EC had higher survival rates, lower epilepsy and mortality rates at one year than the ones who had NC. A 7,4% risk reduction (95% CI, p=0,0001) in the proportion of patients who died or experienced ongoing dependence due to neurosurgical disability was achieved with coiling. However, incidence of late rebleeding was higher in the endovascular group (2,9% versus 0,9% after surgery), and only 58% of coiled aneurysms were totally obliterated compared to 81% clipped aneurysms [31,32].

ISAT cohort was re-examined 5 years later, and embolization with coil was related to a higher risk of recurrent bleeding than clipping and the proportion of survivors who were independent after 5 years did not differ between the two groups (82% vs. 83%). Still, risk of death was significantly lower in the coiled group (14% vs. 11%) [29,33,34].

One thousand, six hundred and forty-four UK patients included in the ISAT trial were followed up for death and clinical outcomes for 10-18 years, using self-reported Rankin scale (Table 1). At 10 years 83% of patients allocated to EC were alive compared to 79% of patients allocated to surgical clipping (odds ratio [OR] 1.35, 95% CI 1.06-1.73). In both groups, the risk of death and rebleeding from the treated aneurysm up to 18 years was very small. Long-term causes of death result mainly of causes other than from the treated aneurysm. There was a small excess of rebleeding risk in the coiling group, which has not resulted in a significantly worse clinical outcome [23].

0	No symptoms
1	No significant disability, despite symptoms; able to perform all usual duties and activities
2	Slight disability; unable to perform all previous activities but able to look after own affairs without assistance
3	Moderate disability; requires some help, but able to walk without assistance
4	Moderately severe disability; unable to walk without assistance and unable to attend to own bodily needs without assistance

5	Severe disability; bedridden, incontinent, and requires constant nursing care and attention
6	Death

Table 1: Modified Rankin Scale [64].

Lin et al. analysed 34899 Hospital discharges with a diagnosis of ruptured or unruptured cerebral aneurysm from 1998 to 2007 identified from the Nationwide Inpatient Survey (NIS), therefore including 5 years before as well as 5 years after publication of the ISAT results. There was an increase in the number of treated aneurysms during this period, being that the trend was towards an increased use of coiling (Figure 2) [8].

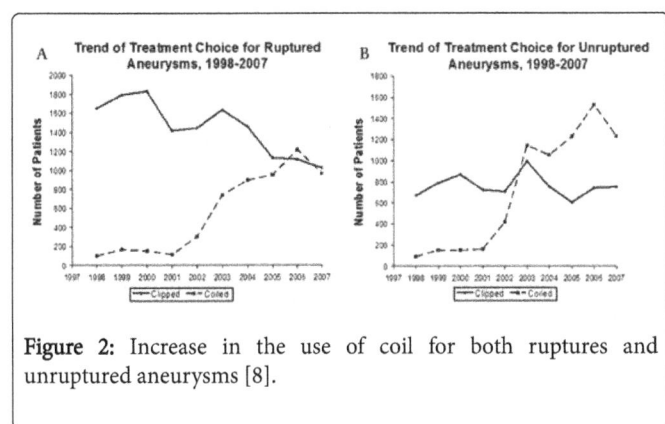

Figure 2: Increase in the use of coil for both ruptures and unruptured aneurysms [8].

A study published in 2011 analysed the national estimates of treatments for RIAs present in the NIS data between 2000-2002 and 2004-2006. There was an increase in utilization of endovascular treatment (3% *vs.* 17%) for intracranial aneurysms and an increase in the proportion of patients receiving any treatment in the post-ISAT period [24].

BRAT: In response to concerns regarding ISAT, in 2002 investigators at the Barrow Neurological Institute in Phoenix launched BRAT. Every patient admitted to the centre with SAH, regardless if it was amenable to NC and EC, was assigned in an alternating fashion to surgical aneurysm clipping or endovascular coil therapy if agreed to participate. Ultimately, 238 patients were assigned to aneurysm clipping and 233 to coil embolization. A large number of patients first assigned to embolization could not be safely treated with coiling and crossed over to aneurysm clipping. Nevertheless, outcomes at one year were better after coil embolization (33,7% of patients assigned to clipping had poor outcome *vs.* 23,2% of the coiling group), what is coherent with the ISAT study [35].

Other studies

A prospective multicentre trial was carried out between 1997 and 2014 to compare the treatment results of RIAs following EC and NC across Middle Europe. Six hundred and 61 cases of RIA were recorded. Two hundred and seventy one cases of SAH underwent EC, 390 underwent NC. Seventeen percent of patients treated with EC suffered from symptomatic Ischemic Stroke compared to 6,7% of the NC group (OR 2.86, 95% CI, p<0,0001). The occlusion rate was significantly better in the NC group versus EC group (OR 11.48, 95% CI, p<0,0001), the rebleeding rate was significantly lower in the NC group (OR 14.90, 95% CI, p<0.0001). Direct mortality was not significantly different

across the two arms of the study. No patient who underwent surgery required retreatment compared to 23 patients in the EC group (p<0.0001). Age and co-morbidities played an important role regarding the decision to retreat [36].

Turek et al. analysed 190 RIAs subjected to EC in the period of 2006-2013 to study the early outcomes and perioperative complications of the technique. Localization of the aneurysm within anterior circulation represented a predictor of negative postoperative outcome. In the case of vertebral-basilar aneurysms, complications are less common. Peri-operative complications included aneurysm rupture (main complication), acute vasospasm, thromboembolism, and prolapse of a coil. Hemiparesis/hemiplegia, dysphasia/aphasia, vasospasm and hydrocephalus could appear as post-procedural complications. Coiling was preferred as a first line treatment of poor-grade patients, especially those with large and inaccessible aneurysms when deciding wether to clip or coil [30].

EC of posterior circulating aneurysms has gained popularity throughout the decades, with several studies demonstrating better outcomes in this technique over surgery [1].

Hospital treatment volumes and availability of both endovascular and neurological intensive care services are important determinants for technique's recommendations [1]. Definite repair was significantly higher in urban teaching Hospitals, comparing to nonteaching Hospitals in a study that took place in the US during 2003 [9]. Better outcomes and lower mortality rates especially for clipping techniques were found in teaching Hospitals and larger Hospitals. Therefore, low volume Hospitals should consider early transfer of SAH patients to high-volume units [37].

Hospital costs of both EC and NC are rising within the years. Expenses vary from country to country, and might be different within the same country what makes it difficult to reach a conclusion concerning the cost-effectiveness of the procedures. Nevertheless, the most recent studies revealed that the NC group demonstrated lower Hospital costs compared to the EC group even considering the superior length of Hospitalization associated to clipping [38].

Unruptured intracranial aneurysm

Unlike patients with SAH, patients with UIA generally experience no neurologic deficits. UIAs are usually asymptomatic and often found incidentally on magnetic resonance imaging (MRI) or CT [39].

The interventional options include NC and EC. Simple observation may be beneficial in some situations, and radiographic follow-up is usually recommended, due to possible aneurysm growth. The relatively benign natural history and the increased detection by non-invasive imaging tests make the treatment option controversial [2].

Few observational and small prospective studies addressed the efficacy of each treatment modality in UIA, and therefore the best treatment choice remains doubtable [39]. The decision towards a procedure is based on the aneurysmal location and size, nature of the neck and presence of tortuous arteries, because these factors were shown to influence prognosis. The risk of intervention increases with age, and a conservative approach is usually considered in the elderly [40]. Decisions regarding optimum manage should balance the probability of short-term and long-term rupture and the risks of the intervention.

The Trial on Endovascular Management of Unruptured Intracranial Aneurysms (TEAM) began in 2006 and was designed to study the long-term efficacy of coiling in prevention of bleeding and clarify if it is beneficial compared to simple observation. However, due to multiple factors this trial was prematurely interrupted and could never reach any conclusions [4].

The International Study of Unruptured intracranial Aneurysms Investigators (ISUIA) and Unruptured Cerebral Aneurysms Study (UCAS) are the most carefully designed large studies on UIA's natural history [2].

ISUIA, first published in 1998, evaluated the natural history of 1937 UIAs influencing contemporary neurosurgical practice. ISUIA analysed two groups: patients with no history of SAH and those with previous SAH who have undergone treatment, because the latter constitutes an independent risk for rupture. Aneurysms of less than 10 mm had a 0,05% risk of rerupture among patients with no history of SAH; the risk became 11 times higher in patients with history of SAH. Aneurysms located in the basilar apex, vertebrobasilar, posterior communicating, and posterior cerebral arteries were more prone to rupture. NC was associated with high morbidity and mortality, and outcome related to EC could not be analysed due to a small number of patients. These data were retrospective and whether the patients were representative was debated [40-42].

A second part of the study was published in 2003, and 4060 patients were analysed prospectively. A smaller cut point for size (<7 mm versus <10 mm) was defined. UIAs <7 mm in diameter had no benefit in treatment, because of the very low rupture risk. Symptomatic UIAs or those with daughter sac constitute exceptions. Risk rates related to EC and NC were higher than in previous studies. Morbidity and mortality rates of NC and EC in patients with no history of SAH from another lesion were 13,7% and 9,3% respectively, whereas in patients with history of SAH the rates were 11% and 7,1% respectively. Location in the posterior fossa and diameter higher than 12 mm were associated with worse outcome after EC. The major drawback in EC was due to incomplete occlusion of lesions [42].

UCAS, a prospective Japanese cohort study published in 2012, analysed 5720 patients who had saccular aneurysms detected on imaging that were ≥ 3 mm. Aneurysms ≥ 7 mm were more prone to rupture, also aneurysms located in the posterior communicating arteries were associated with a higher risk of rupture. Unlike other studies, history of SAH, smoking, presence of multiple aneurysms did not affect the risk of rupture in this study (Table 2) [15].

	Location	Study Type	Number of Patients	Number of aneurysms	Follow-up (months)	Predictors of aneurysm rupture
ISUIA	USA and Europe	Retrospective	1449 untreated	1937	99,6	Aneurysm size and location
ISUIA	USA and Europe	Prospective	4060: 1692 untreated, 1917 NS, 451 EC.	2686	49,2	Aneurysm size and location
Juvela et al	Finland	Retrospective and Prospective	142	181	252	Cigarette smoking, anterior communicating artery location, age
UCAS	Japan	Prospective	5720	2392 surgery, 4305 without early treatment	11660 aneurysm-years	Posterior communicating arteries and age

Table 2: Summary of large cohort studies on Unruptured intracranial aneurysms (UIA) [61].

A meta-analysis from 1990 to 2011 analysed 60 studies harbouring 10845 aneurysms. The majority of studies examining outcomes related to UIA's surgery have been single centre retrospective case series. Clipping of UIAs was associated with 1,7% mortality and 6,7% unfavourable outcomes. Craniotomy with clipping of an UIA provides permanent treatment of the aneurysm, being that recurrence is unusual. Morbidity rates were significantly greater in higher quality studies, and with large or posterior circulation aneurysms [43].

A meta-analysis on the natural history of UIAs published in 2006 integrated 19 studies since 1996. Four thousand seven hundred and five patients were included and several risk factors for aneurysmal rupture were identified. Age >60 years, female sex, Japanese or Finish descent, symptomatic aneurysm, diameter >5 mm and posterior circulation aneurysm were associated with a higher risk of rupture [44].

A retrospective cohort study, published in 2007, using data from 429 USA Hospitals evaluated 2535 treated UIAs. NC was associated with higher morbidity and mortality and longer lengths of stay (7.4 days versus 4.5) [45].

Alshekhlee et al. analysed, over a 7-year period, 21104 cases with admission diagnosis of UIA of which 52,5% were admitted electively. Higher mortality and Hospital complication rates were associated with clipping, what was coherent with anterior studies. However, the location and morphologic characteristics of the aneurysms were not taken into consideration (Table 3) [39].

In 2010, Lindner et al. analysed 304 patients with IAs localised in different areas of the brain and assessed diverse risk factors, such as age, gender, smoking, alcohol intake, hypertension and family preponderance, reaching the conclusion that aneurysms at different sites also differ in risk factors. Rupture of aneurysms in the anterior circulation appeared to be more frequent in patients <55 years of age, posterior communicating aneurysms ruptured more frequently in men, and basilar artery aneurysm rupture is associated with lack of use of alcohol [46].

For aneurysms managed conservatively it is generally recommended imaging follow up to assess aneurysm growth. The likelihood of small aneurysm growth is low. Middle cerebral aneurysm location, size greater than 5 mm, presence of multiple aneurysms and family history of SAH were predictors of growth in a follow-up study by Serial 0,5T

MRA, being that 14 among 130 patients suffered aneurysm growth [47].

Complication	Clip n (%)	Coil n (%)	OR (95%)	P Value
Any event*	312 (8.35)	129 (3.69)	2.37 (1.92, 2.93)	<0.0001
Hospital mortality	60 (1.61)	20 (0.57)	2.83 (1.70, 4.71)	<0.0001
Intracerebral haemorrhage	89 (2.38)	48 (1.37)	1.75 (1.23, 4.49)	<0.0001
Postoperative Stroke	251 (6.71)	102 (2.92)	2.39 (1.89,3.03)	<0.0001
Hydrocephalus	33 (0.88)	44 (1.26)	0.69 (0.44,1.10)	<0.0001
Status epilepticus	4	0	...	<0.0001
Pulmonary	79 (2.11)	29 (0.83)	2.58 (1.68, 3.96)	<0.0001
Cardiac	119 (3.18)	74 (2.12)	1.52 (1.13, 2.04)	<0.0001
Systemic Infection	16 (0.43)	3 (0.09)	5.00 (1.45, 17.20)	<0.0001
Acute Renal Failure	37 (0.92)	32 (0.91)	0.92 (0.57, 1.48)	<0,0001

* Any event included a composite outcome of any mortality, intracerebral haemorrhage, or postoperative stroke

Table 3: Hospital Mortality and Complication rates associated with aneurysm clipping and coiling [39].

Anaesthetic management

Usually, anaesthetic principles for NC are similar to the ones applied to EC of IA. The most common approaches are general anaesthesia and conscious sedation, but no studies comparing these two techniques have been done [1,48].

Monitoring intra-arterial blood pressure and intracranial pressure (ICP), oxygen, carbon dioxide, urine and temperature is important. Slow administration of mannitol (0,25-2 g/kg) is recommended to avoid a transient increase in ICP [49].

Increase in blood pressure is worrisome, because it can motivate aneurysm rupture and ought to be controlled with nicardipine, labetolol, and esmolol to keep systolic blood pressure <160 mmHg [49].

Supervision of the patient with special attention for cardiac function, potential hypovolemia and hyponatremia is of great importance before anaesthesia. Hypovolemia and increased ICP heighten the chance of cerebral vasospasm and possible ischemic events. Albumin has neuroprotective properties and minimal effect on coagulation and is reasonable to treat volume imbalances. Hemodynamic control to avoid aneurysm rerupture and strategies to protect the brain against ischemic injury should be enforced. Nimodipine is recommended for vasospasm prophylaxis. Hyponatremia is a common electrolyte abnormality seen in up to 30% of SAH cases and may benefit from intravenous administration of normal saline solution [49].

General anaesthesia

General Anaesthesia is a popular technique among endovascular and surgical strategies, providing a stationary focal point for surgical manipulation and for visualization target area during the endovascular procedure [49].

Induced hypotension has been used in the past to prevent rerupture, but current data associate decrease in mean arterial pressure with poor outcomes [50].

Propofol and rimifentanil infusion can be used when total IV anaesthesia is considered. Cortical somatosensory (SSEPs) and brainstem auditory evoked potentials (BAEPs) may be used to monitor cerebral function. Volatile anaesthetics interfere with SSEP and BAEP [49].

Conscious sedation

Some centres prefer to use only sedation during the placement of detachable coils in order to monitor the patient's neurologic status during the procedure. However, general anaesthesia is often used [51].

Endovascular coiling

Anticoagulation with heparin is amnistered during the embolization of aneurysms, unlike surgical clipping. If intraprocedure aneurysm rupture occurs, rapid reversal of anticoagulation with protamine is required [1].

When aneurysm obliteration is delayed, antifibrinolytic drugs (aminocaproic acid or tranexamic acid) have been shown to reduce the chance of rebleeding [49]. More than 33% of rebleeds occur in the first three hours after the symptoms, and approximately 50% within the first six hours [52].

Post-operative medication with paracetamol is recommended to relieve pain [30].

Neurosurgical clipping

Intraoperative Hypothermia for Aneurysm Surgery trial (IHAST) analysed 1001 patients of 30 different centres so as to determine wether intraoperative cooling during craniotomy was associated with improved outcomes, but no benefits in long-term morbidity and mortality were achieved [53].

Intraoperative glucose concentrations >129 mg/dl is associated with increased risk of neurological function decline [54].

Temporary clipping is useful to prevent aneurysm rerupture during the procedure. If temporary clipping is expected to exceed 120 minutes, induced hypertension may be considered, but the value of this measure was not established [1].

Discussion

Endovascular coiling and neurosurgical clipping

Diagnosis strategies, imaging surveillance and aneurysm obliteration techniques have undergone multiple changes throughout the years, and algorithms to determine the proper indications for each treatment are continually in transformation. [39,55]. It has been observed an increasing usage of EC in the treatment of RIAs and UIAs in the last decades, and this strategy has overtaken neurosurgery in many Hospitals. Both RIAs and UIAs require special and individualised attention in order to decide which strategy will represent a more beneficial measure.

In general, anaesthetic principles are the same for endovascular and surgical managements. The possibility of rebleeding, hypertension, cerebral edema, DCI, electrolyte abnormalities, hydrocephalus, seizures and cardiopulmonary dysfunction should be considered to guide anaesthetic management [49].

Embolization has the advantage of requiring shorter time of and reduction of surgical complications such as infection [28]. Bare platinum, polymer coated and hydrophilic gel coated coils are some available options to proceed with endovascular treatment, being that no clear differences in outcome have been suggested [21].

Aneurysms initially planned for endovascular treatment are eventually clipped, what doesn't happen the other way round. Also, with certain complications that occur after embolization, surgical therapy may be required to resolve the negative sequel. Therefore, even though endovascular technique is becoming more popular it is not expected to completely substitute surgery [28].

It is remarkable how quickly the attitude is changing in favour of coiling of IA, despite the lack of evidence of superiority over the accepted standard treatment. There is evidence suggesting improvement of clinical outcome and effectiveness of coiling since the ISAT period until nowadays. The former technique is evolving overtime; therefore general outcome described in the past cannot be directly compared to today's [23].

Ruptured intracranial aneurysms

ISAT: ISAT together with technologic advances, increased availability of endovascular procedures and contributed to a shift in the USA practice pattern of cerebral aneurysms [31,56]. However, there are still wide variations in the availability and use of EC, among countries and within countries [31].

Even though ISAT has been a strong driver of change in the management of RIAs (and UIAs), the evidence of the superiority of coiling should not be based on this trial alone. After publication of the results of ISAT, there was a lot of discussion among the neurosurgery community, mainly because of its selection bias, ethical dilemma and poorly chosen primary endpoints. It remains unclear wether the trial can be confidently generalized to all patients since it recruited a small portion of the "universe" of patients with RIAs: 88% of the enrolled patients had a favourable clinical grade, 95% were in the anterior circulation, and 90% were smaller than 10 mm. Also, patients older than 70 years old were not randomized. A total of 9559 patients were screened, but only 2143 enrolled. Selection of good clinical grade patients may be required to avoid masking of the outcomes by poor clinical condition of patients. However, this selection criteria has implications in the generalization of the results. The overall in-Hospital mortality associated to ISAT was 6%, comparing to 26% in-Hospital mortality of SAH in the USA [31,56,57]. Other design issues such as lack of requirements for the proficiency of surgical participants and angiographic control need to be taken into consideration [33]. Recommendations following the interpretation of the trial vary among neurosurgeons and neurointerventionalists communities.

In spite of the fact that most of the IAs covered by the ISAT trial are localised in the anterior circulation, they represent a big percentage of the existing aneurysms, 85% of which are placed in the anterior

circulation [58]. This location represents a negative predictor of postoperative outcome [59]. Aneurysms of the anterior cerebral artery are associated to cognitive impairment, deficits of memory and personality changes, because the surgical techniques used to access aneurysms in this location may require resection of frontal lobe structures [31].

Nevertheless, ISAT was a statistically powerful study whose findings can be applied to patients with rupture of small, anterior circulation aneurysms, with a good World Federation of Neurological Societies grade (Table 4). Various studies analysed NIS, the largest all-payer inpatient care in the US, comparing periods before and after the publication of the ISAT study and concluded that there was an increase in usage of EC comparing to NC in both UIAs and RIAs.

WFNS (World Federation of Neurosurgical Societies)	Glasgow Coma Scale score	Motor deficit
I	15	Absent
II	14-13	Absent
III	14-13	Present
IV	12-Jul	Present or absent
V	06-Mar	Present or absent

Table 4: Subarachnoid hemorrhage scale [65].

At one year, EC was associated with higher survival rates, lower epilepsy and mortality rates comparing to clipping. The difference was likely attributable to the greater incidence of technical complications and longer time needed to secure the aneurysm in NC. Incidence of late rebleeding and partial obliteration was higher in the EC group [32].

The poor outcome rate climbs rapidly with advanced age. The absolute difference between the poor outcome rates after coil embolization and clip occlusion is lower in those <50 years old than it is for those >50 years old (3,3% vs. 10,1%). The advantage of coil embolization could not be assumed for patients <40 years old. Rebleeding rates higher 0,1-0,3% per year after coil embolization comparing to surgical clipping, what may overturn the superiority of coiling in young patients over the years [32].

A 10 year follow-up of a group of UK patients included in the ISAT trial concluded that the small risk excess of rebleeding in the coiling group did not result in a significantly worse clinical outcome. [23] The risk of rebleeding after aneurysm haemorrhage persists for 30 years, therefore it is important to continue the follow up of patients enrolled in the ISAT study [60].

Other studies regarding RIAs

Hammer et al. published in 2016 a prospective, non-randomized trial. The data reached back to 1997, and from that time on endovascular treatment technology suffered noteworthy changes, whereby clipping has not undergone significant changes. Considering the location of the treated IAs there has been a misbalance. In the EC group there was a high rate of treated anterior aneurysms, which are known to be associated with worse outcome. Angiographic visualization is performed after EC, which certainly increases detection of small residuals found post-treatment. On the other hand, occlusion rates for clipping were based on post-operative surgeon reports [36].

In 2012, BRAT was designed to reflect real world practicalities of RIAs in North America, and the conclusions were coherent with the ISAT study.

O'Kelly et al. conducted a nonrandomized and retrospective study using data from the province of Ontario. In order to overcome several limitations associated to the ISAT trial, all patients undergoing repair of RIAs between 1995 and 2004 were analysed. In the adjusted analysis of the entire cohort EC was associated with a significantly increased rate of mortality (hazard ratio 1,25). This study reached to conclusions that disagree with ISAT. Unlike ISAT this study was nonrandomized and retrospective, which limited the ability to measure possible cofounders. The degree of disability could not be directly measured. Similarly to ISAT, the relative expertise of endovascular and neurosurgical practitioners was not assessed [56].

Unruptured intracranial aneurysms

Hospitalizations for clipping and coiling of UIAs in the United States of America from 2001 to 2008 described in the NIS were analysed. In that period it is clear the steady increase in the number of UIAs and the proportion of UIAs treated with EC. The number of UIAs being treated has increased overtime despite its relatively benign natural history. EC was associated with lower morbidity and mortality comparing to NC [61].

Unlike RIAs that have been studied and subjected to a multicentre, randomized, and controlled clinical trial, the study of UIAs is limited to few observational and small prospective studies. There are no randomised clinical trial data regarding management of UIAs, but findings of ISAT may be transposed to UIAs. The number of UIAs treated with EC, overcomes the number of those treated with NC in many Hospitals. Still, the predominant use of the endovascular procedure is not uniform among Hospitals [8,30,39].

EC is likely to be initially less morbid than clipping. The TEAM trial was designed to understand wether EC was associated with lower morbidity than observation. The initial objective was to recruit 2000 patients with UIAs eligible to prophylactic coiling within 3-4 years with a planned follow-up of 10 years. The contrast between the two groups of the trial (intervention versus observation) contributed to the failure of the trial. Also, some neurosurgeons responsible for the decision-making could be reluctant to the endovascular approach what could contribute to an asymmetrical allocation of management. Legal and bureaucratic issues and financial obstacles also contributed to the failure of the trial [4].

ISUIA and UCAS are the most carefully designed large studies regarding UIA's natural history, and guidelines taking into consideration these analyses have been published to better decide the best approach. Imaging control was not required in ISUIA, so it could not address the risk of aneurysms that may change in size overtime. It remains unclear if UCAS can be applied to non-Japanese populations, especially because the incidence rate of SAH is higher in Japan than in Europe or USA.

It has to be balanced if the advantages of the treatment outweigh the potential risks of aneurysm rupture, since UIAs generally have a benign natural history. Decision towards conservative management requires imaging follow-up to control aneurysm growth. Various studies throughout time have concluded that UIAs treated by coiling

have fewer adverse events, lower mortality and shorter Hospital length of stay [8]. Clipping of large aneurysms in a posterior location in older patients is associated with higher rates of morbidity and mortality.

Recent trends

Considering RIAs, several studies have suggested that older patients or patients presenting with low clinical grade carrying anterior circulation aneurysms yield more favourable results with coil embolization rather than clipping [59]. Neurosurgery clipping, even representing a more invasive strategy, has a lower risk of rerupture and better durability, therefore in patients that are able to tolerate this type of surgery (younger patients with good grade aneurysms) this treatment may be preferable [55]. However, data on this matter is still conflicting.

ISAT strongly influenced the change in practice of IAs. However, in real world practice coiling is being offered to types of patients that were not studied in ISAT, and EC of posterior circulating aneurysms has gained popularity over the decades.

Middle cerebral aneurysms are generally treated by clipping not only because of the facilitated access, but also due to specific local angioarchitecture that often requires vascular remodelling of the middle cerebral artery bifurcations, which is better coped with surgery. [59] Van Dijk et al. published in 2011 a study confirming the benefits of surgical clipping in the management of middle cerebral artery aneurysms already mentioned in the literature [62].

Small intracranial aneurysms ($\leq$ 3 mm diameter) represent technical challenges, due to difficulties in obtaining a stable micro catheter position and higher risk rates of perforation related to placing coils in confined spaces. However, with widespread adoption of adjunctive techniques such as balloon and stent successful assisted coiling of small aneurysms has been achieved [63].

Relatively to UIAs, Physicians are able to choose among endovascular, surgical and no treatment of UIA, but the optimum strategy remains unclear. The existent high-quality data is not enough to decide wether intervention is related to better outcome than the natural history without such treatment. In the absence of clinical trial data, decisions regarding treatment or extended follow-up of UIA are based on the natural history. Since the risk of rupture of an UIA is relatively low, the risks associated with the treatment must be even lower.

Guidelines based on ISUIA and UCAS studies have been published recommending observation rather than treatment for aneurysms smaller than 7 mm in patients with no history of SAH, being that those symptomatic or with daughter sac may require treatment. The decision to treat an UIA is not straightforward and aneurysmal factors such as a bigger size and posterior location, whether there is a thrombus within the aneurysm, presence of daughter sac and symptoms; patient factors such as age, sex, comorbidities and family history of SAH ought to be considered. EC is more beneficial than NC for both younger and older patients and for both anterior and posterior circulating aneurysms.

Differences regarding aneurysm's treatment between and within countries mirror the dissimilarities in cost-effectiveness around the world. Hence, it is important to uniform systems of care so as to overcome differences and achieve better results. The risks associated to treatment rely on the surgical and endovascular expertise and caseload of each institution [30].

Regardless of the treatment option, mortality and morbidity associated to treated aneurysms has decreased overtime due to technique evolution, better imaging follow-up and diagnosis. Other factors independent from the aneurysm itself may influence de morbidity and prognosis decay. Therefore, it is crucial to alert the patient for the consequences of smoking, sedentary lifestyle, unhealthy alimentation and salt abuse.

Conclusions

In recent years, multiple publications evaluated the safety of EC and SC. EC is preferred under some circumstances, due to its associated lower morbidity and mortality compared to NC. Nevertheless, the debate about the best choice of treatment is still ongoing and the opinion from the neuroradiology community diverges from the neurosurgery's.

Endovascular treatment has become more popular over the decades in the treatment of anterior and posterior cerebral aneurysms, whereas clipping is usually preferable as the treatment choice of middle cerebral artery aneurysms and very small aneurysms that are often challenging to treat with an endovascular approach.

References

1. Connolly ES Jr, Rabinstein AA, Carhuapoma JR, Derdeyn CP, Dion J, et al. (2012) Guidelines for the management of aneurysmal subarachnoid hemorrhage: a guideline for healthcare professionals from the American Heart Association/american Stroke Association. Stroke 43: 1711-1737.

2. Thompson BG, Brown RD, Amin-Hanjani S, Broderick JP, Cockroft KM, et al. (2015) Guidelines for the Management of Patients With Unruptured Intracranial Aneurysms: A Guideline for Healthcare Professionals From the American Heart Association/American Stroke Association. Stroke 46: 2368-2400.

3. Wardlaw JM, White PM (2000) The detection and management of unruptured intracranial aneurysms. Brain 123: 205-221.

4. Raymond J, Darsaut TE, Molyneux AJ (2011) A trial on unruptured intracranial aneurysms (the TEAM trial): results, lessons from a failure and the necessity for clinical care trials. Trials 12: 64.

5. Stegmayr B, Eriksson M, Asplund K (2004) Declining mortality from subarachnoid hemorrhage: changes in incidence and case fatality from 1985 through 2000. Stroke 35: 2059-2063.

6. Nieuwkamp DJ, Setz LE, Algra A, Linn FH, de Rooij NK, et al. (2009) Changes in case fatality of aneurysmal subarachnoid haemorrhage over time, according to age, sex, and region: a meta-analysis. Lancet Neurol 8: 635-642.

7. Vlak MH, Algra A, Brandenburg R, Rinkel GJ (2011) Prevalence of unruptured intracranial aneurysms, with emphasis on sex, age, comorbidity, country, and time period: a systematic review and meta-analysis. Lancet Neurol 10: 626-636.

8. Lin N, Cahill KS, Frerichs KU, Friedlander RM, Claus EB (2012) Treatment of ruptured and unruptured cerebral aneurysms in the USA: a paradigm shift. J Neurointerv Surg 4: 182-189.

9. Shea AM, Reed SD, Curtis LH, Alexander MJ, Villani JJ, et al., Characteristics of nontraumatic subarachnoid hemorrhage in the United States in 2003. Neurosurgery 61: 1131-1337; discussion 1137-1138.

10. Wagner M, Stenger K (2005) Unruptured intracranial aneurysms: using evidence and outcomes to guide patient teaching. Crit Care Nurs Q 28: 341-354.

11. Austin G, Fisher S, Dickson D, Anderson D, Richardson S, et al. (1993) The significance of the extracellular matrix in intracranial aneurysms. Ann Clin Lab Sci 23: 97-105.

12. van Gelder JM (2003) Computed tomographic angiography for detecting cerebral aneurysms: implications of aneurysm size distribution for the sensitivity, specificity, and likelihood ratios. Neurosurgery, 2003 53: 597-605; discussion 605-606.

13. Perry JJ, Spacek A, Forbes M, Wells GA, Mortensen M, et al. (2008) Is the combination of negative computed tomography result and negative lumbar puncture result sufficient to rule out subarachnoid hemorrhage? Ann Emerg Med 51: 707-713.

14. Maslehaty H, Petridis AK, Barth H, Mehdorn HM (2011) Diagnostic value of magnetic resonance imaging in perimesencephalic and nonperimesencephalic subarachnoid hemorrhage of unknown origin. J Neurosurg 114: 1003-1007.

15. UCAS Japan Investigators, Morita A, Kirino T, Hashi K, Aoki N, et al. (2012) The natural course of unruptured cerebral aneurysms in a Japanese cohort. N Engl J Med 366: 2474-2482.

16. Wiebers DO, Whisnant JP, Huston J 3rd, Meissner I, Brown RD Jr, et al. (2003) Unruptured intracranial aneurysms: natural history, clinical outcome, and risks of surgical and endovascular treatment. Lancet 362: 103-110.

17. Rabinstein AA, Lanzino G, Wijdicks EF (2010) Multidisciplinary management and emerging therapeutic strategies in aneurysmal subarachnoid haemorrhage. Lancet Neurol 9: 504-519.

18. Dorhout Mees SM, Kerr RS, Rinkel GJ, Algra A, Molyneux AJ (2012) Occurrence and impact of delayed cerebral ischemia after coiling and after clipping in the International Subarachnoid Aneurysm Trial (ISAT). J Neurol 259: 679-683.

19. Rincon F, Gordon E, Starke RM, Buitrago MM, Fernandez A, et al. (2010) Predictors of long-term shunt-dependent hydrocephalus after aneurysmal subarachnoid hemorrhage. Clinical article. J Neurosurg 113: 774-780.

20. Murayama Y, Nien YL, Duckwiler G, Gobin YP, Jahan R, et al. (2003) Guglielmi detachable coil embolization of cerebral aneurysms: 11 years' experience. J Neurosurg 98: 959-966.

21. Khan SH, Nichols C, Depowell JJ, Abruzzo TA, Ringer AJ (2012) Comparison of coil types in aneurysm recurrence. Clin Neurol Neurosurg 114: 12-16.

22. Guglielmi G (2009) History of the genesis of detachable coils. A review. J Neurosurg 2009 111: 1-8.

23. Molyneux AJ, Birks J, Clarke A, Sneade M, Kerr RSC (2015) The durability of endovascular coiling versus neurosurgical clipping of ruptured cerebral aneurysms: 18 year follow-up of the UK cohort of the International Subarachnoid Aneurysm Trial (ISAT). The Lancet 385: 691-697.

24. Qureshi AI, Vazquez G, Tariq N, Suri MF, Lakshminarayan K, et al. (2011) Impact of International Subarachnoid Aneurysm Trial results on treatment of ruptured intracranial aneurysms in the United States. Clinical article. J Neurosurg 114: 834-841.

25. Piotin M, Blanc R, Spelle L, Mounayer C, Piantino R, et al. (2010) Stent-assisted coiling of intracranial aneurysms: clinical and angiographic results in 216 consecutive aneurysms. Stroke 41: 110-115.

26. McDougall CG, Johnston SC, Gholkar A, Barnwell SL, Vazquez Suarez JC, et al. (2014) Bioactive versus bare platinum coils in the treatment of intracranial aneurysms: the MAPS (Matrix and Platinum Science) trial. AJNR Am J Neuroradiol 35: 935-942.

27. Lewis SC, Gholkar A, Sellar RJ, Nahser H, Cognard C, et al. (2011) Hydrogel-coated coils versus bare platinum coils for the endovascular treatment of intracranial aneurysms (HELPS): a randomised controlled trial. The Lancet 377: 1655-1662.

28. Birski M, Wałęsa C, Gaca W, Paczkowski D, Birska J, et al. (2014) Clipping versus coiling for intracranial aneurysms. Neurol Neurochir Pol 48: 122-129.

29. Molyneux AJ, Kerr RS, Birks J, Ramzi N, Yarnold J, et al. (2009) Risk of recurrent subarachnoid haemorrhage, death, or dependence and standardised mortality ratios after clipping or coiling of an intracranial aneurysm in the International Subarachnoid Aneurysm Trial (ISAT): long-term follow-up. Lancet Neurol 8: 427-433.

30. Turek G, Lewszuk A, Kochanowicz J, Lyson T, Zielinska-Turek J, et al. (2016) Early outcomes and perioperative complications of endovascular

embolization in patients with aneurysmal SAH. Neurol Neurochir Pol 50: 342-348.

31. Molyneux AJ, Kerr RS, Yu LM, Clarke M, Sneade M, et al. (2005) International subarachnoid aneurysm trial (ISAT) of neurosurgical clipping versus endovascular coiling in 2143 patients with ruptured intracranial aneurysms: a randomised comparison of effects on survival, dependency, seizures, rebleeding, subgroups, and aneurysm occlusion. The Lancet 366: 809-817.

32. Mitchell P, Kerr R, Mendelow AD, Molyneux A (2008) Could late rebleeding overturn the superiority of cranial aneurysm coil embolization over clip ligation seen in the International Subarachnoid Aneurysm Trial? J Neurosurg 108: 437-442.

33. Raymond J, Kotowski M, Darsaut TE, Molyneux AJ, Kerr RS (2012) Ruptured aneurysms and the International Subarachnoid Aneurysm Trial (ISAT): What is known and what remains to be questioned. Neurochirurgie 58: 103-114.

34. Raper DM, Allan R (2010) International subarachnoid trial in the long run: critical evaluation of the long-term follow-up data from the ISAT trial of clipping vs coiling for ruptured intracranial aneurysms. Neurosurgery 66: 1166-1169; discussion 1169.

35. Spetzler RF, McDougall CG, Zabramski JM, Albuquerque FC, Hills NK, et al. (2015) The Barrow Ruptured Aneurysm Trial. J Neurosurg 116: 135-144.

36. Hammer A, Steiner A, Kerry G, Ranaie G, Yakubov E, et al. (2017) Efficacy and Safety of Treatment of Ruptured Intracranial Aneurysms. World Neurosurg 98: 780-789.

37. Andaluz N, Zuccarello M (2008) Recent trends in the treatment of cerebral aneurysms: analysis of a nationwide inpatient database. J Neurosurg 108: 1163-1169.

38. Chang HW, Shin SH, Suh SH, Kim BS, Rho MH, et al. (2016) Cost-Effectiveness Analysis of Endovascular Coiling versus Neurosurgical Clipping for Intracranial Aneurysms in Republic of Korea. Neurointervention 11: 86-91.

39. Alshekhlee A, Mehta S, Edgell RC, Vora N, Feen E, et al. (2010) Hospital mortality and complications of electively clipped or coiled unruptured intracranial aneurysm. Stroke 41: 1471-1476.

40. Brown RD Jr, Broderick JP (2014) Unruptured intracranial aneurysms: epidemiology, natural history, management options, and familial screening. Lancet Neurol 13: 393-404.

41. Tummala RP, Başkaya MK, Heros RC (2005) Contemporary management of incidental intracranial aneurysms. Neurosurg Focus 18: e9.

42. da Costa LB, Gunnarsson T, Wallace MC (2004) Unruptured intracranial aneurysms: natural history and management decisions. Neurosurg Focus 17: p. E6.

43. Kotowski M, Naggara O, Darsaut TE, Nolet S, Gevry G, et al. (2013) Safety and occlusion rates of surgical treatment of unruptured intracranial aneurysms: a systematic review and meta-analysis of the literature from 1990 to 2011. J Neurol Neurosurg Psychiatry 84: p. 42-48.

44. Wermer MJ, van der Schaaf IC, Algra A, Rinkel GJ (2007) Risk of rupture of unruptured intracranial aneurysms in relation to patient and aneurysm characteristics: an updated meta-analysis. Stroke 38: 1404-1410.

45. Higashida RT, Lahue BJ, Torbey MT, Hopkins LN, Leip E, et al. (2007) Treatment of unruptured intracranial aneurysms: a nationwide assessment of effectiveness. AJNR Am J Neuroradiol 28: 146-151.

46. Lindner SH, Bor AS, Rinkel GJ (2010) Differences in risk factors according to the site of intracranial aneurysms. J Neurol Neurosurg Psychiatry 81: 116-118.

47. Miyazawa N, Akiyama I, Yamagata Z (2006) Risk factors for growth of unruptured intracranial aneurysms: follow-up study by serial 0.5-T magnetic resonance angiography. Neurosurgery 58: 1047-1053.

48. Qureshi AI, Suri MF, Khan J, Kim SH, Fessler RD, et al. (2001) Endovascular treatment of intracranial aneurysms by using Guglielmi detachable coils in awake patients: safety and feasibility. J Neurosurg 94: 880-885.

49. Abd-Elsayed AA, Wehby AS, Farag E (2014) Anesthetic management of patients with intracranial aneurysms. Ochsner J 14: 418-425.

50. Hoff RG, VAN Dijk GW, Mettes S, Verweij BH, Algra A, et al. (2008) Hypotension in anaesthetized patients during aneurysm clipping: not as bad as expected? Acta Anaesthesiol Scand 52: 1006-1011.

51. Brisman JL, Song JK, Newell DW (2006) Cerebral aneurysms. N Engl J Med 355: 928-939.

52. Tanno Y, Homma M, Oinuma M, Kodama N, Ymamoto T (2007) Rebleeding from ruptured intracranial aneurysms in North Eastern Province of Japan. A cooperative study. J Neurol Sci 258: 11-16.

53. Todd MM, Hindman BJ, Clarke WR, Torner JC (2005) Mild intraoperative hypothermia during surgery for intracranial aneurysm. N Engl J Med 352: 135-145.

54. Pasternak JJ, McGregor DG, Schroeder DR, Lanier WL, Shi Q, et al. (2008) Hyperglycemia in Patients Undergoing Cerebral Aneurysm Surgery: Its Association With Long-term Gross Neurologic and Neuropsychological Function. Mayo Clin Proc 83: 406-417.

55. Chua MH, Griessenauer CJ, Stapleton CJ, He L, Thomas AJ, et al. (2016) Documentation of Improved Outcomes for Intracranial Aneurysm Management Over a 15-Year Interval. Stroke 47: 708-712.

56. O'Kelly CJ, Kulkarni AV, Austin PC, Wallace MC, Urbach D (2010) The impact of therapeutic modality on outcomes following repair of ruptured intracranial aneurysms: an administrative data analysis. Clinical article. J Neurosurg 113: 795-801.

57. Li H, Pan R, Wang H, Rong X, Yin Z, et al. (2013) Clipping versus coiling for ruptured intracranial aneurysms: a systematic review and meta-analysis. Stroke 44: 29-37.

58. Schievink WI (1997) Intracranial aneurysms. N Engl J Med 336: 28-40.

59. Lanzino G, Murad MH, d'Urso PI, Rabinstein AA (2013) Coil embolization versus clipping for ruptured intracranial aneurysms: a meta-analysis of prospective controlled published studies. AJNR Am J Neuroradiol 34: 1764-1768.

60. Juvela S, Porras M, Poussa K (2000) Natural history of unruptured intracranial aneurysms: probability and risk factors for aneurysm rupture. Neurosurg Focus 8: 379-387.

61. Brinjikji W, Rabinstein AA, Nasr DM, Lanzino G, Kallmes DF, et al. (2011) Better outcomes with treatment by coiling relative to clipping of unruptured intracranial aneurysms in the United States, 2001-2008. AJNR Am J Neuroradiol 32: 1071-1075.

62. van Dijk JM (2011) Surgical clipping as the preferred treatment for aneurysms of the middle cerebral artery. Acta Neurochir (Wien) 153: 2111-2117.

63. Brinjikji W, Lanzino G, Cloft HJ, Rabinstein A, Kallmes DF, et al. (2010) Endovascular treatment of very small (3 mm or smaller) intracranial aneurysms: report of a consecutive series and a meta-analysis. Stroke 41: 116-121.

64. Wilson JT, Hareendran A, Grant M, Baird T, Schulz UG, et al. (2002) Improving the assessment of outcomes in stroke: use of a structured interview to assign grades on the modified Rankin Scale. Stroke 33: 2243-2246

65. Teasdale GM, Drake CG, Hunt W, Kassell N, Sano K, et al. (1988) A universal subarachnoid hemorrhage scale: report of a committee of the World Federation of Neurosurgical Societies (WFNS). J Neurol Neurosurg Psychiatry 51: 1457.

7

Combined Thoracic Epidural with General Anesthesia *vs.* General Anesthesia Alone for Major Abdominal Surgery: Anesthetic Requirements and Stress Response

Alaa M Atia* and Khaled A Abdel-Rahman

Anesthesia Department, Faculty of Medicine, Assiut University, Egypt

***Corresponding author**: Alaa M Atia, Anesthesia Department, Faculty of Medicine, Assiut University, Egypt, E-mail: alaaguhina@yahoo.com

Abstract

Background: There are two components to the anesthetic state, first component is the loss of consciousness and recall, the second component is obtundation of reflex responses to a noxious stimulus, which occurs below the level of cortex. The problem of unexpected awareness has concerned patients and anesthesiologists since the administration of general anesthesia was first described, the incorporation of paralytic agents into the administration of general anesthetics was associated with an epidemic of cases of awareness.

Aim of the study: To determine the effect of epidural bupivacaine on the requirement doses of propofol, fentanyl, and cisatrcurium and on stress response during major abdominal surgery. Patients and methods: This is a randomized, prospective clinical trial, performed in Assiut university hospital in general surgery theatre and department between April 2010 and October 2014. The protocol of the study was approved by our local ethical committee and informed written consent was obtained from all patients. The study included 80 patients of both genders scheduled for major abdominal surgery, age ranged between 18 and 75 years, with ASA physical status between I and III. Patients were divided equally and randomly into two groups to receive general anesthesia or combined general and epidural anesthesia. The induction and maintenance doses of propofol, fentanyl, and muscle relaxants were calculated in addition to hemodynamic changes, fasting blood sugar, serum cortisol, TSH and interleukin-6 level.

Results: Patients received combined general and thoracic epidural anesthesia showed lower requirements of general anesthetics and muscle relaxants, lower intra and postoperative FBS and serum cortisol levelinterleukin-6 level and higher TSH level.

Conclusion: Combined general and thoracic epidural block decrease the need of general anesthesia and muscle relaxants, decrease stress response more than general anesthesia alone during major abdominal surgery.

Keywords: General anesthesia; Abdominal surgery; Thoracic epidural

Introduction

Surgical injury elicits a well-known stress response involving activation of inflammatory, endocrine, metabolic and immunologic mediators. The surgical stress response is believed to be a necessary and beneficial response. However, exaggerated activation of various components of the surgical stress response result in a hypometabolic period, which lasts about 3 days, followed by a hypermetabolic period. As a result of these changes homeostatic disturbance, hemodynamic instability cellular dehydration, capillary leakage and organ dysfunction may occur, leading to a prolonged convalescence period [1].

General anesthesia may limit the perception of sensations due to injury, but does not abolish the response completely as hypothalamus reacts to the noxious stimuli even in the deeper planes of anesthesia (e.g. rise in HR and blood pressure, during sternotomy). All the intravenous agents and volatile anesthetics in normal doses have minor influence on the endocrine and metabolic functions deep levels of general anesthesia may affect the quality of recovery from general anesthesia.

On the contrary the neural blockade by regional anesthesia with local anesthetics have direct influence on endocrinal and metabolic response [2]. The basic mechanism of neural blockade on stress response to surgery is the total prevention of the nociceptive signals from the surgical area from reaching the central nervous system. The inhibitory effect of neural blockade on endocrine and metabolic response to surgery is involved through both afferent and the efferent pathway but differ among the individual endocrine glands [3], the neural blockade are limited by the hemodynamic changes and respiratory derangements when high level of block is needed.

The simultaneous administration of epidural local anesthetics with general anesthetics (IV or inhaled) is frequently used in major abdominal or thoracic surgery. During combined general/epidural anesthesia (CGEA) the noxious stimulus originating from the surgical site is blocked at the spinal level, reducing the requirements of general anesthetics [4].

Proven advantages of CGEA include early recovery from general anesthesia and postoperative analgesia, together with likely decreases in blood loss, cardiac dysrhythmias, or ischemic events and postoperative deep vein thrombosis [5].

The side effects of the technique are related to the dose (hypotension) or site (bradycardia and respiratory distress) of the LA administration and to light general anesthesia, which can result in awareness during surgery [6]. In many settings, the use of CGEA is increasing because of the favorable recovery characteristics that facilitate early hospital discharge [7].

The immunologic and inflammatory responses are largely orchestrated by endogenous mediators referred to as cytokines produced by activated leucocytes, fibroblasts and endothelial cells. Cytokines influence immune cell activity, differentiation, proliferation and survival. They regulate the activity of other cytokines, which may either augment (pro-inflammatory) or attenuate (anti-inflammatory) the inflammatory response. The main cytokines released during surgery are interleukin-1 (IL-1), IL-6 and tumor necrosis factor-α (TNF-α). IL-6 is the main cytokine responsible for production of acute phase proteins in the liver including C-reactive protein, and may activate the hypothalamic-pituitary-adrenal axis [8].

Aim of the Study

To determine the effect of thoracic epidural bupivacaine on the requirement doses of general anesthetic agents and muscle relaxants during major abdominal surgery guided by AAI index and to determine the effect of thoracic epidural block on the stress response to surgery.

Patients and Methods

This study is a randomized, prospective clinical trial, performed in Assiut university hospital in general surgery theater and department between April 2010 and October 2014.

The protocol of the study was approved by our local ethical committee and informed written consent was obtained from all patients.

Patients

The study included 80 patients of both genders scheduled for major abdominal surgery, age ranged between 18 and 75 years, with ASA physical status between I and III.

Exclusion criteria included severe cardiovascular diseases, neuropsychiatric disorders, severe metabolic diseases, drug abuse, any contraindications to neuraxial blockade as hypersensitivity to amide local anesthetics, bleeding or coagulation disorders, infection at injection site...etc.

Study design

Patients fulfilling the inclusion criteria were allocated randomly into two equal groups each of 40 patients.

- The combined group (Group I) received combined total intravenous general anesthesia (TIVA) with thoracic epidural as maintenance anesthesia.
- The general anesthesia group (Group II) received only TIVA as maintenance anesthesia.

All patients were premedicated with ranitidine 150 mg and midazolam 5 mg at the night of the surgery and 2 h before surgery

with sips of water. All patients were monitored non-invasively for heart rate, non-invasive blood pressure, electrocardiogram and oxygen saturation. All Patients were preloaded with 10 mL/kg normal saline (NS). In group I, an epidural catheter was placed between T9-10. Ten mL of bupivacaine 0.1% was administered as a bolus via the epidural route 20 min before induction of anesthesia and then infusion was maintained at 6 mL/h of the same drug concentration.

Patients in both groups received the same technique for induction of anesthesia, bolus dose of fentanyl 2 μg/kg were given intravenously followed by infusion of propofol 1% at a rate of 4 mg/sec. for about 15-20 seconds till the AAI index reached 15-25. Intubation is then performed after I.V cisatracurium 0.15 mg/kg. Ventilation was controlled with a tidal volume of 10 mL/kg and respiratory rate adjusted to maintain end-tidal carbon dioxide between 30-35 mmHg.

After endotracheal intubation, propofol 1% infusion was titrated to maintain AAI index between 15-25 using continuous A-Line ARX index (AAI index) monitoring (AEP monitor/2, Danmeter A/S, Kildemosevej 13, DK-5000 Odense C).

For administration of top-up doses of cisatracurium, one-fifth of the initial dose of cisatracurium was administered once the recovery of T1/T0 of electromyographic response of adductor pollicis muscle to train of four of the ulnar nerve reached 10%.

Inadequate intraoperative analgesia was defined as an increase in SBP and/or HR by >20% of baseline value for >5 min in response. In this case, patients were given bolus doses of fentanyl 0.5 μg/kg.

Fasting and maintenance dose of I.V. crystalloids were calculated as 4 ml/kg for first 10 kg body weight, then 2 ml/kg for the next 10 kg of body weight and 1ml/kg thereafter, blood loss was replaced with 3 ml crystalloid for every 1 ml blood, third space loss were calculated as 6 ml/kg/hour. Packed red blood cells were administered only when hematocrit becomes <24%.

Bradycardia was defined as HR <40 bpm and hypotension as a decrease in SBP <40% of baseline. Hypotension was treated by infusion of NS and, and if necessary, 5 mg ephedrine was given intravenously.

Data collection

Operative date including duration of operation measured from the skin incision to skin closure, blood loss, volume and type of fluid infused were recorded.

At the end of operation, dose requirements of propofol, fentanyl, and cisatracurium were calculated; dose requirements of each drug were calculated by dividing the total amount of the individual drug used by duration of the operation and patient's weight in kilograms, thus giving the individual drug consumption in $mg.kg^{-1}.h^{-1}$[9].

Venous blood sample (5 ml) was withdrawn at baseline, 30 minutes after skin incision and 24 hours postoperatively for detection of fasting blood sugar (FBS), serum cortisol, TSH. Sample for assessment of interleukin 6 was withdrawn at baseline, 6 hours and 24 hours postoperatively.

Data analysis

Statistical analysis was conducted with SPSS 21 for Windows. Data were summarized as mean and SD and number of patients. The sample size was calculated based on that 20% difference in anesthetic doses is significant. Thirty four patients per group were required to demonstrate a 20% difference in anesthetic doses at α=0.05 and power of 90%. To exclude and dropouts, Six more patients were added to each group. The statistical comparisons between groups were analysed with independent t test and Mann- Whitney U, test. P<0.05 was recognized as statistically significant in all the analyses.

Results

Group characteristics

Patients' general characteristics and other pre-operative data were summarized in Table 1. Both groups were comparable to each other as regard age, weight, height, sex, BMI, ASA status, duration of operation, crystalloids and blood infused.

	Group I	Group II	p-value
Sex (male/female)	24/16	27/13	0.485
Age	57.72 ± 9.34	59.92 ± 6.71	0.230
Height	168.42 ± 7.86	169.62 ± 8.01	0.501
Weight	73.07 ± 13.57	75.05 ± 9.2	0.449
ASA (I/II/III)	11/26/3	7/28/5	0.481
Duration of operation (min.)	160.4 ± 40.74	164.72 ± 40.3	0.634
Fluid infused (ml.)	3153.75 ± 326.67	3232.5 ± 293.2	0.260
Blood infused (ml.)	262.5 ± 277.06	337.5 ± 346.91	0.288
Data were represented as mean ± SD unless otherwise indicated			

Table 1: Group characteristics.

Pre- and post-intubation AAI index

Before intubation, induction dose of propofol titrated to a value of AAI index between 15 and 25. Mean pre- and post-intubation AAI index showed no significant differences between both groups (Table 2).

	Group I	Group II	p-value
Pre-intubation AAI index	16.97 ± 1.45	17.5 ± 1.64	0.135
Post-intubation AAI index	21.1 ± 1.75	21.8 ± 1.52	0.06
Data were represented as mean ± SD			

Table 2: Pre- and post-intubation AAI-index.

Hemodynamic Variables

Mean arterial blood pressure: Both groups showed the same pattern as regard mean arterial blood pressure changes. After induction of general anesthesia and before endotracheal intubation mean arterial blood pressure in both groups was significantly lower than baseline value. Immediately after intubation and after skin incision mean arterial blood pressure increased significantly in both groups compared to baseline values (Figure 1).

Mean arterial blood pressure at 1st, 2nd, and more than 2 hours and at the end of operation were significantly lower than baseline values.

Only at skin incision, mean arterial blood pressure was lower in group I compared to group II.

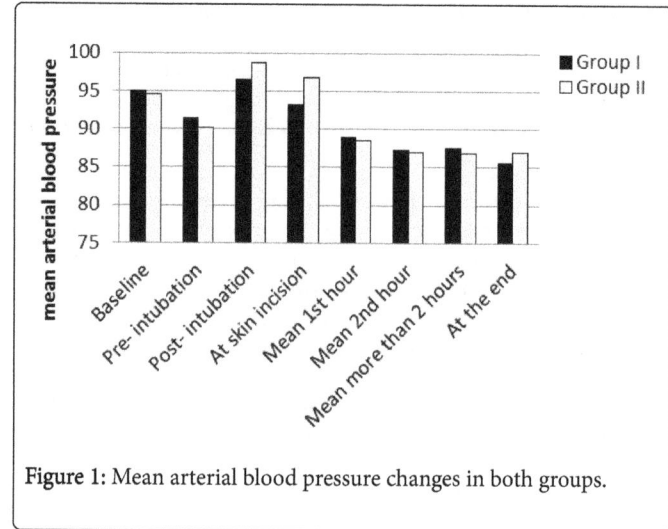

Figure 1: Mean arterial blood pressure changes in both groups.

Heart rate: Heart rate showed higher mean values compared to baseline at after induction, pre and post-intubation and at skin incision in both studied groups (time effect).

Heart rate showed persistently significant lower values in epidural group compared to general anesthesia group after the skin incision till the end of operation (group effect) (Figure 2).

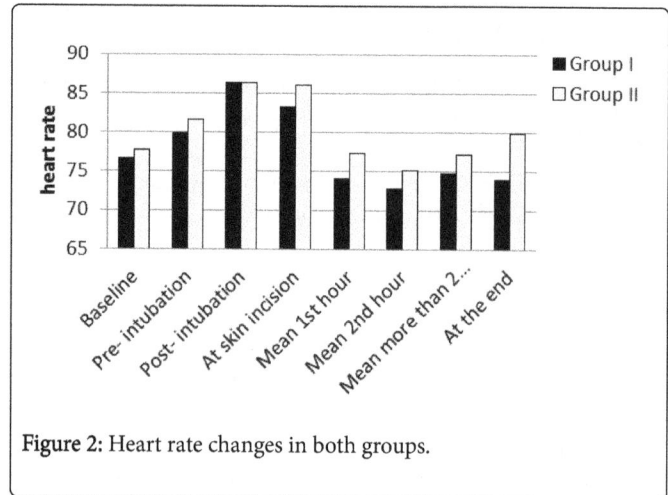

Figure 2: Heart rate changes in both groups.

Induction and maintenance doses of anesthetic agents

In both groups general anesthesia was induced with bolus dose of IV fentanyl 2 μg/kg then propofol was infused at a rate of 4 mg/sec for about 15 to 20 seconds targeting AAI index of 15-25. The total induction dose of propofol required for this AAI index target was significantly lower in epidural group (1.82 ± 0.53 mg/kg) than general anesthesia group (2.94 ± 0.56 mg/kg).

In the same context propofol doses required to maintain the same level of anesthesia were also significantly lower in epidural group compared to general anesthesia group (Table 3).

Increased MAP or HR by more than 20% of the baseline was treated with 0.5 μg fentanyl. Total dose of fentanyl was significantly lower in epidural group compared to general anesthesia group.

Cisatracurium was given at a dose of 0.15 mg/kg to facilitate endotracheal intubation, then top up doses were given guided by the train of four. Maintenance doses of muscle relaxants were significantly lower in epidural group than general anesthesia group.

	Group I	Group II	p-value
Propofol induction dose(mg)	1.82 ± 0.53	2.94 ± 0.56	0.000*
propofol maintenance dose (mg/kg/hr)	4.65 ± 1.21	5.54±1.3	0.002*
Fentanyl (µg)	0.43 ± 0.21	1.09 ± 0.22	0.000*
Cisatracurium maintenance dose (mg/kg/hr)	6.27 ± 2.4	7.83 ± 2.44	0.005*
Data were represented as mean ± SD			
*Significant difference between both groups			

Table 3: Propofol, fentanyl, and cisatracurium doses.

Fasting blood sugar, cortisol and TSH interleukin 6 levels

Baseline values in both groups were comparable to each other. Thirty minutes after skin incision fasting blood sugar, cortisol rose significantly from the baseline while TSH level decreased significantly from the baseline in both groups. After 24 hours significant rise in FBS and cortisol and significant decrease in TSH level still exist.

	Group I	Group II	p-value
Fasting blood sugar			
baseline	93.82 ± 18.74	99.2 ± 16.64	0.181
after 30 minutes	106.94 ± 17.82	119.35 ± 18.42	0.003*
after 24 hours	115.89 ± 16.21	123.15 ± 17.69	0.061
Cortisol level			
baseline	11.96 ± 5.15	13.2 ± 5.96	0.324
after 30 minutes	15.06 ± 5	21.88 ± 5.67	0.000*
after 24 hours	17.81 ± 5.86	25.44 ± 6.14	0.000*
TSH level			
baseline	2.14 ± 0.51	2.01 ± 0.63	0.319
after 24 hours	1.43 ± 0.61	1.14 ± 0.59	0.035*
Interleukin 6 level			
Baseline	7.32 ± 2.04	6.6 ± 2.81	0.193
After 6 hours	11.87 ± 3.99	15.81 ± 4.4	0.000*
After 24 hours	58.01 ± 16.59	66.93 ± 20.06	0.033*
Data were represented as mean ± SD			
*Significant difference between both groups			

Table 4: Fasting blood sugar, cortisol and TSH level.

FBS was significantly higher after 30 minutes of operation but not after 24 hours, while serum cortisol level was significantly higher in the later two times in general anesthesia group compared to combine group. TSH was lower in general anesthesia compared to combined group only after 24 hours.

Interleukin-6 level was significantly higher in group II compared to group I at both postoperative samples (Table 4).

Discussion

We compared the effect of general anesthesia alone or in combination with thoracic epidural block on the consumption of anesthetics and muscle relaxants. Our results showed reduction in induction and maintenance dose of propofol, maintenance dose of fentanyl and atracurium in combined group compared to general anesthesia group.

The use of neuraxial block in combination with general anesthesia was extensively studied. Authors studied the effect of this combination on the anesthetic doses, the hemodynamics, the stress response to surgery, post-operative pain, quality of recovery, and length of hospital stay. Different concentrations and different agents were used. Shono et al. in their study compared the hemodynamic effects, dose of sevoflurane and stress hormones with lidocaine 1% and 2% on 33 patients scheduled for lower abdominal surgery under CGEA with BIS kept between 40-50; with similar hemodynamic and BIS values they reported lower sevoflurane requirements and more suppression of stress hormones with lidocaine 2% more than lidocaine 1% [10].

Kanata et al. studied 35 patients scheduled for lower abdominal surgery, they compared the effect of two different concentrations of epidural bupivacaine (0.2% and 1%) on propofol dose, patients in bupivacaine 1% needed less amount of propofol for unconsciousness, noxious stimuli just above the level of block and at C5 level [11].

Casati et al., found that bupivacaine 0.125% to be more effective than 0.0625% in reducing the isoflurane requirements but not induction dose of thiopental. They also found that addition of fentanyl 2 µg/kg to the lower bupivacaine dose produce the same effect of higher doses of bupivacaine with less hemodynamic effects [12].

Agarwal et al. [9] showed that epidural bupivacaine can reduce the dose requirement of the induction and maintenance dose of propofol, fentanyl and vecuronium during general anesthesia. Moharari et al., also showed that epidural bupivacaine decreases the requirement dose of propofol and fentanyl for maintenance of anesthesia [13].

The mechanism behind this effect of local blocks on the needs for general anesthetic agents is still unclear.

Plasma level of local anesthetic agents was thought to affect the anesthetic needs as i.v. lidocaine infusion has a minimal alveolar concentration (MAC)-sparing effect of 10%~28% [14], Senturk et al., reported reduction in the induction and maintenance doses of propofol with intramuscular lidocaine or bupivacaine [15]. This theory was antagonized by the work of Hodgson and Liu [4] who observed decrease in anesthetic requirements despite matched plasma level of local anesthetic agents in general anesthesia alone and combined general and epidural anesthesia. The afferentation theory proposes that excitatory descending modulation of spinal cord motorneurons can be decreased through decreased afferent input to the brain and that tonic sensory and muscle-spindle activity modulate cerebral activity which maintains the state of wakefulness [16-18]. Decreased pain from the surgical site plays a role in decrease anesthetic requirements [19].

The mechanism behind the reduction in the requirement dose of muscle relaxants is thought to be due to small increase in blood level of local anesthetics which depresses postsynaptic potentiation and increases the neuromuscular block of muscle relaxants [20-22].

Metabolic and endocrinal process occurs as a result of surgery which leads to an increase in plasma levels of stress hormones, such as ACTH, cortisol, TSH [23]. The response is manifested through increased serum level of catabolic hormones and decreased serum level of anabolic hormones which is correlated to the severity of surgical injury [24]. Moreover, the depth of anesthesia may affect this stress response to surgical trauma [25]. Stress hormones such as cortisol, adrenocorticotropic hormone (ACTH), epinephrine, and norepinephrine have been validated to evaluate the magnitude of the surgical stress response [26,27].

Evidences are accumulating that attenuation of this stress response may play an important role in a patients' outcome [28,29].

Epidural blocks were also associated with reduction in postoperative cardiac, pulmonary, coagulation, and infection, which may be closely related to blunting of the stress response. For example, Yeager et al. [30] studied epidural block versus standard general anesthesia in 53 high risk patients, and found a significant reduction in cardiac failure, overall postoperative complications and major infectious complications in epidural group of patients which was also correlated with concurrent, significantly lower urinary cortisol excretion in epidural group. The authors suggested that low serum catecholamines level in the epidural group with subsequent effects of tachycardia, hypertension, and increased myocardial oxygen consumption as the probable mechanism. Decreased incidence of infectious complications and wound healing may be explained by hyperglycemia and hypercatabolic state associated with sympathetic overactivity during periods of stress [31].

Limitations of our study may include the effects of hypotensive events on the level of A-line ARX index and therefore the propofol doses in not thoroughly investigated. Another problem is the difficulty in determining the level of thoracic epidural during general anesthesia. Lastly as we did not determine the plasma concentration level of propofol and with the interaction with propofol and fentanyl, we might use more of one of them instead of other.

Conclusion

Combined general and thoracic epidural block decrease the need for general anesthesia and muscle relaxants, decrease stress response more than general anesthesia alone during major abdominal surgery.

References

1. Kücükakin B, Lykkesfeldt J, Nielsen HJ, Reiter RJ, Rosenberg J, et al. (2008) Utility of melatonin to treat surgical stress after major vascular surgery--a safety study. J Pineal Res 44: 426-431.

2. Simpson PJ, Radford SG, Forster SJ, Cooper GM, Hughes AO (1982) The fibrinolytic effects of anaesthesia. Anaesthesia 37: 3-8.

3. Moore CM, Desborough JP, Powell H, Burrin JM, Hall GM (1994) Effects of extradural anaesthesia on interleukin-6 and acute phase response to surgery. Br J Anaesth 72: 272-279.

4. Hodgson PS, Liu SS (2001) Epidural lidocaine decreases sevoflurane requirement for adequate depth of anesthesia as measured by the Bispectral Index monitor. Anesthesiology 94: 799-803.

5. Rodgers A, Walker N, Schug S, McKee A, Kehlet H, et al. (2000) Reduction of postoperative mortality and morbidity with epidural or spinal anaesthesia: results from overview of randomised trials. BMJ 321: 1493.

6. Domino KB, Posner KL, Caplan RA, Cheney FW (1999) Awareness during anesthesia: a closed claims analysis. Anesthesiology 90: 1053-1061.

7. Senagore AJ, Whalley D, Delaney CP, Mekhail N, Duepree HJ, et al. (2001) Epidural anesthesia-analgesia shortens length of stay after laparoscopic segmental colectomy for benign pathology. Surgery 129: 672-676.

8. Lin E, Calvano SE, Lowry SF (2000) Inflammatory cytokines and cell response in surgery. Surgery 127: 117-126.

9. Agarwal A, Pandey R, Dhiraaj S, Singh PK, Raza M, et al. (2004) The effect of epidural bupivacaine on induction and maintenance doses of propofol (evaluated by bispectral index) and maintenance doses of fentanyl and vecuronium. Anesth Analg 99: 1684-1688.

10. Shono A, Sakura S, Saito Y, Doi K, Nakatani T (2003) Comparison of 1% and 2% lidocaine epidural anaesthesia combined with sevoflurane general anaesthesia utilizing a constant bispectral index. Br J Anaesth 91: 825-829.

11. Kanata K, Sakura S, Kushizaki H, Nakatani T, Saito Y (2006) Effects of epidural anesthesia with 0.2% and 1% ropivacaine on predicted propofol concentrations and bispectral index values at three clinical end points. J Clin Anesth 18: 409-414.

12. Casati L, Fernández-Galinski S, Barrera E, Pol O, Puig MM (2002) Isoflurane requirements during combined general/epidural anesthesia for major abdominal surgery. Anesth Analg 94: 1331-1337.

13. Shariat Moharari R, Samadi A, Imani F, Panahkhahi M, Khashayar P, et al. (2013) The Effect of Epidural Bupivacaine on BIS Levels in the Awake Phase and on the Maintenance Doses of Propofol and Fentanyl During General Anesthesia. Anesth Pain Med 2: 149-153.

14. Himes RS Jr, DiFazio CA, Burney RG (1977) Effects of lidocaine on the anesthetic requirements for nitrous oxide and halothane. Anesthesiology 47: 437-440.

15. Senturk M, Pembeci K, Menda F, Ozkan T, Gucyetmez B, et al. (2002) Effects of intramuscular administration of lidocaine or bupivacaine on induction and maintenance doses of propofol evaluated by bispectral index. Br J Anaesth 89: 849-852.

16. motokizawa F, Fujimori B (1964) Arousal Effect Of Afferent Discharges from Muscle Spindles upon Electroencephalograms In Cats. Jpn J Physiol 14: 344-353.

17. Lanier WL, Iaizzo PA, Milde JH, Sharbrough FW (1994) The cerebral and systemic effects of movement in response to a noxious stimulus in lightly anesthetized dogs. Possible modulation of cerebral function by muscle afferents. Anesthesiology 80: 392-401.

18. Doufas AG, Wadhwa A, Shah YM, Lin CM, Haugh GS, et al. (2004) Block-dependent sedation during epidural anaesthesia is associated with delayed brainstem conduction. Br J Anaesth 93: 228-234.

19. Eappen S, Kissin I (1998) Effect of subarachnoid bupivacaine block on anesthetic requirements for thiopental in rats. Anesthesiology 88: 1036-1042.

20. Usubiaga JE, Standaert F (1968) The effects of local anesthetics on motor nerve terminals. J Pharmacol Exp Ther 159: 353-361.

21. Kordas M (1970) The effect of procaine on neuromuscular transmission. J Physiol 209: 689-699.

22. Nonaka A, Sugawara T, Suzuki S, Masamune T, Kumazawa T (2002) [Pretreatment with lidocaine accelerates onset of vecuronium-induced neuromuscular blockade]. Masui 51: 880-883.

23. Bessey PQ, Lowe KA (1993) Early hormonal changes affect the catabolic response to trauma. Ann Surg 218: 476-489.

24. Davis FM, Laurenson VG, Lewis J, Wells JE, Gillespie WJ (1987) Metabolic response to total hip arthroplasty under hypobaric subarachnoid or general anaesthesia. Br J Anaesth 59: 725-729.

25. Tian K, Kang Y, Deng L, Liu H, Li H, et al, (2014) [Effects of different anesthesia depth on stress response in elderly patients undergoing elective laparoscopic surgery for colorectal cancer]. Nan Fang Yi Ke Da Xue Xue Bao 34: 694-698.

26. Schricker T, Carli F, Schreiber M, Wachter U, Geisser W, et al, (2000) Propofol/sufentanil anesthesia suppresses the metabolic and endocrine response during, not after, lower abdominal surgery. Anesth Analg 90: 450-455.

27. Roizen MF, Horrigan RW, Frazer BM (1981) Anesthetic doses blocking adrenergic (stress) and cardiovascular responses to incision--MAC BAR. Anesthesiology 54: 390-398.

28. Lee TW, Grocott HP, Schwinn D, Jacobsohn E (2003) High spinal anesthesia for cardiac surgery: effects on beta-adrenergic receptor function, stress response, and hemodynamics. Anesthesiology 98: 499-510.

29. Scott NB, Turfrey DJ, Ray DA, Nzewi O, Sutcliffe NP, et al. (2001) A prospective randomized study of the potential benefits of thoracic epidural anesthesia and analgesia in patients undergoing coronary artery bypass grafting. Anesth Analg 93: 528-535.

30. Yeager MP, Glass DD, Neff RK, Brinck-Johnsen T (1987) Epidural anesthesia and analgesia in high-risk surgical patients. Anesthesiology 66: 729-736.

31. Kehlet H (1991) The surgical stress response: should it be prevented? Can J Surg 34: 565-567.

8

Comparative Study between General and Spinal Anaesthesia in Laparoscopic Appendectomy

Ahmed Medhat Ahmed Mokhtar Mehanna[1*] and Atteia Gad Ibrahim[2]

[1]*Lecturer of General Surgery, Ain Shams University, Egypt*

[2]*Lecturer of Anesthesia, Tanta University, Egypt*

*****Corresponding author:** Ahmed Medhat Ahmed Mokhtar Mehanna, Lecturer of General Surgery, Ain Shams University, Egypt, E-mail: drahmedmedhat1@yahoo.com

Abstract

Background: Laparoscopic appendectomy is rapidly increasing in the treatment of acute appendicitis. Spinal anesthesia has some advantages over general anesthesia in providing analgesia and muscle relaxation while avoiding some of the complications of general anesthesia.

Methods: This comparative study was conducted on 80 patients undergoing laparoscopic appendectomy. Surgeries were randomized into two groups. Group (G) was done under General Anesthesia (40 patients) and group (S) Subarachnoid block group (40 patients).

Results: From 1 min to 12 h post-operative there was significant increase in mean heart rate and mean arterial blood pressure in group G than group S. In group (S) 2.5% was converted to open due to shoulder pain and inappropriate level of anesthesia. The operative time between both groups was insignificant. Shoulder pain was found in 5% of group (S). Mean VAS score was significantly lower at 1, 2, 4 and 12 h with significantly less analgesic requirements in group (S).

Nausea was found in 5% of group (G) had and vomiting in 2.5%. No patients of group (S) had back pain. 5% in group (S) had retention and needed urinary catheterization. Early postoperative mobilization was noticed in group (S).

Conclusion: spinal anesthesia using a combination of 0.5% hyperbaric bupivacaine and a fentanyl provided effective anaesthesia for laparoscopic appendectomy with low-pressure CO_2 pneumoperitoneum.

Keywords: Laparoscopy; Laparoscopic appendicitis; Spinal anesthesia; Acute appendicitis

Introduction

Acute appendicitis is one of the most common causes of acute abdominal pain worldwide [1]. The reported lifetime cumulative incidence of acute appendicitis in Western countries is approximately 9%, and some recent reports have suggested that the incidence of acute appendicitis has been increasing in both developed and developing countries [2].

Open appendectomy (OA) was the standard treatment for acute appendicitis and was gradually replaced by laparoscopic appendectomy (LA) after its introduction by Semm in 1983 [3].

Over the last two decades, the laparoscopic approach has rapidly increased in popularity, particularly as published reports have associated laparoscopic appendectomy with earlier recovery, shortened length of hospital stay and decreased infectious complications [4].

Recent evidence suggests that regional anesthesia has a significant role in the care of patients undergoing laparoscopy [5].

Spinal anesthesia is a less invasive anesthetic technique that has lower morbidity and mortality rates, compared with general anesthesia [6].

Spinal anesthesia (SA) has the advantage of providing analgesia and total muscle relaxation in a conscious and compliant patient and an uneventful postoperative recovery. At the same time, it also protects against the potential complications of general anesthesia (GA). Despite these advantages, regional anesthesia is still preferred only for patients who are at high risk for general anesthesia, and the majority of surgeons still prefer doing both open and laparoscopic procedures under GA. Thus, most of the publications and textbooks on laparoscopic surgery cite GA as the only anesthetic option for abdominal laparoscopic surgery. But, lately, occasional reports of laparoscopic surgery being performed under regional anesthesia (spinal or epidural) in selected patients have started coming in [7].

Of the advantages of spinal anesthesia over general anesthesia is that the patient is awake and oriented at the end of the procedure. Second, the absence of general anesthetic side effects (e.g., nausea and vomiting) and less pain experienced due to the effect of neuraxial analgesia. Third, patients that have received spinal anesthesia tend to ambulate earlier than patients receiving general anesthesia. Finally, complications related to intubation and/or extubation is avoided in spinal anesthesia for patients undergoing laparoscopic interventions.

Combining a minimally invasive surgical procedure with a less invasive anesthetic technique appears, theoretically, to further enhance the advantages of the operation [8].

Although many reports of laparoscopic inguinal hernia repair and cholecystectomy under regional anesthesia have been published, few studies have involved regional anesthesia for laparoscopic appendectomy [9].

General anesthesia being the only suitable technique for laparoscopic surgeries needs a relook. Some complications as pressor response to endotracheal intubation, increased release of stress hormones, sore throat, post-operative pain, post-operative nausea and vomiting (PONV) are from the disadvantages of using GA [10].

Patients and Method

This comparative study was conducted in As-Salama hospital in AlKhobar, Saudi Arabia in the period between 1-1-2015 till 1-5-2016. 80 patients in age group ranging from 18-40 years, body mass index<30 kgm/m^2 and ASA physical status I/II were posted for laparoscopic appendectomy after a written informed consent was obtained.

Before the surgical procedures, both anesthetic techniques either general anesthesia or spinal anesthesia were considered for each patient with and patients were randomized by sealed envelopes to receive either general (group G) (40 patients) or spinal anesthesia (group S) (40 patients). Numbered and sealed envelopes were placed in the operating room and only opened at the patients' arrival there.

Patients' preoperative evaluation and preparation were standardized. All patients, who were in spinal anesthesia group, were informed about spinal anesthesia in detail about the possibility of general anesthesia if pain or un-satisfaction from spinal anesthesia during the procedure or discomfort despite administration of intravenous analgesics or sedatives. Patients who failed intraoperative spinal anesthesia or couldn't tolerate shoulder pain were converted to general anesthesia and categorized as cases of spinal anesthesia.

All patients with acute appendicitis undergoing laparoscopic appendectomy were included in this study. Patients with contraindication to laparoscopic appendectomy or converted to open were excluded from this study.

After obtaining baseline vital signs, both groups were preloaded with 10 ml/kg of Ringer lactate *via* a peripheral vein with an 18-gauge intravenous catheter. The patients under both the groups were premedicated 2 mg of midazolam hydrochloride, 4 mg ondanosetron, and 8 mg dexamethasone before the induction of anesthesia.

GA patients

Were induced with iv Propofol 2.5 mg/kg, fentanyl 1 μg/kg and succinyl chlorine 1.5 mg/kg, and intubated with suitable sized cuffed endotracheal tube. Anesthesia was maintained using 2-3% sevoflurane and 50% nitrous oxide in Oxygen and atracurium besylate (0.5 mg/kg) for neuromuscular blocking. Ventilation was controlled with a tidal volume of 6 8 ml/kg, and the ventilatory rate was adjusted to maintain a PaCO$_2$ value of 35-40 mmHg Noninvasive arterial blood pressure, electrocardiography, pulse oximetry and end tidal carbon dioxide (ETCO$_2$) were monitored continuously. Lactated Ringer's solution (3-6 ml/kg/h) was infused throughout surgery. No additional intravenous opioids were injected. At the end of surgery residual neuromuscular

block was reversed by neostigmine 0.05 m/kg and atropine sulphate 0.01 mg/kg intravenously and patient was extubated and transferred to PACU.

SA patients

Patient in a sitting position, under complete aseptic technique at the level of L4-3 or L4-5 lumber interspace vertebrae in the midline approach lumbar puncture was performed using 27 gauge pencil point spinal needle, once flow of clear CSF, 15 mg hyperbaric bupivacian with 25 μg fentanyl in a total volume 3.5 ml injected intrathecally then the patient asked to lie in a supine position and the level of anesthesia was checked to a sensory blockade up to T4. The sensory block level was assessed by the pinprick test using a 24-gauge hypodermic needle, while the motor block level was assessed by the modified Bromage scale. Lactated Ringer's solution (3-6 ml/kg/h) was infused throughout surgery, Oxygen supplementation was given to all the patients at 3 l/min through the nasal cannula. Non-invasive arterial blood pressure, electrocardiography, and pulse oximetry were monitored continuously. Intraoperative incidents (e.g., right shoulder pain, headache, and abdominal discomfort, hypotension, nausea, and/or vomiting) were documented

Intraoperative hypotention more than 20% of the basal measure was managed by intravenous ephedrine sulphate 5 mg increment every 5 min. If any patient experienced pain or discomfort, fentanyl (30-50 μg) can be given and anxiety treated with i.v midazolam 2 mg. At the end of surgery patients transferred to PACU.

All Patients were monitored in the PACU for 30 min by nursing staff for evidence of complications or adverse events.

Surgical technique

Same technique was used for both groups. Patients were positioned supine.

All patients had 3 port technique, one port supraumblical 12 mm, one 5 mm port in infraumblical and one 5 mm port in the supra pubic region. Pneumoperitoneum was established by using closed versus needle technique with carbon dioxide at a maximum intra-abdominal pressure of 12 mmHg to minimize the incidence of shoulder pain. Another modification of the technique was the minimal-if any-tilting of the operating table, i.e., minimal head down and left tilt to minimize diaphragmatic irritation.

Diagnostic laparoscopy was carried out. Then dissection of the meso-appendix did by the use of bipolar cautery (Enseal). Double ligation of the appendix at its base by end loop and cutting the appendix by the help of Enseal. Retrieval of the appendix *via* the 12 mm port with the use of 5 mm lens.

In both the groups, mean ABP, heart rate, SPO$_2$ were recorded at the following points of times,

- Prior to induction.
- After induction in GA group and after subarachnoid block in SA group
- Immediately after pneumoperitoneum
- Every 15 minutes thereafter in both groups
- 1, 2, 4, 8 and 12 h postoperatively

Post-operative pain was analyzed using visual analogue scale (VAS) and assessed at 1, 2, 4 and 12 h. Intensity of pain was assessed by using

10 point VAS representing various intensity of pain from '0' to 10. Diclofenac sodium 75 mg i.v was given when VAS was >4 and the number of ampules administered to each patient during the first 8 h postoperatively was recorded If any patient experienced nausea/vomiting, ondensetron 4 mg was intravenously given. Headache, sore throat, pruritus, or any other neurologic complaint, and urinary retention were monitored.

Post-operative data were recorded including mobilization, and return of bowel sounds. Days of hospital stay were recorded, and the overall cost of both the operations was calculated.

Statistical analysis

Data were collected, revised, coded and entered to the Statistical Package for Social Science (IBM SPSS) version 20. The qualitative data were presented as number and percentages while quantitative data were presented as mean and standard deviations. The comparison between two independent groups with quantitative data and parametric distribution was done by using Independent t-test. The confidence interval was set to 95% and the margin of error accepted was set to 5%. So, the p-value was considered significant as the following: P>0.05: Non significant, P<0.05: Significant and P<0.01: Highly significant.

Results

This study included 80 patients in the age group from (18-40) with mean age 34. Seventy-four patients (92.5%) were males and 6 female (7.5%) patient. There was no statistically significant difference between both studied groups regarding age, sex distribution, mean body mass index (BMI), and the incidence of associated comorbidities (Table 1).

Mean HR	Group (G)	Group (S)	Independent t-test	
	Mean ± SD	Mean ± SD	t	P value
Basal	86 ± 1.77	85 ± 2.57	1.433	0.160
After induction	90 ± 1.05	75 ± 1.75	32.870	<0.001
Pneumo-peritoneum	100 ± 1.25	77 ± 2.05	42839	<0.001
Intra op 15	99 ± 2.47	80 3.17	21.144	<0.001
Intra op 30	95 ± 2.83	85 ± 1.19	14.567	<0.001
Intra op 45	91 ± 2.05	83 ± 2.55	10.935	<0.001
Intra op 60	90 ± 1.27	79 ± 2.07	20.256	<0.001
Post op 1 h	93 ± 3.77	84 ± 1.58	9.846	<0.001
Post op 2 h	94 ± 3.09	85 ± 3.69	8.363	<0.001
Post op 4 h	96 ± 2.33	80 ± 2.83	19.520	<0.001
Post op 8 h	92 ± 1.25	81 ± 2.67	16.686	<0.001
Post op 12 h	89 ± 2.82	83 ± 3.62	5.487	<0.001

Table 1: Comparison between group G and group S regarding mean heart rate at different measuring times.

The previous table shows that there was no statistically significant difference found between group G and group S at basal time but from induction to 12 h post-operative the table shows that there was highly statistically significant increase in mean heart rate in group G than group S with p-value <0.001 (Figure 1).

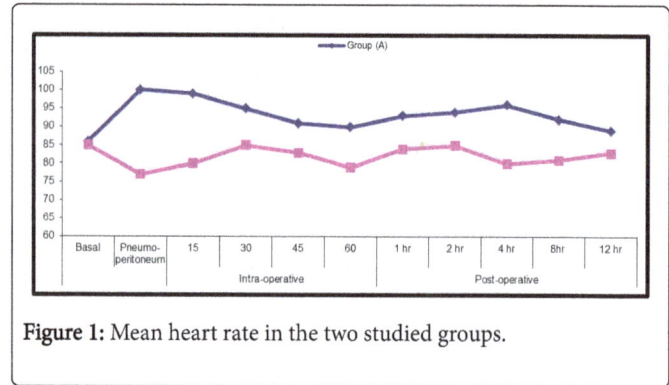

Figure 1: Mean heart rate in the two studied groups.

In both groups, all the cases were completed laparoscopically with no surgical conversion. In the spinal anesthesia group (S) one case (2.5%) was converted to open due to shoulder pain and inappropriate level of anesthesia. The operative time between both groups was statistically insignificant with mean operative time in group (G) 42.36 minutes and in group (S) 44.71 minutes. Intra and post-operative vital data were recorded in Table 2.

Mean ABP	Group (G)	Group (S)	Independent t-test	
	Mean ± SD	Mean ± SD	t	p-value
Basal	100.23 ± 1.25	100.11 ± 2.08	0.221	0.826
Pneumo-peritoneum	95.92 ± 3.18	85.34 ± 3.92	9.374	<0.001
Intra op 15	93.42 ± 2.87	84.7 ± 3.61	8.456	<0.001
Intra op 30	92.22 ± 2.95	86.9 ± 3.69	5.036	<0.001
Intra op 45	91.04 ± 3.45	85.52 ± 4.14	4.581	<0.001
Intra op 60	91.86 ± 4.17	86.21 ± 5.86	3.513	0.002
Post op 1 h	107.76 ± 2.37	92.3 ± 2.8	18.847	<0.001
Post op 2 h	109.65 ± 2.88	94.01 ± 3.31	15.942	<0.001
Post op 4 h	105.22 ± 2.29	96.35 ± 2.72	11.156	<0.001
Post op 8 h	103 ± 2.78	97 ± 2.65	6.986	<0.001
Post op 12 h	101.38 ± 3.38	98.05 ± 3.81	2.924	0.006

Table 2: Comparison between group G and group S regarding mean arterial blood pressure at different measuring times.

The previous table shows that there was no statistically significant difference found between group G and group S at basal time but from induction to 12 h post-operative the table shows that there was highly statistically significant increase in mean arterial blood pressure in group G than group S with p-value <0.01 (Figure 2).

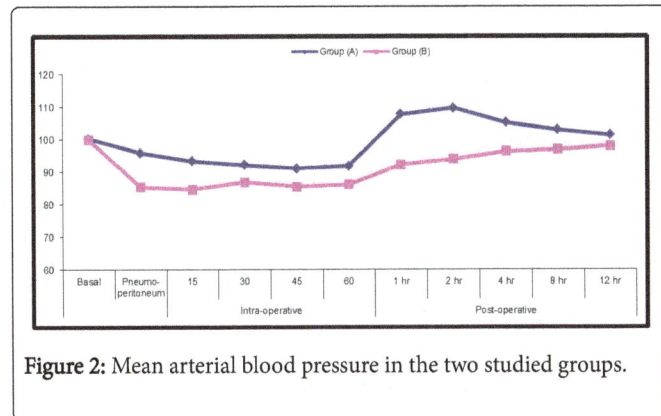

Figure 2: Mean arterial blood pressure in the two studied groups.

As for the pain, we found intra-operative shoulder pain in 2 patients (5%) in group (S), 1 of which was relieved by administration of fentanyl and midazolam injection and the other had to be converted to general anesthesia due to intolerable intraoperative shoulder pain.

As for post-operative pain, VAS score was recorded for both groups with mean score 3.0 ± 0.9 in group (G) and 1.5 ± 0.35 in group (S) at 1 hour post-operative with p-value<0.001. At 2 h postoperative mean score was found 3.2 ± 1.1 in group (G) and 1.9 ± 0.8 in group (S) with p-value<0.001. While it was 3.5 ± 0.88 in group (G) and 2.7 ± 0.95 in group (S) at 4 h with p-value=0.001. At 12 h post-operative the mean score was 2.8 ± 0.75 in group (G) and 2.1 ± 0.36 in group (S) with p-value<0.001. Group (G) needed analgesics ranging from 1 to 3 ampoules diclophenac Na (75 mg) with mean 1.6 ± 0.5 ampoule per patient, while group (S) the need for analgesics was ranging from 0 to 3 ampoules with mean was 0.6 ± 0.29 ampoule per patient with p-value=<0.001.

Two patients (5%) of group (G) had nausea and 1 patient (2.5%) had vomiting. No patients of group (S) had back pain due to the use of small spinal needle. Two patients (5%) in group (S) had retention and needed catheterization by nelaton catheter to evacuate the bladder but none needed further catheterization. Early postoperative mobilization was noticed in group (S) at 11.0 ± 1.3 h as compared to 16.0 ± 2.5 h for group (G) with p-value<0.001. As for the return of bowel sounds, they were heard after mean of 7.3 ± 2.1 h in group (G) and 6.8 ± 1.3 h in group (S) with p-value=0.371. Group (G) had a higher mean cost of the operation and hospital stay due to the use of anesthetic drugs and more pain killers but it was statistically non-significant.

Discussion

General anesthesia is the most commonly used and the most acceptable form of anesthesia for laparoscopic procedures. Some patients are more prone to the risks of general anesthesia than others (smokers, asthmatic patients etc.). Basal atelectasis, rise in the airway pressure, hypercapnia and post-operative nausea and vomiting are from the risks of general anesthesia. Spinal anesthesia offers a safer alternative to general anesthesia with some advantages over the general anesthesia group in pain management and hence in the recovery of the patients and their return to work.

Although not enough is written about the comparison between general and spinal anesthesia in laparoscopic appendectomy, some papers were discussing this comparison in laparoscopic cholecystectomy so the comparison with them might not be as effective

in some items like shoulder pain due to the difference in the operative fields.

In our study 7.5% of the spinal group (S) of patients showed bradycardia, which was similar to Gurudatta and Arif in their study of spinal anesthesia in lower abdominal surgeries found that 12% of the patients had bradycardia [10], while Mehta et al. compared general and spinal anesthesia in laparoscopic cholecystectomy and found no evidence of bradycardia [11]. 5% of group (S) patients had hypotension (>20% fall in BP) in our study, while it was 24% in Gurudatta and Arif paper [10], 30% in Mehta et al. (>30% fall in BP) [11], 18.21% in Sinha et al. study discussing laparoscopic surgeries under spinal anesthesia [12].

Post-operative pain as measured by the VAS score was in favor of group (S) throughout the post-operative period (1, 2, 4, 12 h) with p-value= <0.001, while Gurudatta and Arif's study [10], and Bessa et al. study found that the difference was non-significant after 6 h 8 but Imbelloni et al. showed significant difference at 2, 4, 6 h but non-significant difference at 12 h in his study comparing general and spinal anesthesia in laparoscopic cholecystectomy [13].

The mean number of analgesic ampoules needed was significantly lower in the spinal anesthesia group 0.6 ± 0.29 ampoules/patient as compared to 1.6 ± 0.5 ampoules /patient the general anesthesia group. Bessa et al. did a study and compared general and spinal anesthesia in laparoscopic cholecystectomy and also found significantly lower values being 0.5 to 1.1 [8].

Shoulder pain was recorded in 2 cases (5%) of group (S) which was less than that reported by Gurudatta and Arif 24% [10], and Van Zandart et al. 25% in a study of laparoscopic cholecystectomy under spinal anesthesia [14], and this pain was relieved by sedation administration in 1 patient and the other was converted to GA. In postoperative period shoulder pain was found in 2 cases in both groups (2.5%) and resolved after 5-6 h with the aid of analgesia.

Other complications as PONV were in 3 cases (7.5%) of group (G) and none of group (S) compared to 32% and 8% respectively in Gurudatta and Arif study [10]. As for urinary retention, 2 patients (5%) of group (S) suffered from it and needed catheterization although Imbelloni et al. showed no cases of retention [13].

Early post-operative mobilization and the return of bowel sounds were in favor of the spinal anesthesia group over the general anesthesia group mostly due to better pain control outcome. The mean h for postoperative mobilization was 16.0 ± 2.5 h for group (G) and was 11.0 ± 1.3 h for group (S) which was significant on statistical level p-value <0.001. On the other hand, bowel sounds were heard earlier in group (S) after mean of 6.8 ± 1.3 h as compared to 7.3 ± 2.1 h in group (G) but it was non-significant statistically.

Conclusion

Using a combination of 0.5% hyperbaric bupivacaine and a fentanyl provided effective anaesthesia for laparoscopic appendectomy with low-pressure CO_2 pneumoperitoneum. It offers better pain management for the patients, earlier recovery and less operating room costs. We recommend an increasing use of spinal anaesthesia for laparoscopic appendectomy especially in patients with risks for general anesthesia.

References

1. Andersson M, Rubér M, Ekerfelt C, Hallgren HB, Olaison G, et al. (2014) Can new inflammatory markers improve the diagnosis of acute appendicitis? World J Surg 38: 2777-2783.

2. Kong VY, Bulajic B, Allorto NL, Handley J, Clarke DL (2012) Acute appendicitis in a developing country. World J Surg 36: 2068-2073.

3. K Semm (1983) Endoscopic appendectomy, Endoscopy 15: 59-64.

4. Masoomi H, Mills S, Dolich MO, Ketana N, Carmichael JC, et al. (2012) Comparison of outcomes of laparoscopic versus open appendectomy in children: data from the Nationwide Inpatient Sample (NIS), 2006-2008. World J Surg 36: 573-578.

5. Collins LM, Vaghadia H (2001) Regional anaesthesia for laparoscopy. Anesthesiol Clin North America 19: 43-55.

6. Lennox PH, Vaghadia H, Henderson C, Martin L, Mitchell GW (2002) Small-dose selective spinal anesthesia for short-duration outpatient laparoscopy: Recovery characteristics compared with desflurane anesthesia. Anesth Analg 94: 346-350.

7. Sinha R, Gurwara AK, Gupta SC (2009) Laparoscopic Cholecystectomy Under Spinal Anesthesia: A Study of 3492 Patients. J Laparoendosc Adv Surg Tech A 19: 323-327.

8. Bessa SS, El-Sayes IA, Abdel-Baki NA, El-Saiedi MK, Abdel-Maksoud MM (2010) Laparoscopic Cholecystectomy Under Spinal Versus General Anesthesia: A Prospective, Randomized Study. J Laparoendosc Adv Surg Tech A 20: 515-520.

9. Jun GW, Kim MS, Yang HJ, Sung TY, Park DH, et al. (2014) Laparoscopic appendectomy under spinal anesthesia with dexmedetomidine infusion. Korean J Anesthesiol 67: 246-251.

10. Gurudatta KN, Arif M (2014) A Clinical Study of Comparison between General Anesthesia and Spinal Anesthesia for Lower Abdominal Laparoscopic Surgeries. Sch J App Med Sci 2(3D): 1127-1133.

11. Mehta PJ, ChavedaHR, Wadwana AP (2010) Comparative analysis of spinal vs general anaesthesia for laparoscopic cholecystectomy; A controlled prospective randomized trial. Anaes Essays Res 4: 91-95.

12. Sinha R, Gurwara AK, Guptha SC (2008) Laparoscopic surgery using spinal Anesthesis. J of society ofLaparoendoscopic Surgeons 12: 133-138.

13. Imbelloni LE , Fornasari M , Fialho JC , Sant'Anna R , Cordeiro JA (2010) General Anesthesia versus Spinal Anesthesia for Laparoscopic Cholecystectomy Rev Bras Anestesiol 60: 217-227.

14. Van Zundart AAJ, Stultiends G, Jakimowiez JJ, Peak DL (2007) Laparoscopic cholecystectomy under segmental thoracicl anesthesia & feasibility study. Br J Anaesth 98: 682-686.

9

Comparative Study between Intravenous Ketamine and Lidocaine Infusion in Controlling of Refractory Trigeminal Neuralgia

Mona Mohamed Mogahed*, **Atteia Gad Anwar and Rabab Mohamed Mohamed**

Faculty of Medicine, Tanta University, Egypt

*Corresponding author: Mona Mohamed Mogahed, Faculty of Medicine, Tanta University, Tanta, Egypt, E-mail: monamogahedfr@hotmail.com

Abstract

Background: Trigeminal neuralgia (TN) is considered one of the most debilitating disorders. Several medications such as anticonvulsants are available to provide relief from pain. In this study we used either ketamine which acts as an antagonist to N-methyl-d-aspartate receptors, or lidocaine which can block sodium channels in controlling of refractory trigeminal neuralgia.

Aim: The primary outcome of the study was the pain score (The NRS) for pain assessment during the 12-week study period. The secondary outcomes were (1) Amount of analgesic medications (2) Frequency of pain (3) descriptors of pain.

Methods: This study was conducted on 100 adult patients (aged 20-70 years) with refractory trigeminal neuralgia. Patients were enrolled into two groups each group contain 50 patients. In group I (ketamine group), patients underwent ketamine infusion protocol which consisted of 3 sessions of ketamine infusion in a dose of 0.4 mg/Kg over 30-45 minutes in 250 mL of 5% dextrose solution, and each session was performed consecutively every 4 days. In group II (lidocaine group), patients underwent lidocaine infusion protocol which consisted of 3 sessions of lidocaine infusion in a dose of 5 mg/kg over 30-45 minutes in 250 mL of 5% dextrose solution, and each session was performed consecutively every 4 days.

Results: Our results showed that both groups were comparable regarding age, gender and site of pain. A significantly longer duration of pain relief was noticed in group I when compared to group II at 2 weeks, 1 month, 2 months and 3 months (3.11 ± 2.01, 3.15 ± 1.23, 4.23 ± 1.12, 4.50 ± 1.02) p<0.001. Immediately after infusion, 12 h and at 24 h pain relief was highly significant decreased in lidocaine group when compared to ketamine group (1.27 ± 1.11, 1.67 ± 1.48, 2.35 ± 1.25) p<0.001. At 48 h there was decrease in pain scores in both groups when compared to pre infusion values but without any statistical significance (3.25 ± 1.24, 3.56 ± 1.25) p=0.216. The analgesic consumption was significantly decreased in ketamine group. Complications were minor and self-controlled.

Conclusion: The infusion of either ketamine or lidocaine controls pain in refractory trigeminal neuralgia and decreases anticonvulsant consumption with minimal post- infusion complications but with the upper hand to ketamine.

Keywords: Refractory trigeminal neuralgia; Ketamine; Lidocaine; Infusion therapy; Neuropathic pain

Introduction

Trigeminal neuralgia is considered one of the most incapacitating disorders characterized by paroxysms of brief, intense, and stabbing pain affecting one or more divisions of the trigeminal nerve [1]. Treatment guidelines, published from the European Federation of Neurologic Societies, and the American Academy of Neurology, recommend carbamazepine or oxcarbazepine as the first pharmacological choice treatment of TN and baclofen as the second choice. However, some patients may become unresponsive to medication despite of adequate treatment. Also, sometimes, patients cannot tolerate the medications side effects and discontinue, although recommended treatments have achieved sufficient reduction of their pain [2].

Ketamine has an analgesic effect. It exerts its analgesic action both centrally and peripherally at many sites and mediated through multiple receptors. Ketamine also inhibits serotonin and dopamine reuptake and inhibits voltage-gated sodium and potassium channels [3].

Lidocaine has been also used to relieve several types of neuropathic pain, including post herpetic neuralgia [4] and intractable TN [5,6]. This therapeutic effect is due to dose dependent sodium channels block [7,8] both peripherally and centrally [9].

Patients and Methods

This randomization blind study was conducted on 100 adult patients (aged 20-70 years) with intractable trigeminal neuralgia, from the outpatient pain management unit, Tanta University Hospital, after approval of the ethics committee and obtaining verbal and written informed consent from each patient from May 2015 to July 2016. All patients' data was confidential with secret codes were used for the current study.

Subjects were randomly assigned to treatment sequence *via* a computer-generated randomization list. A randomization list was prepared in sealed envelopes for each patient. Before each procedures, both techniques either ketamine infusion or lidocaine infusion were considered for each patient and patients were received either ketamine (group I) (50 patients) or lidocaine (group II) (50 patients). Numbered and sealed envelopes were placed in the outpatient room and only opened upon the patients' arrival there. Investigator A was responsible for solution preparation according to the randomization list. Investigator B, who was blind to the treatment, was responsible for clinical examination and treatment administration. At the end of each treatment investigator B had to record data and enclose the forms in envelopes that remained closed until the end of the study.

Patients were only included if their mean daily pain intensity was >4 on a 10-point Numercal Rating Scale (NRS) (where 0=no pain and 10=worst pain imaginable) over a period more than one month while on standard treatments which include: physical therapy, pharmacologic therapy with NSAIDs, benzodiazepines, anticonvulsants or antidepressants.

Exclusion criteria were history of drug or alcohol abuse, severe psychiatric disease, previous cardiac arrhythmia, abnormal ECG, angina pectoris, a history of apoplexy, renal impairment, pregnancy, lactation, insufficient pulmonary function or allergy to the study drugs. On the study day, patients were placed in a quiet room and were monitored with a 3-lead ECG, pulse oximeter, and a noninvasive blood pressure (NIBP) monitoring.

A peripheral intravenous line was inserted for fluid and drug administration. Oxygen (4 L/min) was given *via* a nasal cannula and then our patients were included into one of two groups. In group I, ketamine infusion technique, the patients were planned to receive ketamine infusion in a dose of 0.4 mg\Kg over 30-45 minutes in 250 mL of 5% dextrose solution, and this session was performed consecutively every 4 days for 3 sessions. All patients were fasted for 8 h prior to each session. Each session of ketamine infusion was taken at the same time in the day. Midazolam was administered with ketamine in a dose of 2 mg to attenuate the potential central nervous system adverse effects.

Patients were determined to have recovered completely from ketamine infusion if they were fully awake, attained full orientation to time, place, and person, and were not in need of treatment for central nervous system adverse effects. On complete recovery, the patients were discharged from the recovery unit after the end of each session of ketamine infusion with an accompanying reliable person.

In group 2, lidocaine infusion technique, patients underwent lidocaine protocol which consisted of 3 sessions of lidocaine infusion in a dose of 5 mg/kg over 30-45 minutes in 250 mL of 5% dextrose solution, and each session was performed consecutively every 4 days. Patients were fasted for 8 h prior to each session. Each session of lidocaine infusion was taken at the same time in the day for each session.

The primary outcome of the study was the pain score (The NRS) for pain assessment during the 12-week study period. The secondary outcomes were (1) Amount of analgesic medications (2) Frequency of pain (3) descriptors of pain. All were measured at the following periods, just before the initiation of infusion directly after infusion therapy, at 12 h, 24 h, 48 h, 1 week, 2 weeks, 1 month, 2 months, 3 months. Central nervous system adverse effects were assessed with close monitoring of ECG, BP, oxygen saturation, and an open question about discomfort at the end of each session.

Statistical analysis

Sample size calculation was performed before patients' recruitment. Based on a previous reports; 100 patients was calculated for 90% power, α=0.05, β=0.1, using sample size software (G*Power Version 3.00.10, Germany). Descriptive and analytic. The full detailed form is: SPSS 20, IBM, Armonk, NY, United States of America.

Quantitative data were expressed as mean ± standard deviation (SD). Qualitative data were expressed as frequency and percentage. Independent-samples t-test of significance was used when comparing between two means. Chi-square (χ^2) test of significance was used in order to compare proportions between two qualitative parameters. A one-way analysis of variance (ANOVA) when comparing between more than two means.

Results

Our results showed that both groups were comparable regarding age, gender and site of pain Table 1. A significantly longer duration of pain relief was noticed in group I when compared to group II at 2 weeks, 1 month, 2 months and 3 months (3.11 ± 2.01, 3.15 ± 1.23, 4.23 ± 1.12, 4.50 ± 1.02. p<0.001). Immediately after infusion, 12 h and at 24 h pain relief was highly significant decreased in lidocaine group when compared to ketamine group (1.27 ± 1.11, 1.67 ± 1.48, 2.35 ± 1.25) p<0.001. At 48 h there was decrease in pain scores in both groups when compared to pre infusion values but without any statistical significance in between (3.25 ± 1.24, 3.56 ± 1.25) p=0.216 (Figure 1 and Table 2).

		Group I	Group II	P
Age (Years) (Mean ± SD)		55.21 ± 12.25	60.14 ± 16.21	0.089
Weight (Kg) (Mean ± SD)		60.23 ± 21.22	62.12 ± 11.02	0.577
Sex	**Male (%)**	27 (54)	30 (60)	0.545
	Female (%)	23 (46)	20 (40)	
Location of neuralgia	**1st trigeminal branch (%)**	5 (10)	4 (8)	0.893
	2nd trigeminal branch (%)	20 (40)	22 (44)	
	3rd trigeminal branch (%)	25 (50)	24 (48)	
P value: comparison between G I & G II				

Table 1: Characteristics of the study population.

	Before the initiation of IT	Directly after infusion therapy	12:00	24:00	48:00	1 week	2 weeks	1 month	2 months	3 months
P	0.655	0.001*	0.001*	0.001*	0.216	0.109	0.001*	0.001*	0.001*	0.001*
G I	7.33 ± 1.25	6.92 ± 2.35	6.88 ± 1.12	4.11 ± 1.11	3.25 ± 1.24	3.15 ± 2.0	3.11 ± 2.01	3.15 ± 1.23	4.23 ± 1.12	4.50 ± 1.02
P 1		0.243	0.061	0.001*	0.001*	0.001*	0.001*	0.001*	0.001*	0.001*
G II	7.21 ± 1.42	1.27 ± 1.11	1.67 ± 1.48	2.35 ± 1.25	3.56 ± 1.25	3.75 ± 1.45	6.95 ± 1.33	6.78 ± 1.24	7.11 ± 1.21	7.22 ± 1.28
P 2		0.001*	0.001*	0.001*	0.001*	0.001*	0.347	0.109	0.705	0.971
P value: comparison between GI & GII (T test)										
P1: comparison in G I (ANOVA)										
P2: comparison in G II (ANOVA)										

Table 2: NRS score before and after infusion therapy.

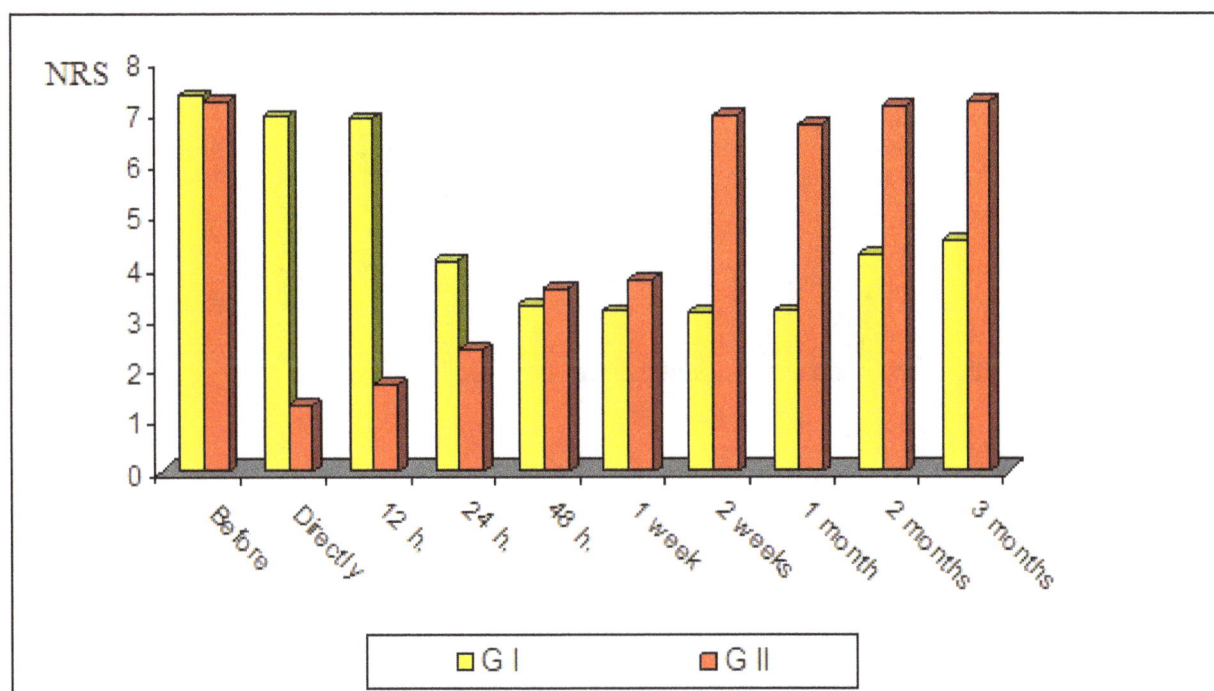

Figure 1: NRS score before and after infusion therapy.

Frequency of pain, allodynia (pain to light touch) pain score and pin prick pain score. Tables 3-5 showed the same pattern with significantly decrease in the number of attacks in lidocaine group immediately after infusion and during 12 h and 24 h follow up period (1.21 ± 0202, 1.56 ± 0.52, 1.23 ± 1.03) p<0.001 (Figures 2 and 3). Anticonvulsant therapy (carbamazepine) requirements significantly decreased in lidocaine group immediately after infusion and continued up to one week follow up period p<0.001 in ketamine group anticonvulsant therapy started to be significantly decreased at 2 h and continued to be significant during the whole follow up period. When comparing the both groups together, significantly fewer patients used anticonvulsants in ketamine group at 2 weeks, 1 month, 2 months and 3 months. Twelve patients succeeded to stop anticonvulsant therapy in ketamine group during the follow up period, while in lidocaine group nobody succeeded to stop medication Table 6 and Figure 4.

	Before the initiation of IT	Directly after infusion therapy	12:00	24:00	48:00	1 week	2 weeks	1 month	2 months	3 months
P	0.737	0.001*	0.001*	0.001*	0.625	0.209	0.001*	0.001*	0.001*	0.001*
G I	7.12 ± 0.21	4.15 ± 1.2	2.25 ± 1.2	2.0 ± 1.0	2.20 ± 1.01	2.35 ± 1.33	1.21 ± 1.29	1.29 ± 1.31	2.28 ± 1.0	2.42 ± 1.58
P 1		0.001*	0.074	0.001*	0.001*	0.001*	0.001*	0.001*	0.001*	0.001*
G II	7.11 ± 0.01	1.21 ± 0.02	1.56 ± 0.52	1.23 ± 1.03	2.30 ± 1.03	2.65± 1.02	4.27 ± 1.02	4.29 ± 1.11	6.85 ± 1.01	6.94 ± 1.21
P 2		0.001*	0.001*	0.001*	0.001*	0.001*	0.347	0.179	0.072	0.323
P: comparison between GI & GII, P1: comparison in G I, P2: comparison in G II										

Table 3: Frequency of pain.

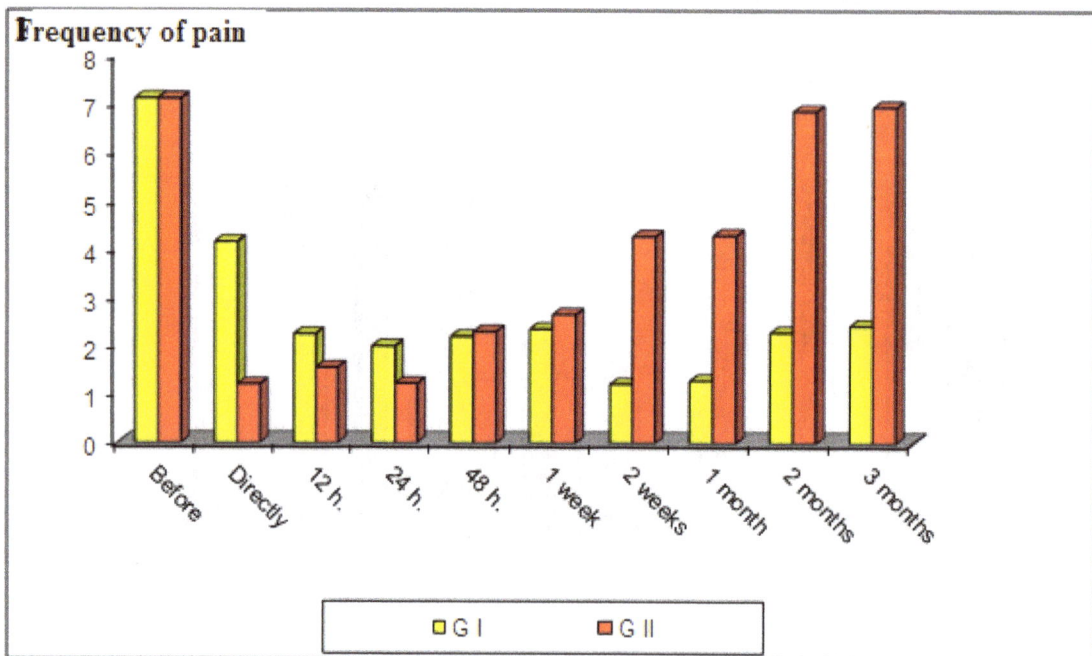

Figure 2: Frequency of pain.

	Before the initiation of IT	Directly after infusion therapy	12:00	24:00	48:00	1 week	2 weeks	1 month	2 months	3 months
P	0.110	0.001*	0.001*	0.001*	0.091	0.086	0.001*	0.001*	0.001*	0.001*
G I	6.58 ± 1.2	6.11 ± 2.0	6.03 ± 2.1	4.10 ± 0.12	3.20 ± 0.23	3.35 ± 1.01	3.10 ± 2.0	3.10 ± 1.0	4.01 ± 1.0	4.44 ± 1.14
P 1		0.157	0.110	0.001*	0.001*	0.001*	0.001*	0.001*	0.001*	0.001*
G II	7.0 ± 1.40	1.16 ± 1.01	1.06 ± 1.01	2.07 ± 1.22	3.50 ± 1.22	3.75 ± 1.28	6.54 ± 1.30	6.60 ± 1.36	7.10 ± 1.06	7.20 ± 1.29
P 2		0.001*	0.001*	0.001*	0.001*	0.001*	0.092	0.150	0.688	0.459

P: comparison between GI & GII, P1: comparison in G I, P2: comparison in G II

Table 4: Allodynia pain NRS score.

	Before the initiation of IT	Directly after infusion therapy	12:00	24:00	48:00	1 week	2 weeks	1 month	2 months	3 months
P	0.993	0.001*	0.001*	0.001*	0.250	0.116	0.001*	0.001*	0.001*	0.001*
G I	7.02 ± 1.0	6.74 ± 2.30	6.64 ± 1.10	4.0 ± 1.10	3.23 ± 1.20	3.10 ± 2.01	3.0 ± 2.02	3.13 ± 1.20	4.20 ± 1.12	4.15 ± 1.0
P 1		0.432	0.074	0.001*	0.001*	0.001*	0.001*	0.001*	0.001*	0.001*
G II	7.01 ± 1.30	1.20 ± 1.10	1.60 ± 1.30	2.30 ± 1.21	3.51 ± 1.22	3.65± 1.41	5.54 ± 1.30	6.67 ± 1.21	7.0 ± 1.32	7.21 ± 1.25
P 2		0.001*	0.001*	0.001*	0.001*	0.001*	0.347	0.179	0.969	0.435

P: comparison between GI & GII, P1: comparison in G I, P2: comparison in G II

Table 5: Pinprick hyperalgesia NRS score.

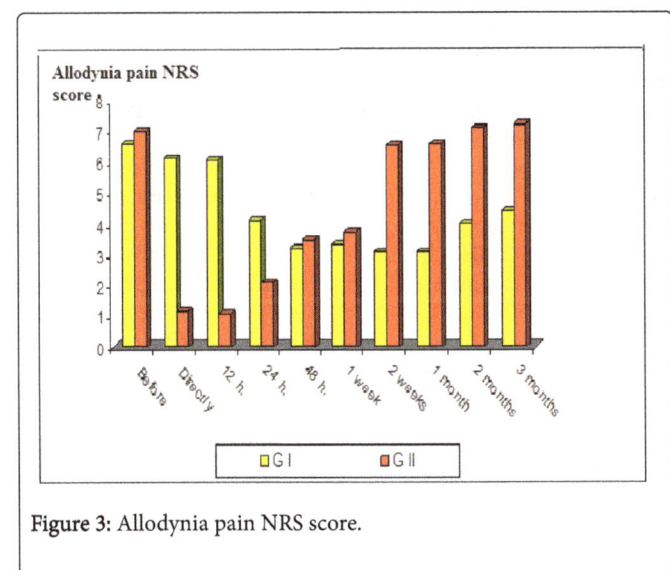

Figure 3: Allodynia pain NRS score.

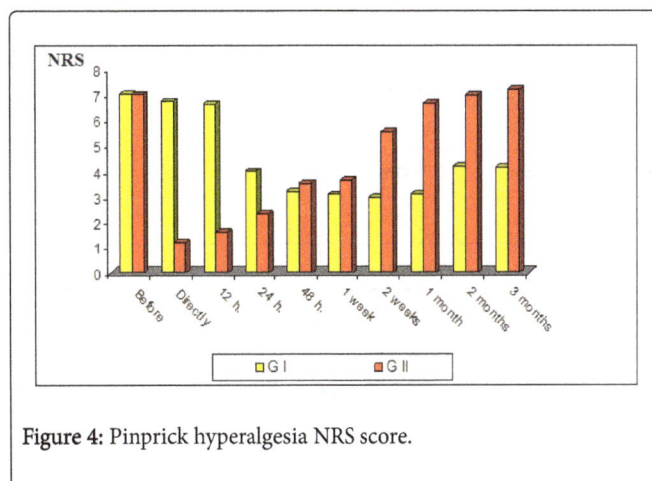

Figure 4: Pinprick hyperalgesia NRS score.

	Before the initiation of IT	Directly after infusion therapy	12:00	24:00	48:00	1 week	2 weeks	1 month	2 months	3 months
P	1.0	0.001*	0.001*	0.001*	0.250	0.606	0.001*	0.001*	0.001*	0.001*
G I	1800 ± 0	658.6 ± 213.65	324.7 ± 195.84	315.6 ± 157.85	337.7 ± 154.36	324.8 ± 145.6	172.6 ± 120.6	162.3 ± 95.68	368.7 ± 84.69	341.5 ± 75.95
P 1		0.432	0.074	0.001*	0.001*	0.001*	0.001*	0.001*	0.001*	0.001*
G II	1800 ± 0	214.6 ± 98.63	203.7 ± 84.65	195.7 ± 79.68	322.5 ± 158.9	310.8 ± 124.7	621.5 ± 214.6	603.9 ± 127.6	1747.8 ± 352.4	1785.9 ± 365.7
P 2		0.001*	0.001*	0.001*	0.629	0.001*	0.347	0.179	0.297	0.773

P: comparison between G I & G II, P1: comparison in G I, P2: comparison in G II

Table 6: Amount of analgesic medications.

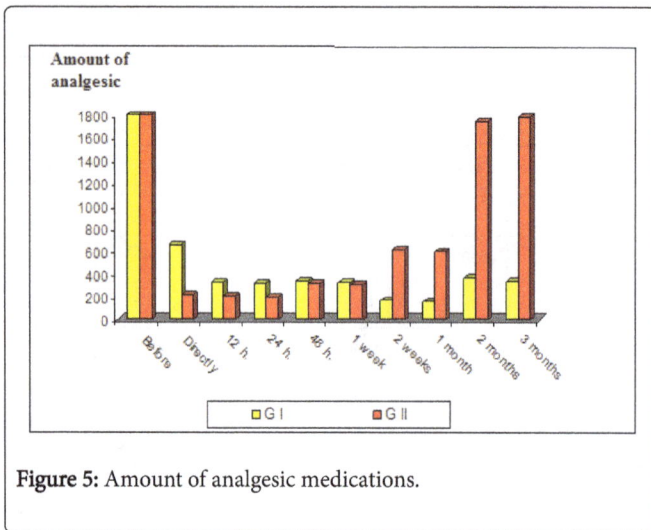

Figure 5: Amount of analgesic medications.

No serious adverse effects were reported during or after the infusion procedure. Number of responders and patient satisfaction were significantly better in group I compared to group II. Ten patients developed adverse effects (Paresthesia, Dysarthria, Dizziness, Headache, Nausea, Blurred vision) in ketamine group versus 6 patients in lidocaine group without any statistical significance p=0.297 (Table 7, 8 and Figure 5).

No. of responders	Group 1	Group 2	X^2	P-value
Responders (%)	26 (52%)	11 (22%)	9.652	0.002*
* =significant				

Table 7: Responders and patient satisfaction No. (%).

Side effects of study drugs	Group 1		Group 2		P-value
	N	%	N	%	
AEs	4	8	8	16	0.218
Tiredness	1	2	2	4	0.558
Feeling drank	1	2	3	6	0.307
Headache	2	4	5	10	0.239
Nausea	3	6	1	2	0.307
Paresthesia	2	4	3	6	0.646
Dry mouth	4	8	2	4	0.399
Fear	1	2	0	0	0.315
Euphoria	1	2	0	0	0.315
Dizziness	5	10	3	6	0.461
Dysarthria	1	2	3	6	0.307

Table 8: Side effects of study drugs.

Discussion

In this study, we compared ketamine infusion versus lidocaine infusion in management of intractable trigeminal neuralgia by 3 consecutive infusion sessions every 4 days. We found that ketamine infusion had a better analgesic outcome for the treatment of neuropathic pain without serious central nervous system adverse effects for up to 3 months, a time which may be adequate to support its long-term effect. The long-lasting effect of ketamine is due to ketamine itself and its metabolite nor ketamine which is produced *via* N-demethylation, resulting in small concentrations of both in blood and tissue [10]. Our study did not include a placebo group because of the ethical dilemma concerning withheld treatment in this population.

Thirty percent were not satisfied with ketamine infusion. A possible explanation may be related to the presence of different pain mechanisms other than NMDA-dependent pathway of ketamine infusion. In randomized clinical trials assessing efficacious medications (eg., antidepressants, gabapentin, and pregabalin) for neuropathic pain, typically <50% of patients experience satisfactory pain relief [11]. It has been suggested that 10-15% of patients with neuropathic pain are really rebellious to all forms of pharmacotherapy [12,13].

The response rate in this study was analyzed by definition of a 50% reduction in NRS score compared with baseline [14], but we think that any reduction of pain compared with baseline might be meaningful to the participants who had been unresponsive to 1800 mg/day oxycarbamazepine (600 mg/8 h) with presence of multiple side effects of tegeratol. In our study 70% of participants in ketamine group had a reduction of >30% of the NRS score, which was similar to that of satisfaction , this percent begin directly after infusion and increase gradually to 40%, 50% and reach about more than 60% during the period of study, this high percent mainly present in the period from 2 days until 1 month, after that the improvement is still present by about more than 50% till the end of the study i.e. 3 months (26 patients developed decrease in pain score >50%).

Also in our study we observed that lidocaine achieved a significant decrease in pain intensity directly after infusion and then increased gradually till 2 weeks, which is considered a long period despite the fact that lidocaine's half-life is 1.6 h [15] (only 11 patients developed decrease in pain score >50%).

Infusion of both anesthetics significantly reduced the pin-prick areas of hyperalgesia and allodynic area as compared with baseline but the analgesic effect of lidocaine was significantly weaker and shorter as compared with ketamine infusion. Ketamine acts as an antihyperalgesic and antiallodynic compound in pain management [16], Patients with TN suffer from allodynia and hyperalgesia is thought to be involved with NMDA receptors [17,18].

The central hyperalgesia, on the other hand, is related to sodium channels located at the ends of mechanoreceptors, in the spinal cord, and in dorsal root ganglia [19]. Boas et al. reported a decrease of central pain with the use of intravenous lidocaine, demonstrating a potential therapeutic value of lidocaine in the treatment of syndromes of intractable neuropathic pain [20]. Lidocaine infusion is an inexpensive and relatively easily administered treatment that has been safely used with very few side effects [21]. The analgesic effects of lidocaine may be observed in patients with diabetic neuropathy, post herpetic neuralgia and in several neuropathic disorders, such as complex regional syndrome type I and II and post-stroke pain [22]. The mechanism of "electric pain" is supposed to be peripheral nociceptor hyper excitability over sodium channels [17,18], and this descriptor also had a significant response to ketamine infusion but less than lidocaine group. This finding is in accordance with a previous report that suggests that ketamine acts as a pain modulator, targeting sodium channels as well as NMDA receptors [19].

In our study we also observed that frequency of pain is significantly decreased in ketamine infusion group directly after infusion till the end of the study, but in the other group the frequency of pain is significantly decreased mainly in the 1st 48 h and then increase gradually till the end of the study. An experimental study in neuropathic rats showed that intravenous, but not intrathecal or regionally applied, lidocaine yields dose dependent suppression of allodynia associated with nerve injury. Amusingly, the effects last longer than plasma concentrations of lidocaine; however, the mechanism of these prolonged effects remains unknown [23] Similar to this, Attal et al. showed that lidocaine reduced VAS for 6 hrs after the injection and a subgroup of patients experienced prolonged analgesia for up to 7 days in patients with central pain [24]. Furthermore, Arai et al. [25] claimed that in some patients, who suffered from trigeminal neuralgia and had pain relief after receiving lidocaine and magnesium, the therapeutic result continued for nearly one year, which is not the case in our study, this difference is explained by adding magnesium to lidocaine. Although the drug half-life of is only 120 mins, the analgesia provided by systemic lidocaine is prolonged, may be extending over days or even weeks [24]. This may be caused by the action of intravenous lidocaine in the central and peripheral nervous system. Using ketamine for neuropathic pain may be associated with the occurrence of central nervous system adverse effects such as dizziness, dysphoria, and hallucinations [26]. So in the present study, midazolam was administered with ketamine with dose of 1 mg given if there is any adverse effects was present, This might explain why none of the patients in the present study complained of unacceptable adverse effects such as hallucinations or dysphoria.

We chose to use the dose of 5 mg/kg lidocaine over 30 to 45 mins because in this dose lidocaine does not affect the peripheral conduction and acts at hyper excitable neurons without affecting normal nerve conduction, showing good effects on neuropathic pain (Lidocaine between 1.5 and 5.0 mg/kg proved effective dose to suppress ectopic discharge without blocking nerve conduction) [27,28]. As regards safety profiles, intravenous lidocaine and ketamine has been used to relieve several kinds of neuropathic pain without producing major adverse effects [29] similarly, in our study, lidocaine and ketamine infusions caused minor side effects, and during the infusions all the patients were hemodynamically stable with good oxygen saturation.

Conclusion

Ketamine infusion associated with more analgesic effect and lesser anticonvulsant therapy requirementsthan lidocaine infusion in refractory trigeminal neuralgia with minimal post-infusion complications. We think that the short period of follow up is a limitation in our study, however, this is not affecting the validity of our results nevertheless further studies with longer follow up periods may be warranted.

References

1. Zakrzewska JM (2002) Diagnosis and differential diagnosis of trigeminal neuralgia. Clin J Pain 18: 14-21.

2. Cruccu G, Gronseth G, Alksne J, Argoff C, Brainin M, et al. (2008) American Academy of Neurology Society; European Federation of Neurological Society AAN-EFNS guidelines on trigeminal neuralgia management. Eur J Neurol 15: 1013-1028.

3. Kohrs R, Durieux ME (1998) Ketamine: teaching an old drug new tricks. Anesth Analg 87: 1186-1193.

4. Nalamachu S, Morley-Forster P (2012) Diagnosing and managing postherpetic neuralgia. Drugs Aging 29: 863-869.

5. Arai YC, Hatakeyama N, Nishihara M, Ikeuchi M, Kurisuno M, et al. (2013) Intravenous lidocaine and magnesium for management of intractable trigeminal neuralgia: a case series of nine patients. Journal of Anesthesia 27: 960-962.

6. Souza MF, Kraychete DC (2014) The analgesic effect of intravenous lidocaine in the treatment of chronic pain: a literature review. Rev Bras Reumatol 54: 386-392.

7. Przeklasa MA, Kocot KM, Dobrogowski J, Wiatr M, Mika J (2016) Intravenous lidocaine infusions in a multidirectional model of treatment of neuropathic pain patients. Pharmacol Rep 68: 1069-1075.

8. Tanelian DL, Brose WG (1991) Neuropathic pain can be relieved by drugs that are use-dependent sodium channel blockers: lidocaine, carbamazepine, and mexiletine. Anesthesiology 74: 949-951.

9. Lauretti GR (2008) Mechanisms of analgesia of intravenous lidocaine. Rev Bras Anestesiol 58: 280-286.

10. Grant IS, Nimmo WS, Clements JA (1981) Pharmacokinetics and analgesic effect of i. m. and oral ketamine. Br J Anaesth 53: 805-810.

11. Finnerup NB, Attal N, Haroutounian S, McNicol E, Baron R, et al. (2015) Pharmacotherapy for neuropathic pain in adults: a systematic review and meta-analysis and updated NeuPSIG recommendations. Lancet Neurol 14: 162-173.

12. Vranken JH (2009) Mechanisms and treatment of neuropathic pain. Cent Nerv Syst Agents Med Chem 9: 71-78.

13. Harden RN (2005) Chronic neuropathic pain. Mechanisms, diagnosis, and treatment. Neurologist 11: 111-122.

14. McQuay HJ, Tramèr M, Nye BA (1996) A systematic review of antidepressants in neuropathic pain. Pain 68: 217-227.

15. JE Heavner (2007) Local anesthetics. Curr Opin Anaesthesiol 20: 336-342.

16. Visser E, Schug SA (2006) The role of ketamine in pain management. Biomed Pharmacother 60: 341-348.

17. Jensen TS, Baron R (2003) Translation of symptoms and signs into mechanisms in neuropathic pain. Pain 102: 1-8.

18. Baron R (2006) Mechanisms of disease: Neuropathic pain—a clinical perspective. Nat Clin Pract Neurol 2: 95-106.

19. Oliveira CMB, Issy AM, Sakata RK (2010) Lidocaína por via venosa intraoperatória. Rev Bras Anestesiol 60: 325-332.

20. Boas RA, Covino BG, Sahnarian A (1982) Analgesic responses to IV lidocaine. Br J Anesth 54: 501-505.

21. Kandil E, Melikman E, Adinoff B (2016) Lidocaine Infusion: A Promising Therapeutic Approach for Chronic Pain. J Anesth Clin Res 8: 697.

22. Tremont-Lukats IW, Hutson PR, Backonja MM (2006) A randomized, double-masked, placebo-controlled pilot trial of extended IV lidocaine infusion for relief of ongoing neuropathic pain. Clin J Pain 22: 266-271.

23. Gierthmühlen J, Binder A, Baron R (2014) Mechanism-based treatment in complex regional pain syndromes. Nature Reviews Neurology 10: 518-528.

24. Attal N, Rouaud J, Brasseur L, Chauvin M, Bouhassira D (2004) Systemic lidocaine in pain due to peripheral nerve injury and predictors of response. Neurology 6: 218-225.

25. Arai YC, Hatakeyama N, Nishihara M, Ikeuchi M, Kurisuno M, et al. (2013) Intravenous lidocaine and magnesium for management of intractable trigeminal neuralgia: a case series of nine patients". J Anesthesia 27: 960-962.

26. Kohrs R, Durieux ME (1998) Ketamine: Teaching an old drug new tricks. Anesth Analg 87: 1186-1193.

27.   Wallace MS, Dyck JB, Rossi SS, Yaksh TL (1996) Computer-controlled lidocaine infusion for the evaluation of neuropathic pain after peripheral nerve injury. Pain 66: 69-77.

28.   Ferrante FM, Paggioli J, Cherukuri S, Arthur GR (1996) The analgesic response to intravenous lidocaine in the treatment of neuropathic pain. Anesthesia and Analgesia 82: 91-97.

29.   Tremont-Lukats IW, Challapalli V, McNicol ED, Lau J, Carr DB (2005) Systemic administration of local anesthetics to relieve neuropathic pain: a systematic review and meta-analysis. Anesth Analg 6: 1738-1749.

30.   Hadzic A, Kerimoglu B, Loreio D, Karaca PE, Claudio RE, et al. (2006) Paravertebral blocks provide superior same-day recovery over general anesthesia for patients undergoing inguinal hernia repair. Anesth Analg 102:1076-1081.

31.   Kehlet H (1991) The surgical stress response: should it be prevented? Can J Surg 34: 565-567.

32.   Mitchell P, Kerr R, Mendelow AD, Molyneux A (2008) Could late rebleeding overturn the superiority of cranial aneurysm coil embolization over clip ligation seen in the International Subarachnoid Aneurysm Trial? J Neurosurg 108: 437-442.

Comparison between General Anesthesia and Epidural Anesthesia in Inguinal Herniorrhaphy Regarding the Incidence of Urinary Retention

Seyed Mohammad Mireskandari[1], Kasra Karvandian[1], Yashar Iranpour[1], Sanaz Shabani[1], Afshin Jafarzadeh[1], Shahram Samadi[1], Jalil Makarem[1], Negar Eftekhar[1] and Jayran Zebardast[2]

[1]Department of Anesthesiology & Critical Care, Imam khomeini Hospital Complex, Tehran University of Medical Sciences, Tehran, Iran

[2]Department of Electronic Learning in Medical Education, Statistics Expert, Deputy of Universality affairs , Imam Khomeini Hospital, Tehran University, of medical sciences, Tehran , Iran

*Corresponding author: Seyed Mohammad Mireskandari, Department of Anesthesiology & Critical Care, Imam khomeini Hospital Complex, Tehran University of Medical Sciences, Tehran, Iran, E-mail: mireskandari@sina.tums.ac.ir, mmireskandari@yahoo.com

Abstract

Background: Inguinal herniorrhaphy is among the most common type of surgeries in adults. One of the important side effects of herniorrhaphy is post-operative urinary retention (UR). The incidence of urinary retention after herniorrhaphy may vary depending on the method of anesthesia.

Methods: This is a double blind randomized clinical trial conducted on 80 patients undergoing inguinal hernia repair. Half of the cases were generally anesthetized (GA) and the other half underwent continues lumbar epidural anesthesia (EA). The epidural catheter was inserted before the procedure and remained for 24 hours post-operative period. The need for urinary catheterizing either in post anesthetic care unit (PACU) or in ward was compared between two groups, beside the incidence of urination in, the mean interval between the end of surgery and first urination. Also the duration of the surgery, length of PACU admission, surgeon and patients satisfaction with the method of their anesthesia was compared between the groups.

Results: The incidence of urination in PACU was one patient (2.5%) in EA and 5 patients (12.5%) in GA (P=0.09). The mean interval between the end of surgery and first urination was 3.40 ± 2.30 in EA and 3.06 ± 2.50 in GA (P=0.2). The incidence of urinary retention in PACU was 4 patients (10%) in EA and one patient (2.5%) in GA (P=0.1).

Conclusion: According to this study the incidence of urinary retention is not higher in epidural anesthesia compared with general anesthesia according to statistical significance.

Keywords: Urinary retention; General anesthesia; Epidural anesthesia; Inguinal hernia repair

Introduction

Inguinal herniorrhaphy is among the most common type of surgeries in adults [1-5]. The cause of this event is abdominal wall defect due to loss of strength in inguinal area [1-5]. The patients undergoing hernia repair surgeries are in older ages and choosing appropriate method of anesthesia is very important for them, because they may have some underlying disease [1,3]. The policy of most medical centers is short period of admission and early discharge for this type of surgery and because of that this centers are trend to employ regional methods of anesthesia obviating the risks of general anesthesia [1,6-13]. One of the important side effects of herniorrhaphy is post-operative urinary retention (UR) [13,14]. Postoperative urinary retention is defined as any situation in which patient develops with voiding difficulty and the incidence of this problem may increase in advanced age [15-19]. On the other hand UR may be side effect of the method of anesthesia [19-22]. There is no double blind clinical trial in literature comparing the incidence of UR between general and epidural anesthesia, which are both two common methods of anesthesia for herniorrhaphy. In this study we compared the incidence of UR in

patients undergoing herniorrhaphy either with general or epidural anesthesia.

Methods

This is a double blind randomized clinical trial which is conducted on eighty patients undergoing herniorrhaphy in Imam Khomaini General Hospital between March 2014 and March 2015. The patients were otherwise healthy subjects with unilateral or bilateral inguinal hernia which were scheduled for surgical intervention. All of the patients aged between 30- 50 years old. The cases were randomly assigned into two age and sex matched groups by using code numbers kept in sealed envelopes by a secretory not involved in the study, the codes were computer random generated. One group underwent herniorrhaphy by general anesthesia (GA) and the other group underwent herniorrhaphy by epidural anesthesia (EA). Inclusion criteria was need for inguinal hernia repair surgery and exclusion criteria was any underlying disease that needs special anesthetic consideration, age lower than thirty and higher than fifty, any history of previous urinary retention for any cause and history of benign prostatic hypertrophy in males, any anatomical problem in lumbar spine that makes epidural anesthesia difficult, obesity with body mass index higher than 30, and patient`s refusal for epidural anesthesia. Any event of hemodynamic instability during the procedure and in PACU was considered to exclude the patient from study. Institutional ethics committee and patients informed consent was obtained before the study.

According to similar studies the incidence of UR was 8-15 percent post-operative period [15-19], and with this data we considered 10 pilot cases: $n = Z^2_{1-\frac{\alpha}{2}} \, pq/d^2$

α=0.05

Z1-α/2=1.961150776

d=0.18

p=0.08

n=9

And with the result of pilot study the sample size was determined for this clinical trial, by considering no incidence of UR in GA and 20 percent in EA according to previous studies and estimating 10 percent loss to follow up: $n = (\left(Z_{1-\frac{\alpha}{2}}\right) + Z_{1-\beta})^{\frac{2}{pq}}/((P_1 - P_2))$

α=0.05

β=0.2

Z1-a/2=1.96

Z1-B=0.84

p1=0

p2=0.2

n=36

All the patients voided before performance of anesthesia. In GA after premedication with midazolam (0.02 μg/kg) and fentanyl (2 μg/kg), induction of anesthesia was performed by NA-thiopental (5 mg/kg) and atracurium (0.6 mg/kg) and proper size of endotracheal tube was applied for all patients. The anesthesia was maintained by 1.2-1.5% isoflurane. Fentanyl and atracurium were repeated in 30 minutes intervals as needed. At the end of the procedure the muscle relaxant reversed in the operative room and patients were extubated before transferring to post anesthetic care unit (PACU). In EA epidural anesthesia performed for all patients by the same anesthesiologist in sitting position and at the L3-L4 level. All Epidural Kits were no 18, provided by Sepanomed Medical Company. Bupivacaine 0.5% (15-20 ml) was administered in the beginning and after achieving the desired level of epidural anesthesia all patients received intravenous sedation by midazolam (2 mg). Epidural injection was repeated in one hour interval as needed. At the end of the surgery the patients were transferred to PACU by remaining the epidural catheter in place. The administered intravenous fluid in both groups was exactly recorded [23,24].

The study one site double blinded because neither the patient and nor the nurse who collected the data were informed about the details of the study. The same nurse, who completed the data sheets for all patients, visited them in the surgery ward when all the patients were ready for discharge, she used anesthetic and PACU sheets to complete the data beside a brief interview with the patients. The length of

hospital staying was recorded for each patient, too. All the interventions in PACU including urinary catheterization was recorded in data collection sheet, this sheet also included patient's age, sex, the extent of surgery (unilateral or bilateral herniorrhaphy), duration of the surgery, length of PACU admission, time of first urination in PACU, and patients satisfaction with the method of their anesthesia. We also asked the surgeon to indicate in his operation report whether he was satisfied with the method of anesthesia or not. The patients were discharged from PACU according to Alderete's PACU discharge scoring system [25]. The first episode of urination was recorded by time in their chart either in PACU or in surgery ward. For those patients who had UR, and needed urinary catheterization, several ward visits by an anesthesiologist, who was not involved in the research team, was considered and either the time of first urination or any episodes of urinary catheterization was recorded in their chart too.

At the end of the study data were entered in SPSS software version 16 (SPSS Inc., Chicago, IL, USA), as cod sheet and master sheet. Student's t test and chi-square test were employed for data analysis. The power of this study was 99% and P value ≤ 0.05 was considered statistically significant.

Results

Forty individuals recruited in each study group in this clinical trial as defined. There was no incidence of hemodynamic instability during the surgery and post-operative period in both groups.

There were 38 (95%) male and 2 (5%) female patients in GA, and 39 (97.5%) male and 1 (2.5%) female patients in EA (P=0.6).

The mean age of the patients was 47.55 ± 6.9 and 48.10 ± 5.9 in GA and EA respectively (P=0.7).

The mean weight of the patient was 78.52 ± 12.58 Kg in GA and 79.65 ± 13.00 Kg in EA (P=0.4).

The extent of surgery was also statistically identical in both groups, in GA 36 (90%) patients had bilateral inguinal hernia and in EA 35 (87.5%) patients had bilateral inguinal hernia (P=0.7).

The mean amount of intravenous fluid administered was 1.45 ± 6.2 liter and 1.40 ± 0.20 liter in GA and EA respectively (P=0.2).

The length of PACU staying was 0.9 ± 0.39 hour for GA and 1.29 ± 0.56 hours for EA (P=0.004).

The period of hospital staying was 1.44 ± 0.62 days for GA and 1.43 ± 0.63 for EA (P=0.9).

The interval between adequate level of anesthesia and start of operation was 26.37 ± 2.34 minutes for EA and 14.32 ± 1.96 minutes for GA (P=0.001) (Table 2).

	GA	EA	P value
Bilateral inguinal hernia	36 (90%)	35 (87.5%)	(P=0.7)
Intravenous fluid (L)	1.45 ± 6.2	1.40 ± 0.20	(P=0.2)
PACU staying (hrs.)	0.9 ± 0.39	1.29 ± 0.56	(P=0.004)
Hospital staying (day)	1.44 ± 0.62	1.43 ± 0.63	(P=0.9)
Interval between anesthesia & operation (minutes)	14.32 ± 1.96	26.37 ± 2.34	(P=0.001)

Interval between operation & first urination (hrs.)	3.06 ± 2.50	3.40 ± 2.30	(P=0.2)
First urination in PACU	5 (12.5%)	1 (2.5%)	(P=0.09)
Urinary retention	1 (2.5%)	4 (10%)	(P=0.1)
Patient`s satisfaction	38 (95%)	37 (92.5%)	(P=0.6)
Surgeon`s satisfaction	38 (95%)	38 (95%)	(P=0.9)

Table 2: Compared variables between two groups.

The mean interval between conclusion of operation and first episode of urination was 3.06 ± 2.50 hours for GA and 3.40 ± 2.30 hours for EA (P=0.2).

About 5 patients in GA (12.5%) and 1 patient in EA (2.5%) had their first episode of post-operative urination in PACU (P=0.09).

The incidence of urinary retention was 1 (2.5%) patient in GA and (4%) patients in EA (P=0.1).

Thirty eight (95%) patients had satisfaction with the method of their anesthesia in GA and thirty seven (92.5%) patients in EA (P=0.6).

The surgeon was satisfied with the condition provided by anesthesia in 38 (95%) cases in GA and the same number in EA (P=0.9).

Discussion

Nowadays, inguinal hernioplasty is generally a widely performed surgery in Iranian population. Day surgery of this type of surgery has been significantly expanded in last decay, because by application of it`s less interference on patients daily activity and a faster it`s faster recovery [1- 5]. To aim early ambulation of patients and sufficient pain control many centers prefer to apply regional techniques of anesthesia for this procedure especially in older population. Many studies are designed to confirm that regional methods of anesthesia including neuraxial blocks are acceptable or even preferable methods of anesthesia in this setting [6-13]. UR may delay discharge and in recent years different studies were designed to purpose a method of anesthesia for herniorrhaphy that may have lower incidence of urinary retention [13]. Previous studies compared the incidence of post-operative UR in general and regional anesthesia and most of these studies showed that the incidence of UR was much more in regional anesthesia [19-22], but some studies refused to confirm this result [23,24].

This randomized clinical trial was conducted on 80 patients in two equal, age and sex matched study groups which were similar with respect to demographic characteristics and showed no statistically significant difference. The extent of herniorrhaphy (P=0.7), the mean length of operation (P=0.3) and hospitalization (P=0.9) was statistically similar in both groups, too. The same result was obtained in previous studied comparing neuraxial block and general anesthesia for inguinal herniorrhaphy (Table 1) [13].

	GA	EA	P value
Age	47.55 ± 6.9	48.10 ± 5.9	0.7
Sex (F/M)	2/38	1/39	0.6

Mean Weight	78.52 ± 12.58	79.65 ± 13.00	0.4

Table 1: Demographic characteristic of groups.

As expected according to previous studies the mean period of PACU admission was longer in EA group, (P=0.004). The mean interval between proper level of anesthesia and start of operation was longer in EA, due to time consumption for performing epidural procedure (P=0.001). By applying spinal and epidural techniques patients benefit from avoiding muscle relaxants and endotracheal intubation, but they will experience slow recovery of motor and sensory function, longer PACU admission period [11,13].

There was no study in literature to compare the incidence of UR between EA and GA in herniorrhaphy, but according to the studies comparing different methods of regional anesthesia with general anesthesia the incidence of post-operative UR was higher by applying neuraxial blocks [19-22]. This is because of that neuraxial local anesthetic injection blocks detrusor muscle that causes bladder over distention, and as a result urinary retention develops [26]. But some studies refused to confirm this event [23,24]. In this study we detected UR in 10% of patients in EA and 2.5% of patients in GA, this finding was not statistically significant (P=0.1) and this is in the setting that the amount of administered intravenous fluid was similar in both groups (P=0.2). Among the patients in EA one patient (2.5%) and in GA five patients (12.5%) had voluntary urination in PACU (P=0.09) which was not statistically important. The interval between conclusion of operation and first episode of urination was longer in EA but this was not statistically significant. This result may be justifiable because all we know that general anesthesia may lead to urinary retention due to bladder atony as a result of muscle relaxation and interfering with autonomic regulation of detrusor muscle tone [27].

Both patients and surgeons satisfaction from the method of anesthesia was identical in the two study groups and it was not statistically significant (P=0.9).

It seems that employing epidural anesthesia will not result in higher incidence of UR in comparison with GA in inguinal herniorrhaphy surgery. And beside acceptable hemodynamic condition and feasibility of its performance we can consider using epidural anesthesia for herniorrhaphy surgery to obviate risks of general anesthesia, and to benefit from its post-operative analgesic properties, especially in older subjects [1,28-30]. The brief elongation of recovery period and anesthesia establishment is acceptable due to several advantages of neuraxial methods for herniorrhaphy [1,13,28-30].

We suggest further studies by using quantified methods like measuring bladder contents with ultrasound in larger number of cases to confirm this result.

References

1. Su Y, Zhang Z, Zhang Y, Li H, Shi W (2015) Efficacy of ropivacaine by the concentration of 0.25%, 0.5%, and 0.75% on surgical performance, postoperative analgesia, and patient's satisfaction in inguinal hernioplasty: a randomized controlled trial. Patient Prefer Adherence 9: 1375-1379.

2. Saeed M, Andrabi WI, Rabbani S, Zahur S, Mahmood K, et al. (2015) The impact of preemptive ropivacaine in inguinal hernioplasty--a randomized controlled trial. Int J Surg 13: 76-79.

3.   Palumbo P, Amatucci C, Perotti B, Zullino A, Dezzi C, et al. (2014) Outpatient repair for inguinal hernia in elderly patients: still a challenge? Int J Surg 12 Suppl 2: S4-7.

4.   Yasuo S, Kenichi Y, Ueno N, Arimoto A, Hosono M, et al. (2015) Topic: Inguinal Hernia - Unsolved problem in the daily practice. Hernia 19 Suppl 1: S293-304.

5.   Wang YC, Huang CS, Uen Y, Tan WB, Tang SW, et al. (2015) Topic: Inguinal Hernia - Recurrences: incidence, approach, follow up. Hernia 19 Suppl 1: S281-286.

6.   Tomak Y, Erdivanli B, Sen A, Bostan H, Budak ET, et al. (2016) Effect of cooled hyperbaric bupivacaine on unilateral spinal anesthesia success rate and hemodynamic complications in inguinal hernia surgery. J Anesth 30: 26-30.

7.   Srivastava U, Kumar A, Saxena S, Neeraj, Sehgal DR (2007) Comparison of local, spinal and general anaesthesia for inguinal hernia repair. J Anaesthesiol Clin Pharmacol 23:151-154.

8.   Varshney PG, Varshney M, Bhadoria P (2008) Comparison of total intravenous anaesthesia, spinal anaesthesia and local block for day care inguinal herniorrhaphy. Internet J Anesthesiol 22: 9.

9.   Ozgün H, Kurt MN, Kurt I, Cevikel MH (2002) Comparison of local, spinal, and general anaesthesia for inguinal herniorrhaphy. Eur J Surg 168: 455-459.

10. Kato T, Sasaki H (2015) Comparison of Postoperative Analgesic Effects between 0.25% Levobupivacaine and 0.5% Levobupivacaine Local Instillation in Inguinal Hernia Repair. Masui 64: 973-977.

11. Burney RE, Prabhu MA, Greenfield ML, Shanks A, O'Reilly M (2004) Comparison of spinal vs general anesthesia via laryngeal mask airway in inguinal hernia repair. Arch Surg 139: 183-187.

12. Kehlet H, Aasvang E (2005) Groin hernia repair: anesthesia. World J Surg 29: 1058-1061.

13. Bakota B, Kopljar M, Baranovic S, Miletic M, Marinovic M, et al. (2015) Should we abandon regional anesthesia in open inguinal hernia repair in adults? Eur J Med Res 20: 76.

14. Mohammadi-Fallah M, Hamedanchi S, Tayyebi-Azar A (2012) Preventive effect of tamsulosin on postoperative urinary retention. Korean J Urol 53: 419-423.

15. Baldini G, Bagry H, Aprikian A, Carli F (2009) Postoperative urinary retention: anesthetic and perioperative considerations. Anesthesiology 110: 1139-1157.

16. Buckley BS, Lapitan MC (2010) Drugs for treatment of urinary retention after surgery in adults. Cochrane Database Syst Rev: CD008023.

17. Madani AH, Aval HB, Mokhtari G, Nasseh H, Esmaeili S, et al. (2014) Effectiveness of tamsulosin in prevention of post-operative urinary

18. retention: a randomized double-blind placebo-controlled study. Int Braz J Urol 40: 30-36.

18. Cheong KX, Lo HY, Neo JX, Appasamy V, Chiu MT (2014) Inguinal hernia repair: are the results from a general hospital comparable to those from dedicated hernia centres? Singapore Med J 55: 191-197.

19. Sung KH, Lee KM, Chung CY, Kwon SS, Lee SY, et al. (2015) What are the risk factors associated with urinary retention after orthopaedic surgery? Biomed Res Int 2015: 613216.

20. Lamonerie L, Marret E, Deleuze A, Lembert N, Dupont M, et al. (2004) Prevalence of postoperative bladder distension and urinary retention detected by ultrasound measurement. British Journal of Anesthesia 92: 544-546.

21. Ringdal M, Borg B, Hellström AL (2003) A survey on incidence and factors that may influence first postoperative urination. Urol Nurs 23: 341-346, 354.

22. Lau H, Lam B (2004) Management of postoperative urinary retention: a randomized trial of in-out versus overnight catheterization. ANZ J Surg 74: 658-661.

23. Bødker B, Lose G (2003) Postoperative urinary retention in gynecologic patients. International Urogynecology Journal and Pelvic Floor Dysfunction 14: 94-97.

24. Izard J P, Sowery RD, Jaeger MT, Siemens DR (2006) Parameters affecting urologic complications after major joint replacement surgery. Can J Urol 13: 3158-3163.

25. Phillips NM, Street M, Kent B, Haesler E, Cadeddu M (2013) Post-anaesthetic discharge scoring criteria: key findings from a systematic review. Int J Evid Based Healthc 11: 275-284.

26. Kamphuis ET, Ionescu TI, Kuipers PW, de Gier J, van Venrooij GE, et al. (1998) Recovery of storage and emptying functions of the urinary bladder after spinal anesthesia with lidocaine and with bupivacaine in men. Anesthesiology 88: 310-316.

27. Darrah DM, Griebling TL, Silverstein JH (2009) Postoperative urinary retention. Anesthesiol Clin 27: 465-484.

28. Amato B, Compagna R, Della Corte GA, Martino G, Bianco T, et al. (2012) Feasibility of inguinal hernioplasty under local anaesthesia in elderly patients. BMC Surg 12 Suppl 1:S2.

29. Kehlet H, Bay Nielsen M (2005) Anaesthetic practice for groin hernia repair--a nation-wide study in Denmark 1998-2003. Acta Anaesthesiol Scand 49: 143-146.

30. Hadzic A, Kerimoglu B, Loreio D, Karaca PE, Claudio RE, et al. (2006) Paravertebral blocks provide superior same-day recovery over general anesthesia for patients undergoing inguinal hernia repair. Anesth Analg 102:1076-1081.

Comparison of Different Bupivacaine and Fentanyl Combinations When used with a Single Shut Spinal Block for Labor Analgesia

Aslan Bilge*, Arıkan Müge, Gedikli Ahmet, Kısa Karakaya Burcu, Moraloğlu Özlem

Zekai Tahir Burak Education and Research Hospital, Turkey

Corresponding author: Aslan Bilge, Zekai Tahir Burak Education and Research Hospital, Turkey, E-mail: drbilgeaslan@hotmail.com

Abstract

Background: Single-shot spinal analgesia with bupivacaine plus a short-acting opioid is an effective technique for pain control in labor, and it is particularly useful in the active phase. We compared the effects of adding two different doses of fentanyl (15 µg or 25 µg) to intrathecal bupivacaine, and to evaluate the impacts on duration of labor analgesia, newborn, and side effects.

Method: One hundred and five multiparous healty women in advanced labor (cervical dilatation ≥ 7 cm, and pain score >5), requesting labor analgesia were included in the study. They were randomly allocated into three groups. Group I received 2.5 mg bupivacaine; Group II received 2.5 mg bupivacaine plus 15 µg fentanyl; Group III received 2.5 bupivacaine plus 25 µg fentanyl intrathecally. The patients' demo figure characteristics, hemodynamic parameters, pain scores (by using visual analogue scale - VAS), analgesic requirements, duration of analgesia (the time from intrathecal injection to the return of pain >4), fetal Apgar scores (at 1st and 5th min), and maternal and neonatal side effects were recorded. We used analysis of variance (ANOVA), post hoc test with Bonferroni adjustment, and chi-square test for statistical analysis; the analyses were performed using the SPSS-16 software. Given a significant level of 0.05, overall and pair-wise comparisons were made.

Results: The mean VAS scores were significantly lower in Group II than in the other two groups at 5, 15, 30 min, and 1 h (P<0.001). There was no difference among Group I and Group III. The VAS scores were significantly higher in the Group III than in the other two groups at 2 (P=0.005) and 3 h (P<0.001). The incidence of adverse events was similar in all three groups. There was no difference in Apgar scores at 1 min, but Apgar score at 5 min was higher in Group 2 (P=0.02).

Conclusion: In this study, we found that 2.5 mg of bupivacaine plus 15 µg fentanyl is more preferable option for SSA.

Keywords: Analgesia; Labor; Single shut spinal block; Fentanyl

Introduction

The combined spinal-epidural (CSE), and epidural techniques are considered as the most effective methods for providing labor analgesia. Single Shut Spinal (SSS) block is not routinely preferred due to its limited duration of action, but it is an effective method, especially in advanced stages of labor.

In our department, we prefer single dose spinal analgesia (SSA) with hyperbaric bupivacaine and fentanyl for pain control in advanced labor.

In this study, we aimed to compare the effects of adding two different doses of fentanyl (15 µg or 25 µg) to intrathecal bupivacaine, and to evaluate the impacts on duration of labor analgesia, newborn, and side effects.

After approval of the Local Ethics Committee of Zekai Tahir Burak Hospital, informed consent forms were obtained from each patients. This prospective, double-blinded, randomized study was performed from February 2015 to March 2016. 105 multiparous healty women in advanced labor (cervical dilatation ≥ 7 cm, and pain score >5),

American Society of Anesthesiologist (ASA) grade I, and consenting for labor analgesia were included in the study (Figure 1).

Patients with a history of allergic reactions to any study drug, with any contraindication to regional anesthesia, with pre-eclampsia, eclampsia, gestational hypertension, diabetes mellitus, cardiac problems or bleeding diathesis were excluded.

The patients were randomly allocated into three groups according to a computer-generated randomization table: Group I received 2.5 mg of bupivacaine, Group II received 2.5 mg of bupivacaine+15 µg fentanyl, Group III received 2.5 mg of bupivacaine+25 µg fentanyl intrathecally.

In our study, the patient as well as the anesthesiologist administering the drug did not know which drug was used. The drug was prepared by another anesthesiologist who was not directly involved in the study.

Before the initiation of analgesia, the following parameters: Maternal age, height, weight, gestational age, cervical dilatation, use of oxytocin and parity were recorded. Baseline pain score was assessed by using visual analogue scale (VAS) (VAS; 10 cm; 0=no pain and 10=worst imaginable pain) before the SSA. An intravenous (i.v.) access was achieved in every parturient, and preloading was done with 10 ml/kg body weight of lactated Ringer's solution.

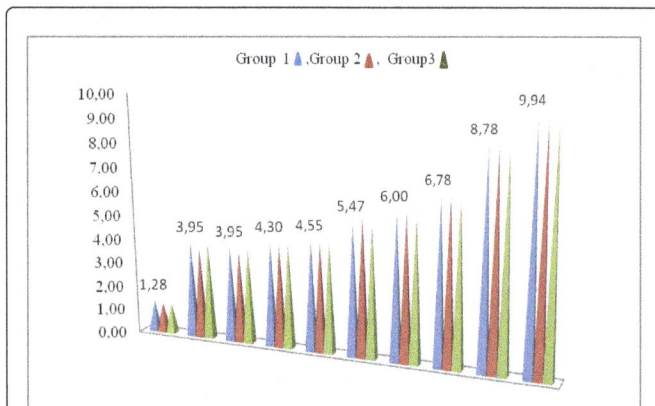

Figure 1: Dilatation (cm) (The change in each groups over time were studied with Friedman Test. The change in time within each groups were significant p<0.001 but no difference between groups).

The SSA was performed with parturients in left lateral position, under all aseptic precautions at L2-L3 or L3-L4 level using a 25-gauge Whitacre spinal needle. After the correct position of the tip in the intrathecal space was confirmed by observation of free flow of cerebrospinal fluid (CSF), the prefilled study drug was injected intrathecally. The parturient was turned supine, and a wedge was placed under the right buttock to prevent aortocaval compression.

Maternal blood pressure, heart rate, respiratory rate, oxygen saturation were measured noninvasively by a blinded observer every 5 min, and recorded.

VAS were eveluated every 5 min and then every 30 min until the delivery. The duration of analgesia (the time from intrathecal injection to the return of pain >4), and analgesic requirements were recorded. If the VAS score is 4 after spinal injection, 25 mg of petidine is intravenously (i.v) administered.

Side effects, such as hypotension, nausea-vomiting, bradycardia, shivering, pruritus, tachycardia were also recorded and treated.

The weights of the newborns as well as one-minute and five-minute Apgar scores were recorded.

Results

A total of 105 laboring women were accepted and participated throughout the study. The demofigure data is shown in Table 1. The three groups were comparable in terms of demofigure variables, gestational age, cervical dilatation, oxytocin assisted, and membran ruptured.

The baseline VAS scores were not significantly different among the groups (Figure 1). In all patients, VAS scores were significantly lower at all time intervals compared to baseline. The mean VAS scores were significantly lower in Group II than in the other two groups at 5, 15, 30 min, and 1 h (P<0.001). However; there was no difference among Group I and Group III. The VAS scores were significantly higher in the Group III than in the other two groups at 2 (P=0.005) and 3 h (P<0.001) (Table 2 and Figure 2).

	Group I (n=35)	Group II (n=35)	Group III (n=35)	P-value
Age (years), mean ± SD	23,74 ± 3.42	24,14 ± 4.11	25.31 ± 3.96	0.12
Height (cm), mean ± SD	161,94 ± 12.76	165,11 ± 10.45	163.33 ± 10.45	0.72
Weight (Kgs), mean ± SD	76,05 ± 6.34	74,51 ± 8.12	72.64 ± 7.87	0.41
Gestational age (weeks), mean ± SD	38,71 ± 1.13	39,43 ± 1.04	38.24 ± 1.36	0.07
Cervical Dilation (cm), mean ± SD	7,45 ± 0.71	7,11 ± 0.55	7.0 ± 0.58	0.65
Oxytocin assisted, n (%)	16 (45.71 %)	17 (48.57 %)	15 (42.85 %)	0.81
Membrane ruptured, n (%)	9 (25.71 %)	8 (22.86 %)	10 (28.57 %)	0.78
Data were expressed as mean ± standard deviation (mean ± SD), or patient number and percentage (n, %).				

Table 1: The demographic details and obstetric parameters of the study groups.

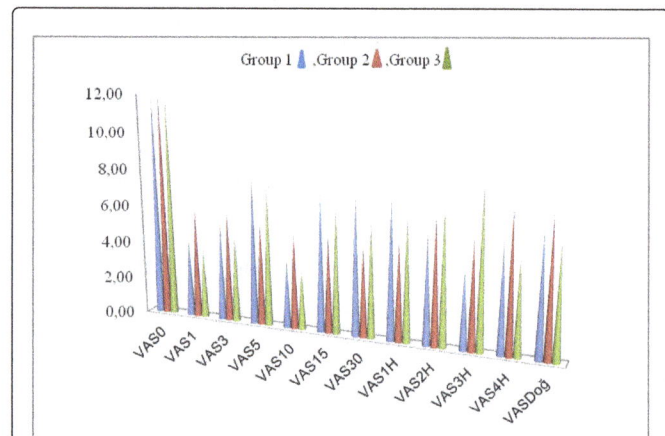

Figure 2: The mean Visual Analog Scale (VAS: 0-10 point) score (Generally group 2 VAS score was showed better decrease and more stable. The group 3 VAS score was showed a further decrease when the baby removed from the mother).

VAS	Group I (n=35)	Group II (n=35)	Group III (n=35)	P-value
Before Spinal	8,25 ± 1.38	7,61 ± 1.87	8.12 ± 1.27	0.728
5 minutes	1,23 ± 0.69	0.22 ± 0.63	1.29 ± 0.71	<0.001*
10 minutes	0,11 ± 0.32	0.08 ± 0.29	0.11 ± 0.32	0.886
15 minutes	1.06 ± 0.68	0.08 ± 0.28	1.03 ± 0.78	<0.001*
30 minutes	1.06 ± 0.68	0.00 ± 0.00	0.94 ± 0.63	<0.001*
1 hours	1.11 ± 0.83	0.22 ± 1.01	1.03 ± 0.78	<0.001*

2 hours	0.91 ± 1.52	0.92 ± 1.73	1.40 ± 1.09	0.005 #
3 hours	0.26 ± 0.61	0.28 ± 0.70	1.69 ± 0.83	<0.001 #

Data were expressed as mean ± standard deviation (mean ± SD), or patient number and percentage (n, %). VAS: Visual Analogue Scale. * VAS scores were significantly lower in Group II than the other groups (P<0.001). # VAS scores were significantly higher in the Group III than in the other two groups at 2 (P=0.005) and 3 h (P<0.001).

Table 2: The mean visual analog scale (VAS) score.

On comparing heart rates and mean blood pressure all groups showed changes over time, but there was no significant difference in the three groups.

The incidence of adverse events was similar in all three groups. There was no difference in Apgar scores at 1 min, but Apgar score at 5 min was higher in Group 2 (P=0.02) (Table 3).

	Group I (n=35)	Group II (n=35)	Group III (n=35)	P-value
Additional analgesic, n (%)	6 (%21)	3 (%8.57)	4 (%11.43)	0.73
Hypotension, n (%)	2 (%5.71)	2 (%5.71)	3 (%8.57)	0.64
Bradycardia, n (%)	1 (%2.86)	0	1 (%2.86)	0.68
Nausea/Vomiting, n (%)	1 (%2.86)	1 (%2.86)	3 (%8.57)	0.61
Pruritis, n (%)	3 (%8.57)	4 (%11.43)	4 (%11.43)	0.70
Apgar 1 minutes	7.85 ± 0.72	7.77 ± 0.47	7.88 ± 0.64	0.95
Apgar 5 minutes	9.92 ± 0.44	10.00 ± 0.00	9.85 ± 0.56	0.02*

Data are represented as mean ± SD or number (%).* P value <0.05; vs. Group II and Group III.

Table 3: Adverse events and Apgar scores.

Discussion

The mean VAS scores were significantly lower in Group II than in the other two groups at 5, 15, 30 min, and 1 h (P<0.001). Moreover; Apgar score at 5 min was higher in Group II.

The most commonly used neuroaxial block methods for labor analgesia are epidural and CSE, but SSA has some advantages, such as providing an effective and rapid analgesia. This method is popular due to its simplicity. Especially, the hospitals where are insufficient equipment and personnel like ours.

Tarek AbdElBarr et al. [1] concluded that single dose spinal analgesia is a good alternative to epidural analgesia in controlling labour pain, because spinal compared to epidural is more easy performed, faster, less expensive, and provide effective analgesia.

Minty et al. examines the safety and efficacy of single dose spinal analgesia for controlling labour pain, and they concluded that single-dose spinal anaesthesia is useful alternative to epidural analgesia for appropriately selected patients [2]. The advantage of our study was that all pregnant women were multiparous and the cervical openings reached 6-7 cm when they arrived at the hospital. Therefore, the analgesia of a single dose of intrathecal injection provided adequate anesthesia until the baby was born [2-10].

Otokwala et al. showed that low dose spinal bupivacaine either alone or in combination with fentanyl is safe for labour analgesia, but the combination of bupivacaine (2.5 mg) with fentanyl (25 µg) provided much more prolonged pain relief [3].

Anabaha et al. suggested that low-dose intrathecal bupivacaine (2.5 mg), and intrathecal opioids (25 µg of fentanyl and 0.2 mg of morphine) can provide sufficient pain relief without reducing ambulation in labouring parturients [4].

Viitanen et al. studied 671 multiparous women who received spinal analgesia with low dose bupivacaine and fentanyl during labor, and they concluded that single-shot spinal block is an usable method of pain relief in multiparous women in active labour [5]. The combination of an opioid and a local anesthetic for intrathecal analgesia during labour has been well documented in previous studies across the world [8-10].

We, therefore, compared two different combinations of bupivacaine and fentanyl. In this study, we found that 2.5 mg of bupivacaine plus 15 µg fentanyl is more preferable option for SSA.

References

1. Tarek AbdElBarr, Nirvana A. Elshalakany, Yasser M Shafik (2014) Single dose spinal analgesia: Is it a good alternative to epidural analgesia in controlling labour pain? Egyptian Journal of Anaesthesia 30: 241–246.

2. Minty RG, Kelly L, Minty A, Hammett DC (2007) Single-dose intrathecal analgesia to control labour pain: is it a useful alternative to epidural analgesia? Can Fam Physician 53: 437–442.

3. Otokwala JG, Fyneface-Ogan S, Mato CN (2013) Comparative effects of single shot low dose spinal bupivacaine only and bupivacaine with fentanyl on labour outcome. Niger J Med 22: 279-285.

4. T Anabaha, A Olufolabia, J Boydc, R Georgec (2015) Low-dose spinal anaesthesia provides effective labour analgesia and does not limit ambulation. Southern African Journal of Anaesthesia and Analgesia 21: 19–22.

5. Viitanen H, Viitanen M, Heikkila M (2005) Single-shot spinal block for labour analgesia in multiparous parturients. Acta Anaesthesiologica Scandinavica 49: 1023-1029.

6. Zapp J, Thorne T (1995) Comfortable labor with intrathecal narcotics. Mil Med 160: 217-219.

7. Viscomi CM, Rathmell JP, Pace NL (1997) Duration of intrathecal labor analgesia: early versus advanced labor. Anesth Analg 84: 1108–1112.

8. Hess PE, Vasudevan A, Snowman C, Pratt SD (2003) Small dose bupivacaine-fentanyl spinal analgesia combined with morphine for labor. Anesth Analg 97: 247–252.

9. Cascio M, Pygon B, Bernett C, Ramanathan S (1997) Labour analgesia with intrathecal fentanyl decreases maternal stress. Can J Anaesth 44: 605–609.

10. Campbell DC, Camann WR, Datta S (1995) The addition of bupivacaine to intrathecal sufentanil for labor analgesia. Anesth Analg 81: 305–309.

Comparison of the Effectiveness of Unimodal Opioid Analgesia with Multimodal Analgesia in the Management of Postoperative Pain in Patients Undergoing Surgery under Spinal Anesthesia-Double Blind Study

Madhu Mala[*], **Prabha Parthasarathy and Raghavendra Rao**

Department of Anaesthesiology, Bangalore Medical College, Karnataka, India

[*]**Corresponding author:** Madhu Mala, Assistant Professor, Department of Anaesthesiology, Bangalore Medical College, BMCRI, KR market, Bangalore, Karnataka 560002, India, E-mail: drmadhumala@gmail.com

Abstract

Objective: To evaluate the efficacy and safety of opioid analgesic alone or in combination with a Non-steroidal Anti-inflammatory Drug (NSAID) in management of post-operative pain after regression of spinal anesthesia.

Methods: In this double-blind study, 120 patients who underwent infra-umbilical surgeries under spinal anesthesia were chosen for the study and were randomly allocated into 4 groups of 30 each. Each group received Tramadol 100 mg or Pentazocine 30 mg or Tramadol 100 mg+Piroxicam 20 mg or Pentazocine 30 mg+Piroxicam 20 mg intramuscularly, 30 minutes after the end of the surgery. The primary efficacy end points were the total duration of post-operative analgesia and the intensity of pain relief in different groups, as assessed by VAS. Level of sedation and incidence of side effects were observed as secondary outcomes.

Results: The mean VAS scores of the patients in Pentazocine group was lower, hence better pain relief, than Tramadol group at all time periods. The mean VAS score of the patients in Pentazocine+Piroxicam was lower than Tramadol+Piroxicam group.

In the inter-group comparison of VAS, between all 4 groups, it was observed that VAS, pain score was least for Pentazocine+Piroxicam group and highest for Tramadol group. In this comparison, it was observed that the Ramsay sedation score was highest for Pentazocine group and least for Tramadol group.

In multimodal group, Pentazocine+Piroxicam had longer duration of action compared to Tramadol+Piroxicam group, p<0.0001. As far as the adverse effects were concerned, the addition of Piroxicam to Tramadol and Pentazocine reduced the incidence of side effects compared to individual agents

Conclusion: Combining an Opioid and an NSAID, like Tramadol or Pentazocine with Piroxicam, provides better post-operative pain relief than giving an opioid alone.

Keywords: Multimodal analgesia; Tramadol; Pentazocine; Piroxicam; Post-operative pain relief

Introduction

Spinal anesthesia is the most common method of anesthesia used in our day-to-day practice; it is efficient, easy and economical and provides intense anesthesia and analgesia in the intra operative period. It is ideal for infra-umbilical surgeries lasting for 1 to 2 hours. The duration of analgesia lasts for a period of 2 to 3 hours and at the end of which, patient experiences severe pain and requires a rescue analgesic at the earliest. Various modalities and adjuvants have been added intrathecally to increase the duration of spinal anesthesia and hence post-operative analgesia but it comes with the disadvantage of continual motor block also. This increases the time for ambulation, leading to increased duration of hospital stay and hence increase costs. Infra umbilical surgeries like Inguinal hernias, Varicose veins and elective caesarean sections which routinely last for around 45 minutes to 1 hour will benefit from a good post-operative pain relief in place

after the regression of spinal anesthetic block. Cesarean delivery patients have even more compelling reasons to treat postoperative pain, as they present with unique challenges; such as, a higher risk for thromboembolic events, which may also be precipitated by immobility from inadequate pain control or excessive sedation associated with the use of opioids [1].

Various rescue analgesics have been used to treat post-operative pain relief; NSAIDs are the main stay of this treatment. NSAIDs inhibit the synthesis of prostaglandins both in the spinal cord and at the periphery, thus diminishing the hyperalgesic state after surgical trauma. NSAIDs are useful as the sole analgesic after minor surgical procedures and may have a significant opioid-sparing effect after major surgery [2].

NSAIDs have many adverse effects like nausea and present a significant GI bleeding risk, along with a risk of a variety of renal complications, and myocardial infarction and other serious cardiovascular complications [3]. In addition, NSAIDs also has ceiling effects, and no therapeutic advantage is gained after increasing dosage beyond those recommended [4]. The recent guidelines issued by numerous professional medical societies, recommend NSAIDs at the lowest effective dose and shortest possible period, in view of the associated gastrointestinal, renal, and cardiovascular toxicity.

Opioids, which have a dual mode of action on opioid and monoaminergic receptors, comprise another group of analgesic drugs that are efficacious against both nociceptive and neuropathic pain. Among the opioids, Tramadol has fewer side effects, such as constipation, respiratory depression, and sedation, compared with the typical strong opioids. Tramadol is now considered to be a first-line analgesic for many musculoskeletal indications [5]. Opioids used as a mode of pain relief, require continuous monitoring and lead to nausea, vomiting, constipation and pruritus. Hence, opioids can impede recovery and early rehabilitation; a problem that is of increasing concern with the rapid rise in the number of ambulatory surgeries.

Pain has a multifactorial origin; hence it may be difficult to achieve effective pain control with a single drug [6]. Currently, the American Society of Anesthesiologists Task Force on Acute Pain Management advocates the use of multimodal analgesia [7]. The complex humoral and neuronal response that occurs with surgery requires a balanced approach for perioperative pain management [8].

As such, one approach for multimodal analgesia is the use of regional anesthesia and analgesia to inhibit the neural conduction from the surgical site to the spinal cord and decrease spinal cord sensitization. Spinal cord sensitization that has been well described and demonstrated in animal studies is challenging to demonstrate in humans [9].

Hence, a combination of both an NSAID and an opioid using the synergestic analgesic effects can be used to combat post-operative pain. Moreover, when used in combination the dose requirement of individual drugs also proportionately comes down and so does the side effects.

Combination therapy of analgesics from different groups is advantageous in targeting both peripheral and central pain pathways and hence, helps in production of analgesia at lower and more tolerable doses of the constituent drugs. Combination therapies can have a positive influence on the ability of individual components to minimize pain, with better tolerability and reduced recovery time [10,11]. This combination therapies, now termed as Multimodal Analgesia is the call of the day with ever increasing numbers of ambulatory or day care surgeries. It may be a combination of two or more modalities of analgesia like-Opioids, NSAIDs and COX 2 selective inhibitors, NMDA antagonists, Alpha-2 Adrenergic agonists, GABA mimetic drugs, Glucocorticoids, Cholinergic drugs, regional nerve blocks and last but not the least Local anaesthetic infiltrations at wound site [12,13].

NSAIDs offer an opioid-sparing strategy in which the opioid activity can be potentiated by NSAIDs. This activity is due to an increased conversion of arachidonic acid to 12-lipoxygenase products, which in turn augments the effects of opioids on K+ channels [14]. Tramadol is an atypical, centrally acting analgesic, as a result of its combined effect as opioid agonist and serotonin and noradrenaline reuptake inhibitor [15,16].

Pentazocine is a synthetically prepared, Benzomorphan class of opioid. It is a strong analgesic with weak narcotic antagonist activity. It is advocated for the relief of moderate to severe pain. Pentazocine has a low abuse potential and is not controlled by narcotic regulations.

Therapeutic trials comparing pentazocine with other strong analgesics have shown it to possess a strong analgesic effect when given intramuscularly and a lesser analgesic effect when administered orally at a dose of 50 mg. Pentazocine produces side-effects similar to those associated with the morphine-like analgesics, and as with these analgesics the effects are exaggerated in ambulatory patients [17].

Piroxicam is a Non-Steroidal Analgesic and anti-inflammatory Drug. It is similar in potency to indomethacin and superior in action than aspirin and ibuprofen. It has an extended half-life of about 40 hours and is suitable for once daily administration. It has been used effectively for both acute and chronic pain. The most frequently reported side effects are only gastro-intestinal and even these have occurred less frequently than with aspirin or indomethacin [18].

Various studies were conducted to compare the efficacy of NSAIDs and opioids. Cepeda et al. compared the efficacy of Ketorolac vs. Morphine. They found that Ketorolac was more effective than morphine. These results contrast with clinical experience and consensus recommendations that opioids are more effective than NSAIDs for moderate-to-severe acute pain [19,20].

Therefore, we designed a randomised controlled double blinded study, first to compare the analgesic efficacy of an NSAID and an opioid in a head-to-head trial by determining the proportion of subjects who obtained adequate postoperative pain relief 30 min after analgesic administration, and second to determine whether the opioid-sparing effect of NSAIDs decreases the risk of opioid side effects, by comparing opioid requirements and side effects in patients who received Tramadol or Pentazocine plus Piroxicam or Tramadol or Pentazocine alone .

Materials and Methods

This prospective, randomised, double blind control study was conducted after the Ethical Committee clearance of Bangalore Medical College and Research Institute, in Victoria and Vani Vilas Hospital, over a period of 12 months from June 2014 to June 2015. 120 patients, of ASA I and II, aged 18-65 yrs, undergoing uni-lateral inguinal hernia, Varicose Veins and elective Caesarean sections under spinal anesthesia were chosen for the study. Patients with any contra indications for spinal anesthesia were excluded from the study. So were patients with peptic ulcer disease or opioid drug abuse. Using a sealed envelope method, (double blind and random) patients were randomly allocated into 4 groups of 30 each Patients demographic data, history and clinical examination findings were recorded. No premedication was given in any of the groups.

Spinal anesthesia in the L2-L3 or L3-L4 interspace was provided by 2 cc of 0.5% Bupivacaine Heavy. A single anesthesiologist was responsible for administration of the. The duration and level of motor block and sensory block was noted. Intraoperative monitoring of vital signs- heart rate, blood pressure, SpO_2 was done. 30 minutes after the end of the surgery, all patients received intramuscular (i.m.) injections of 2 ml each, in either buttock.

Group T patients received Tramadol 100 mg, 2 ml im in one buttock and 2 ml normal saline in the other buttock, Group P patients received Pentazocine 30 mg 2 ml im in one buttock and 2 ml normal saline in the other buttock. Group Tp patients received Tramadol 100 mg, 2 ml in one buttock and Piroxicam 20 mg 2 ml in the other buttock. Group Pp patients received Pentazocine 30 mg 2 ml in one buttock and Piroxicam 20 mg 2 ml in the other buttock.

Normal saline i.m. was given for uniformity of the drug administration in all 4 groups, to avoid any kind of bias, since it is a double blind study. The intramuscular injections were given 30 minutes after the end of the surgery. Level of sensory block at the time of study drug administration was noted. All patients had a sensory level of T8 to T10. The average duration of the surgeries chosen for the study was around one hour.

The syringes containing the drugs were prepared by an anaesthesiologist, identified with a progressive number. Drug administration 30 min after the end of surgery was done by an anaesthesiologist unaware of the content of the syringe and he was responsible for the monitoring of the patients in the following 6 hrs.

Control of postoperative pain was assessed using a Visual Analog Scale (VAS) and sedation assessed by Ramsay Sedation Score (RSS) in the immediate postoperative period, at 30 mins, 1st, 2nd, 4th and 6th hour in the postoperative period. Analgesic duration of action was determined from the interval between drug administration and patient's request for rescue analgesia (VAS>4). All patients were trained to use VAS. Injection Diclofenac 75 mg i.m. was the rescue analgesic given.

Patients were also closely observed for the occurrence of any side effects of the drug administered. Any incidence of Nausea or vomiting was treated with Injection Ondansetron, 4 mg, i.v.

Statistical analysis

Sample size: For power of study as 80%, and confidence limit 95%, to detect a 30% difference in duration of analgesia, minimum sample size required was 25 in each group. Total sample size was taken as 120.

Data obtained were entered into a predesigned sheet and analyzed with the Statistical Package for Social Sciences version 20. Means ± standard deviation (SD) were calculated for the quantitative variables, and the difference between two independent groups was compared using unpaired Student's t-test. The level of significance was set at $P \leq 0.05$.

Results

The results were compared within opioid groups alone (unimodal analgesia) or opioids in combination with NSAIDs (multimodal analgesia) and then all 4 groups were compared with each other for inter group, group variance.

All groups were comparable in the demographic variables, types of surgeries and also average duration of surgery. None of the patients had sensory regression below T 10 at the time of drug administration (Table 1).

	Group T	Group P	Group Tp	Group Pp
Age (yrs)	28 ± 6.3	30 ± 4.8	29 ± 5.7	30 ± 5.2
Height (cms)	158 ± 2.4	160 ± 1.3	157 ± 3.7	159 ± 2.6
Weight (kg)	78 ± 5.0	76 ± 4.9	82 ± 3.5	80 ± 2.8
Inguinal hernia	16	18	15	18
Varicose vein	7	4	7	6
Caesarean section	7	8	8	6
Duration of surgery (mins)	64 ± 6.8	66 ± 4.9	65 ± 5.3	67 ± 5.0

Table 1: The mean VAS scores of the patients in Pentazocine (P) group was lower when compared to Tramadol (T) group at all time periods, p<0.001. The mean VAS scores of the patients in Pentazocine+Piroxicam (Pp) was lower when compared to Tramadol+Piroxicam group (Tp) at all time periods, p<0.001. In the Inter-group comparison of VAS, between all 4 groups, it was observed that VAS was lowest for Pentazocine +Piroxicam (2.71) group and highest for Tramadol group (5.83), p<0.001.

In this (Figures 1-3) comparison, it was also observed that the Ramsay sedation scores were highest for Pentazocine group (2.83) and lowest for Tramadol group (1.61), p<0.001.

When the duration of post-operative pain relief was compared, it was observed that, in unimodal group, pentazocine had longer duration of action compared to tramadol.

In multimodal group; Pentazocine+Piroxicam had longer duration of action compared to Tramadol+Piroxicam group, p<0.0001.

The mean RSS of the patients in Pentazocine group was higher when compared to Tramadol group at all time periods (Figure 4).

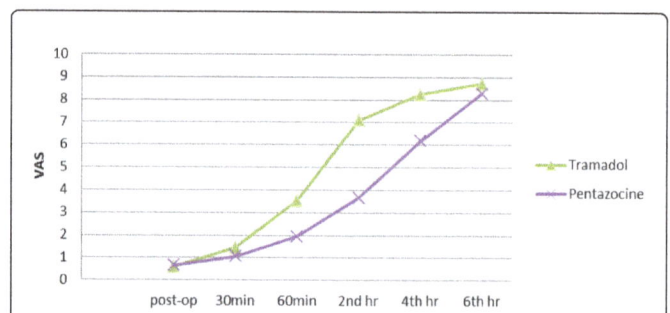

Figure 1: Visual Analog Scale comparision between unimodel analgesia groups.

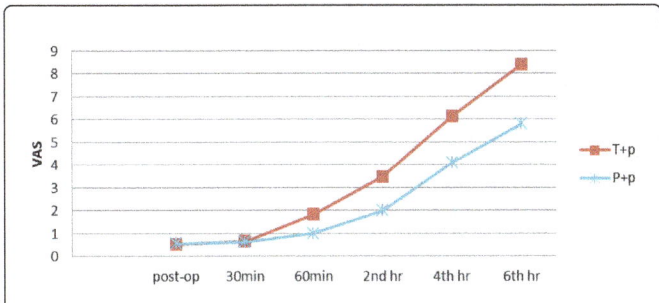

Figure 2: Visual Analog Scale comparision between multimodel analgesia groups.

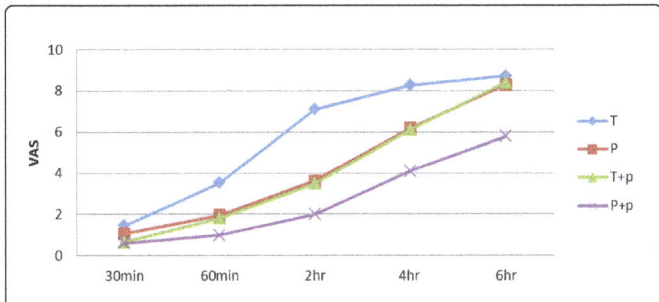

Figure 3: Visual Analog Scale comparision between unimodel and multimodel analgesia groups.

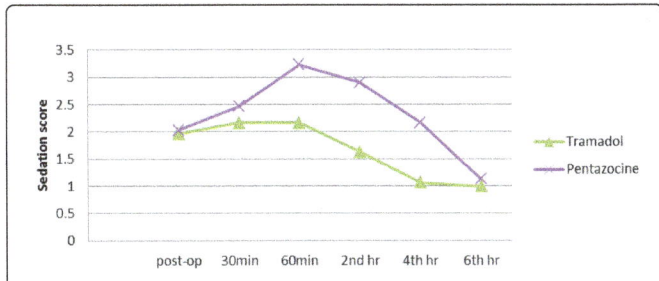

Figure 4: Ramsay sedation score comparision in unimodel analgesia groups.

The mean RSS of the patients in Pentazocine+Piroxicam (Pp) was higher when compared to Tramadol+Piroxicam group (Tp) at all time periods (Figure 5).

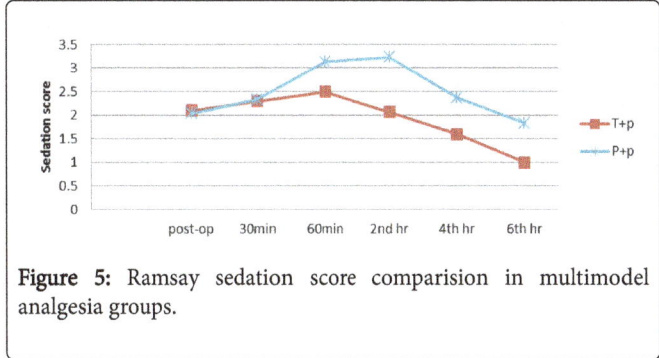

Figure 5: Ramsay sedation score comparision in multimodel analgesia groups.

Inter-group comparison of Ramsay sedation score. In the comparison, it was observed that the sedation scores were highest for Pentazocine group (2.83) and lowest for Tramadol group (1.61) (Figure 6).

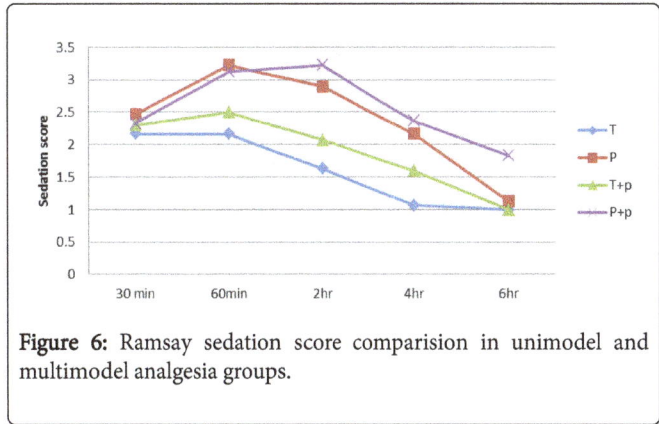

Figure 6: Ramsay sedation score comparision in unimodel and multimodel analgesia groups.

Inter-group comparison of duration of action. In unimodal group, pentazocine had longer duration of action compared to tramadol. In multimodal group, Pentazocine+Piroxicam had longer duration of action compared to Tramadol+Piroxicam group. In the comparison, it was observed that Pentazocine+Piroxicam group (7.31 hours) had the longest duration of action and Tramadol group (2.53 hours) had the lowest duration of action (Table 2 and Figures 7 and 8).

Parameters	Unimodal Analgesia Groups			Multimodal Analgesia Groups		
Groups	Tramadol Group (T) N=30	Pentazocine Group (P) N=30	P-value	Tramadol+Piroxicam group(Tp) N=30	Pentazocine+Piroxicam group (Pp) N=30	P-value
Duration of action (hrs) Mean(SD)	2.53 (0.50)	4.08 (0.37)	<0.0001	5.35 (0.55)	7.31 (0.54)	<0.0001

Table 2: Comparision between Unimodal and Multimodal Analgesia Groups.

As far as the adverse effects were concerned, the addition of Piroxicam to Tramadol and Pentazocine reduced the incidence of side effects compared to individual agents.

The incidence of adverse effects was higher with Pentazocine and Pentazocine+Piroxicam as compared to Tramadol and Tramadol +Piroxicam.

It was also observed that the combination of Pentazocine +Piroxicam had lower incidence of side effects compared to Pentazocine group and the combination of Tramadol+Piroxicam group had lower incidence of adverse effects compared to Tramadol (Table 3).

Discussion

The World Health Organization and International Association for the Study of Pain have recognized pain relief as a human right [21]. Poorly managed postoperative pain can lead to complications and prolonged rehabilitation [22]. Uncontrolled acute pain is associated with the development of chronic pain with reduction in quality of life [23].

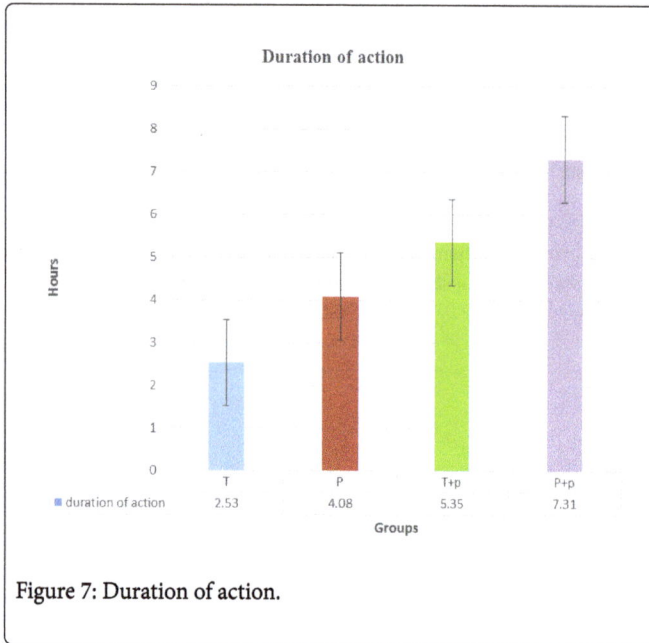

Figure 7: Duration of action.

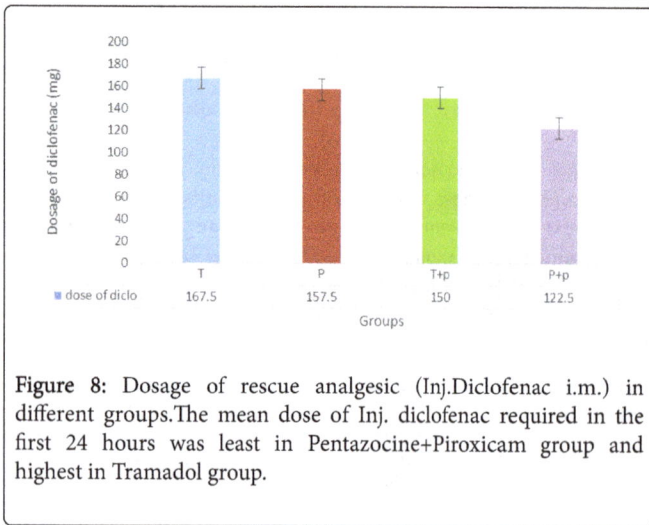

Figure 8: Dosage of rescue analgesic (Inj.Diclofenac i.m.) in different groups.The mean dose of Inj. diclofenac required in the first 24 hours was least in Pentazocine+Piroxicam group and highest in Tramadol group.

Adverse drug effects	Tramadol$_{100}$	Pentazocine$_{30}$	Tramadol$_{100}$ + Piroxicam$_{20}$	Pentazocine$_{30}$ + Piroxicam$_{20}$
Headache	-	-	-	-
Nausea	2(6.6%)	5(16.6%)	3(10%)	3(10%)
Vomiting	2(6.6%)	7(23%)	2(6.6%)	5(16.6%)
Abdominal pain	-	-	-	-
Vertigo	-	1(3.3%)	-	-
Diarrhea	-	-	-	-
Rashes	-	-	-	-
Pruritis	-	-	-	-
Drowsiness	-	-	-	2(6.6%)
Dry mouth	-	-	-	-
Bleeding	-	-	-	-
Anxiety/agitation	-	-	-	1(3.3%)
Psychotic symptoms	-	-	-	-
Respiratory depression	-	-	-	-
Sweating	-	2(6.6%)	-	-

Table 3: Adverse drug effects.

In a study that assessed patients' postoperative pain experience and the status of acute pain management in a random sample, approximately 80% of patients said they experienced acute pain after surgery.

The authors concluded that; despite an increased focus on pain management programs and the development of new standards for pain management, many patients continue to experience intense pain after surgery [24]. To address the under treatment of postoperative pain and the limitations of opioid monotherapy, a strategy known as multimodal pain management was introduced in the early 1990s [25,26].

This approach simultaneously administers two or more analgesic agents with different mechanisms of action. Principles of a multimodal strategy include control of postoperative pain to allow early mobilization, early enteral nutrition and attenuation of the perioperative stress response through the use of regional anesthetic techniques and a combination of analgesic agents (i.e., multimodal analgesia) [27].

To achieve a maximum short-term and long-term benefits from multimodal analgesic therapies, the pain management would be initiated as a preventive in the preoperative period continued in the early postoperative period and extended into the postcharge period for 3-7 days [28,29].

In our study, control of post-operative pain was better with multimodal analgesia as compared to monotherapy.

Among the Multimodal groups, the combination of Pentazocine +Piroxicam achieved better control of post-operative pain and had longer duration of action as compared to the combination of Tramadol +Piroxicam. Among the Unimodal groups, Pentazocine had a longer duration of action and offers better pain control as compared to Tramadol.

The mean consumption of rescue analgesic (Inj.diclofenac) was lower in the Pentazocine+Piroxicam group compared to other groups. The incidence of adverse effects was higher with Pentazocine alone than Pentazocine+Piroxicam also higher in Tramadol alone than Tramadol+Piroxicam group.

The value of NSAIDs in minor, moderate, or severe postoperative pain is well documented [30,31], but their efficacy is too small to be the sole analgesic in more severe pain states, although they represent an ideal alternative component in the multimodal approach to postoperative pain treatment.

So far, only one such study is available. It demonstrates improved analgesia by fixed-dose combination with piroxicam and opioid after total hip replacement [32]. The combination of systemic NSAID with a central neural block with bupivacaine and/or opioids has been studied in major abdominal [33] and thoracic surgery [34], in which additional treatment with piroxicam 20-40 mg daily did not improve analgesia during rest, cough, or mobilization during an otherwise effective epidural low-dose bupivacaine-opioid regimen After cesarean section the combination of low-dose epidural morphine and intramuscular diclofenac provided analgesia superior to either drug alone [35].

Combination of systemic NSAID with intraarticular bupivacaine may reduce pain and analgesic requirements [36].

Limitations

The possible confounding influence of the spinal analgesia agent (bupivacaine) on the observed analgesic effects of all agents studied was a limitation of our study.

Conclusion

A multimodal approach combining pentazocine or tramadol with an NSAID, such as Piroxicam, offers better control of pain in the postoperative period than when the opioid is given alone.

Though Pentazocine offers better pain control and acts longer, it is associated with higher incidence of adverse effects compared to tramadol. However, the addition of an NSAID to opioid not only decreases the adverse effects but also has an opioid sparing action.

References

1. Pan PH (2006) Post cesarean delivery pain management: multimodal approach. Int J Obstet Anesth 15: 185-188.

2. American Society of Anesthesiologists Task Force on Acute Pain Management (2004) Practice guidelines for acute pain management in the perioperative setting: an updated report by the American Society of Anesthesiologists Task Force on Acute Pain Management. Anesthesiology 100: 1573-1581.

3. McCarberg B, Tenzer P (2013) Complexities in the pharmacologic management of osteoarthritis pain. Curr Med Res Opin 29: 539-548.

4. Mercadante S (2001) The use of anti-inflammatory drugs in cancer pain. Cancer Treat Rev 27: 51-61.

5. Schug SA (2007) The role of tramadol in current treatment strategies for musculoskeletal pain. Ther Clin Risk Manag 3: 717-723.

6. Vanderah TW (2007) Pathophysiology of pain. Med Clin North Am 91: 1-12.

7. Ashburn MA, Caplan RA, Carr DB (2004) Practice guidelines for acute pain management in the perioperative setting. An updated report by the American Society of Anesthesiologists task force on acute pain management. Anesthesiology 100: 1573-1581.

8. Kehlet H, Dahl JB (2003) Anaesthesia, surgery, and challenges in postoperative recovery. Lancet 362: 1921-1928.

9. Woolf CJ (2007) Central sensitization: uncovering the relation between pain and plasticity. Anesthesiology 106: 864-867.

10. Rawal N, Macquaire V, Catala E, Berti M, Costa R, et al. (2011) Tramadol/paracetamol combination tablet for postoperative pain following ambulatory hand surgery: a double-blind, double-dummy, randomized, parallel-group trial. J Pain Res 4: 103-110.

11. Raffa RB (2001) Pharmacology of oral combination analgesics: rational therapy for pain. J Clin Pharm Ther 26: 257-264.

12. Buvanendran A, Kroin JS (2009) Multimodal analgesia for controlling acute postoperative pain. Curr Opin Anaesthesiol 22: 588-593.

13. Garimella V, Cellini C (2013) Postoperative pain control. Clin Colon Rectal Surg 26: 191-196.

14. Brunton LL, Chabner BA, Knollmann BC (2011) Goodman and Gilman's The Pharmacological Basis of Therapeutics. (12thedn). New York, McGraw Hill.

15. Raffa RB, Friderichs E, Reimann W, Shank RP, Codd EE, et al. (1992) Opioid and nonopioid components independently contribute to the mechanism of action of tramadol, an 'atypical' opioid analgesic. J Pharmacol Exp Ther 260: 275-285.

16. [Authors not listed] (2005) Australian and New Zealand College of Anaesthetists (ANZCA). Acute Pain Management: Scientific Evidence. (2ndedn). Melbourne, Australian and New Zealand College of Anaesthetists.

17. Brogden RN, Speight TM, Avery GS (1973) Pentazocine: A Review of its Pharmacological Properties, Therapeutic Efficacy and Dependence Liability. Drugs 5: 6-91.

18. Brogden RN, Heel RC, Speight TM, Avery GS (1981) Piroxicam: A Review of its Pharmacological Properties and Therapeutic Efficacy. Drugs 22: 165-187.

19. Cepeda MS, Vargas L, Ortegon G, Sanchez M, Carr DB (1995) Comparative analgesic efficacy of patient-controlled analgesia with ketorolac versus morphine after elective intra-abdominal operations. Anesth Analg 80: 1150-1153.

20. Carr DB, Jacox AK, Chapman CR, Fields HL, Heidrich G, et al. (1992) Acute pain management: Operative or medical procedures and trauma, Clinical Practice Guideline. (950034thedn). Rockville, Agency for Health Care Policy and Research.

21. Brennan F, Carr DB, Cousins M (2007) Pain management: a fundamental human right. Anesth Analg 105: 205-221.

22. Kehlet H, Holte K (2001) Effect of postoperative analgesia on surgical outcome. Br J Anaesth 87: 62-72.

23. Kehlet H, Jensen TS, Woolf CJ (2006) Persistent postsurgical pain: risk factors and prevention. Lancet 367: 1618-1625.

24. Apfelbaum J, Chen C, Mehta S, Gan T (2003) Postoperative pain experience: results from a national survey suggest postoperative pain continues to be undermanaged. Anesth Analg 97: 534-540.

25. Kehlet H, Dahl JB (1993) The value of "multimodal" or "balanced analgesia" in postoperative pain treatment. Anesth Analg 77: 1048-1056.

26. White PF (2008) Multimodal analgesia: its role in preventing postoperative pain. Curr Opin Investig Drugs 9: 76-82.

27. Ulufer Sivrikaya G (2012) Multimodal Analgesia for Postoperative Pain Management, Pain Management-Current Issues and Opinions.

28. Bisgaard T (2006) Analgesic treatment after laparoscopic cholecystectomy: a critical assessment of the evidence. Anesthesiology 104: 835-846.

29. White PF, Kehlet H, Neal JM, Schricker T, Carr DB, et al. (2007) The role of the anesthesiologist in fast-track surgery: from multimodal analgesia to perioperative medical care. Anesth Analg 104: 1380-1396.

30. Dahl JB, Kehlet H (1991) Non-steroidal anti-inflammatory drugs: rationale for use in severe postoperative pain. Br J Anaesth 66: 703-712.

31. Mather LE (1992) Do the pharmacodynamics of the nonsteroidal anti-inflammatory drugs suggests a role in the management of postoperative pain? Drugs 44: 1-12.

32. Gore M, Sadosky A, Zlateva G, Clauw D (2010) Initial use of pregabalin, patterns of pain-related pharmacotherapy, and healthcare resource use among older patients with fibromyalgia. Am J Manag Care 16: S144-153.

33. Mogensen T, Vegger P, Jonsson T, Matzke AE, Lund C, et al. (1992) Systemic piroxicam as an adjunct to combined epidural bupivacaine and

morphine for postoperative pain relief--a double-blind study. Anesth Analg 74: 366-370.

34. Bigler D, Meller J, Kam-Jensen M, Berthelsen P, Hjortso NC, et al. (1992) Effect of piroxicam in addition to continuous thoracic epidural bupivacaine and morphine on postoperative pain and lung function after thoracotomy. Acta Anaesthesiol Scand 36: 647-650.

35. Sun HL, Wu CC, Lin MS, Chang CF, Mok MS (1992) Combination of low-dose epidural morphine and intramuscular diclofenac sodium in postcesarean analgesia. Anesth Analg 75: 64-68.

36. Smith I, Shively RA, White PF (1992) Effects of keterolac and bupivacaine on recovery after outpatient arthroscopy. Anesth Analg75: 208-212.

37. Feld JM, Hoffman WE, Stechert MM, Hoffman IW, Ananda RC (2006) Fentanyl or dexmedetomidine combined with desflurane for bariatric surgery. J Clin Anesth 18: 24-28.

38. Ibraheim OA, Abdulmonem A, Baaj J, Zahrani TA, Arlet V (2013) Esmolol versus dexmedetomidine in scoliosis surgery: study on intraoperative blood loss and hemodynamic changes. Middle East J Anaesthesiol 22: 27-33.

39. Unlugenc H, Gunduz M, Guler T, Yagmur O, Isik G (2005) The effect of pre-anaesthetic administration of intravenous dexmedetomidine on postoperative pain in patients receiving patient-controlled morphine. Eur J Anaesthesiol 22: 386-391.

13

Controlled Hypotensive Anesthesia in Children Undergoing Nasal Surgery

Sabry Mohamed Amin*, **Mohamed Gamal Elmawy and Rabab Mohamed Mohamed**

Departments of Anesthesiology and Surgical Intensive Care, Faculty of Medicine, Tanta University, Egypt

***Corresponding author:** Sabry Mohamed Amin, Assistant professor, Departments of Anesthesiology and Surgical Intensive Care, Faculty of Medicine, Tanta University, Egypt, E-mail: sabry_amin@yahoo.com

Abstract

Background: The nasal surgery in pediatric patient's caries a major challenge to both anesthesiologist and surgeon. The surgeon faces small nostrils and narrow nasal passages. The anesthesiologist has to produce condition which facilitate the surgery, decrease the operative time by minimize the intraoperative bleeding to allow better visualization this can be achieved by controlled hypotensive anesthesia which is the key issue in the success of nasal surgery in pediatric age group.

Patient and methods: Seventy pediatric patients aged 8-12 years scheduled for elective nasal surgery under general anesthesia. Patients were classified into two equal groups (35 patients per group) according to study drugs used. Group (D): The patients in this group received dexmedetomidine 0.5 µg/kg as loading dose over 10 minutes followed by 0.2-0.5 µg/kg/h as maintenance infusion after induction of anesthesia but before surgery. Group (E): The patients in this group received esmolol 0.5 mg/kg as loading dose over 10 minutes followed by 100-300 µg/kg/min as maintenance infusion after induction of anesthesia but before surgery. Measurements: Heart rate, Mean Arterial blood Pressure, Quality of surgical field, duration of surgery, duration of anesthesia, Aspartate aminotransferase (AST), alanine aminotransferase (ALT), blood urea, serum creatinine, adverse events and postoperative analgesia.

Results: There were no significant differences between groups as regards to demographic data, duration of surgery, and duration of anesthesia. The MABP and HR were significantly decreased after infusion of study drugs till the end of surgery with no differences between both groups in all times of measurements. The quality of surgical field was comparable between both groups in all times of measurements. There were no changes in blood urea, serum creatinine, AST, and ALT.

Conclusion: Our study demonstrated that both dexmedetomidine and esmolol are safe and effective agents for inducing controlled hypotension in pediatric patients undergoing nasal surgery with no reported complications.

Keywords: Nasal surgery; Hypotensive anesthesia; Hypotensive drugs; Esmolol; Dexmedetomidine

Introduction

The anesthetist is an important member of the nasal surgery. The technique of anesthesia plays an important role in success of surgery as the anesthesiologist has to produce conditions which facilitate surgery by inducing immobile bloodless surgical field while maintaining organ perfusion.

A dry surgical condition is needed for nasal surgery; major complications can occurred as result of poor visualization of the nasal and paranasal structures. So the anesthesiologist should use different physical and pharmacologic methods to minimize the bleeding in the operative field.

Major bleeding and poor visualization of the nasal and paranasal structures leads to serious complications include but not limited to optic nerve damage, dural injury, and meningitis have been reported for functional endoscopic sinus surgery under general or local anesthesia [1].

The anesthetists should make an optimum surgical condition to avoid the threat of serious complications which result from poor visibility [2].

Deliberated hypotensive anesthesia is used to induce dry surgical field which allow better visualization of the surgical site and decrease the amount of intraoperative blood loss [3].

Functional endoscopic sinus surgery was done safely in children using hypotensive anesthesia without any adverse events although the blood pressure was reduced up to 25% below baseline [4].

Deliberated hypotensive anesthesia can be done using different drugs which include direct vasodilator, alpha blocker, beta blocker, combined alpha and beta blocker [5].

Reflex increase in the heart rate as result in decrease in blood pressure may increase the surgical site bleeding making its wisdom to use beta-blocker to enable good control of heart rate.

Esmolol is short acting, highly selective beta one antagonist used by intravenous route as bolus and continuous infusion to induce controlled hypotension with very short half-life. The total clearance of esmolol from the body was 3 times of cardiac output and 14 times of hepatic blood flow [6].

Dexmedetomidine is a specific and selective α_2 agonist has anesthetic-sparing properties, anxiolytic, sedative, decrease perioperative opioid consumption, prolong postoperative analgesia and maintain hemodynamic stability [7].

The aim of our study was to compare surgical condition in children undergoing nasal surgeries under general anesthesia combined with dexmedetomidine or esmolol to induce controlled hypotension. The primary outcomes of this study are the quality of surgical field and hemodynamic changes while the duration of surgery, time to first analgesic request and postoperative complications were the secondary outcomes.

Patients and Methods

After approval of the ethics committee and obtaining written informed consent from patient's guardian, this study was carried out on seventy pediatric patients aged 8-12 years prepared for nasal surgery under general anesthesia in the otorhinolaryngology department, Tanta University Hospital.

All patients' data were confidential with secret codes and was used for the current study only.

Any unexpected risk appears during the course of the study was cleared to the guardian of the patient and the ethical committee on time and the proper measures were taken to minimize or overcome these risks. The approval code of ethics committee was 30830/03/16.

The randomization of this study was done by using simple method of sealed numbered envelopes. A blind person who did not share in patients' care read the number, open the envelopes and made group classification. A blind anesthesiologist who not participates in the patients' follow up will be responsible for preparation of study drugs. Both attendant anesthesiologist and surgeon were blind to pharmacological intervention and group's classification.

Inclusion criteria

Pediatric patients aging 8-12 years of both sex with ASA I and II scheduled for elective nasal surgery during general anesthesia.

Exclusion criteria

Refusal of patients' guardian to participate in the study, patients with disorder of coagulation, thrombocytopenia, patients on anticoagulant therapy, and patients with congenital heart disease. Figure 1 shows the patients flow diagram.

Anesthetic management

Preoperative preparation: All patients underwent preoperative assessment by history taking, clinical examination and laboratory investigations (which include complete blood count, liver function test, renal function test, prothrombin time and INR, bleeding and coagulation time).

Clear fluids were allowed up to 2 h before operation while solid food was omitted 6 hours before anesthesia. All patients received orally 0.5 mg/kg of injectable midazolam mixed with juice 30 min before anesthesia to facilitate parent's separation. Emla cream was applied to patients' skin 30 min before induction of anesthesia.

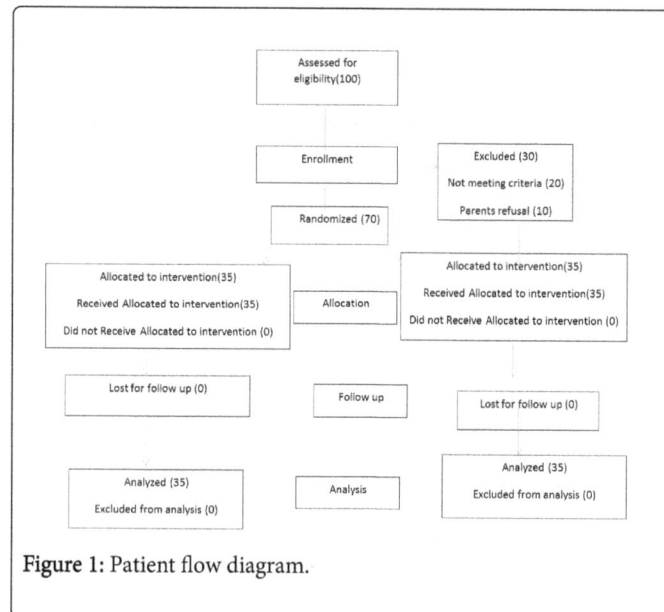

Figure 1: Patient flow diagram.

Intraoperative management: On arrival to operating room two intravenous lines were inserted at site of emla cream and secured. One for study drug infusion and the other for fluid infusion and other medications.

Anesthesia was induced by fentanyl 1 µg/kg, propofol 2 mg/kg and rocuronium 0.6 mg/kg, the patients were ventilated by face mask for 3 min then; airway was secured by suitable size cuffed endotracheal tube by direct laryngoscope. Tracheal intubation was confirmed by observation of chest wall movement, chest auscultation and appearance of square wave of capnography. The patients' lungs were mechanically ventilated. The ventilation was adjusted and controlled by the respiratory rate and tidal volume to maintain normocarbia ($ETCO_2$ between 32-35 mmHg).

Maintenance of anesthesia: Isoflurane 1 to 1.5 vol. % in O_2 was used for anesthesia maintenance and top up dose of rocuronium 0.01 mg/kg was given every 30 minutes. Patients were attached to monitor displaying ECG, HR, NIBP, $ETCO_2$ and O_2 saturation. All patients received 5% dextrose in 0.9% saline at rate 5 ml/kg/hour.

Folly catheter was inserted for urinary bladder decompression and to observe urine output. Following induction of anesthesia all patients received topical application of epinephrine 1/1000 to nasal mucosa with cotton for 10 min, after removal of the cotton the surgeon infiltrates 1 ml of lidocaine and epinephrine 1/100000 submucosally. Patients were positioned supine with head up 30 degrees to facilitate venous drainage.

Signs of inadequate anesthesia (increases in MAP or increases in HR greater than the baseline by 20% or more) were treated with additional fentanyl 1 µg/kg and recorded. Nitroglycerine was infused as a rescue hypotensive agent if these target levels could not be achieved with the uppermost dose. The primary endpoint was MAP 20-25% below baseline value before beginning of surgery in both groups, while secondary endpoints included: occurrence of tachycardia, and the need to use rescue hypotensive agent.

Decrease in MAP below baseline by 30% was considered hypotension and treated with ephedrine 5 mg. HR below 60 beats/

minute was considered as bradycardia and treated with atropine 0.01 mg/kg.

The infused drugs in both groups was stopped 10 minutes before anticipated end of surgery to allow the pressure to rise to detect bleeding point and to make effective hemostasis.

During placement of nasal pack, intravenous (IV) 15 mg/kg of paracetamol and 1 mg/kg of tramadol were given intramuscular to control postoperative pain in both groups.

For prophylaxis against postoperative nausea and vomiting (PONV) metoclopramide 0.15 mg/kg combined with dexamethasone 0.15 mg/kg were administered at the end of surgery. In case of PONV ondansetron 0.1 mg/kg was given.

After surgery was completed, isoflurane was stopped, residual muscle relaxant was antagonized with atropine 0.02 mg/kg and neostigmine 0.05 mg/kg, awake extubation of the endotracheal tube was done after insertion of suitable size oral airway and suction of the oropharynx.

After extubation the patients were transferred to postanesthesia care unit for close monitoring of conscious level, hemodynamic parameter and oxygen saturation postoperatively.

Randomization

The randomization of this study was done by using simple method of sealed numbered envelopes. A blind person who did not share in patients' care read the number, open the envelopes and made group classification. A blind anesthesiologist who not participates in the patients' follow up will be responsible for preparation of study drugs.

The process of inclusion in the study went on until the required number of patients was reached. All operating room anesthesiologists, surgeons, and nurses were blinded to randomization, and preparations.

Patients classification

Patients were classified randomly into two equal groups (35 patients per group) according to study drugs used.

Group D: Dexmedetomidine (Precedex®, Meditera, 200 μg/2 mL) 0.5 μg/kg in diluted 20 ml of normal saline was given over 10 minutes as loading dose followed by continuous infusion 0.2-0.5 μg/kg/h after induction of anesthesia but before surgery, in order to maintain the mean arterial blood pressure 20-25% below baseline value.

Group E: Esmolol (Brevibloc®, Eczacibasi, 100 mg/10mL) 0.5 mg/kg diluted in 20 ml of normal saline was given over 10 min as loading dose followed by continuous infusion 100-300 μg/kg/min after induction of anesthesia but before surgery, in order to maintain the mean arterial blood pressure 20-25% below baseline value.

Measurements

- Demographic data: age, weight, sex, ASA classification.
- Heart rate and mean arterial blood Pressure (as baseline, after intubation, then every 5 minutes after study drugs infusion till the end of operation).
- Quality of surgical field (by the operating surgeon every 15 minutes): with a predefined scale adapted from Fromme et al. (Table 1) [8].
- Aspartate aminotransferase (AST), alanine aminotransferase (ALT), blood urea and creatinine were analyzed before surgery, and in day one and day two after surgery.
- Duration of surgery.
- Duration of anesthesia.
- Adverse events.
- Postoperative analgesia according to FLACC scores [9].

Score	Definition
0	No bleeding.
1	Slight bleeding - no suctioning of blood required
2	Slight bleeding - occasional suctioning required. Surgical field not threatened
3	Slight bleeding - frequent suctioning required. Bleeding threatens surgical field a few seconds after suction is removed.
4	Moderate bleeding - frequent suctioning required. Bleeding threatens surgical field directly after suction is removed
5	Severe bleeding - constant suctioning required. Bleeding appears faster than can be removed by suction. Surgical field severely threatened and surgery not possible.

Table 1: Average category scale (ACS) for assessment of intra-operative surgical field.

The postoperative pain was evaluated by a chef nurse blind to study by using FLACC scale Table 2 graded from 0 to 10 (0=no pain, 10=the worst possible pain) at 2 hours, 4 hours, 6 hours, 8 hours, 12 hours, and 18 hours after recovery.

Intravenous paracetamol 15 mg/kg was given as rescue analgesic every 6 hour as long as pain scores less than 5.

Tramadol 1 mg/kg was given intravenously if the pain scores more than 5.

The time to first dose of analgesia and total amount of tramadol used were recorded.

Statistical analysis

The sample size was calculated depending on the primary outcome of this study. Power analysis identified 32 patients per group, required to detect 15% difference between groups with a power 80% and a significant level of 0.05.

Criteria	Score 0	Score 1	Score 2
Face	No particular expression or smile	Occasional grimace or frown, withdrawn, uninterested	Frequent to constant quivering chin, clenched jaw
Legs	Normal position or relaxed	Uneasy, restless, tense	Kicking, or legs drawn up
Activity	Lying quietly, normal position, moves easily	Squirming, shifting back and forth, tense	Arched, rigid or jerking
Cry	No cry (awake or asleep)	Moans or whimpers; occasional complaint	Crying steadily, screams or sobs, frequent complaints
Consolability	Content, relaxed	Reassured by occasional touching, hugging or being talked to, distractible	Difficult to console or comfort
The Face, Legs, Activity, Cry, Consolability scale or FLACC scale is a measurement used to assess pain for children between the ages of 2 months-7 y or individuals that are unable to communicate their pain. The scale is scored between a range of 0-10 with 0 representing no pain while 10 representing the worst pain. The scale has 5 criteria which are each assigned a score of 0, 1 or 2.			

Table 2: FLACC scale.

To avoid potential errors, 35 patients were included in each group. Medcalc program version 3.5; was used for sample size calculation.

The primary outcomes of this study are the quality of surgical field and changes in the hemodynamic parameters while duration of surgery, time to first analgesic request and postoperative complications were the secondary outcomes.

Student's t-test was used to compare the demographic data, hemodynamic parameters, duration of surgery, duration of anesthesia, Time to first analgesic request, and total amount of tramadol consumption. Mann-Whitney-U test was used for nonparametric measurements including quality of surgical field and pain score. $P<0.05$ was considered significant.

Results

Seventy children aged 8-12 years underwent nasal surgery had completed this study were divided into two equal groups.

There were no statistically significant differences between both groups as regards to demographic data, duration of surgery, duration of anesthesia, and types of surgeries $P>0.05$ (Table 3).

Variables	Group D: N=35	Group E: N=35	P value
Age (yr.)	10.5 ± 2.05	10.8 ± 1.55	0.2
Weight (kg)	32.6 ± 2.65	34.5 ± 1.45	0.7
Sex (M/F)	22/13	20/15	
Duration of anesthesia (min)	106.15 ± 45.25	108.25 ± 43.35	0.7
Duration of surgery (min)	92.55 ± 7.15	90.65 ± 6.55	0.8
Tramadol consumption (mg)	14.28 ± 8.15	25.15 ± 12.55	0.02
Time to first analgesic request (h)	9. 45 ± 2.65	4. 55 ±0.55	0.01
All data expressed as mean ± SD			

Table 3: Demographic data; duration of surgery, duration of anesthesia , tramadol consumption; time of first analgesic requirement.

There were no statistically significant differences between both groups as regards to heart rate and mean arterial blood pressure values throughout the study period ($p>0.05$) and the values of HR and MABP were decreased significantly after infusion of the study drugs till the end of surgery when compared to base line values $p<0.05$ (Tables 4 and 5).

Time	Group D: N=35	Group E: N=35	P1
T0	110.55 ± 6.92	112.25 ± 7.45	0.54
T1	115.35 ± 7.55	118.56 ± 6.65	0.65
T2	102.55 ± 6.52	100.56 ± 6.25	0.54
T3	82.35 ± 5.55	80.43 ± 5.25	0.62
T4	78.42 ± 4.65	80.48 ± 4,25	0.72
T5	76.55 ± 5.52	78.35 ± 4.42	0.45

T0=base line, T1=after intubation, T2=5 min after drugs infusion, T3=15 min after drug infusion, T4=30 min after drugs infusion, T5=60 min after drugs infusion. All data expressed as mean ± SD

Tables 4: Changes in HR (beat/min) in both groups.

Time	Group D: N=35	Group E: N=35	P1
T0	62.65 ± 4.5	65.55 ± 5.60	0.53
T1	70.55 ± 5.35	72.25 ± 3.55	0.62
T2	60.55 ± 3.65	62.45 ± 5.42	0.52
T3	58.65 ± 4.45	60.55 ± 3.34	0.65
T4	60.42 ± 4.54	62.44 ± 3.33	0.45
T5	62.62 ± 5.52	60.44 ± 3.545	0.7

T0=base line, T1=after intubation, T2=5 min after drugs infusion, T3=15 min after drugs infusion, T4=30 min after drugs infusion, T5=60 min after drugs infusion. All data expressed as mean ± SD

Table 5: Changes in MABP (mmHg) in both groups.

Both groups were comparable with no statistically significant differences as regards to the quality of surgical field in all times of measurements p>0.05, the score ranged between 1-3 with majority of patients had score 1 (Table 6).

Predefined scale	Group D: N=35	Group E: N=35	P
0	0	0	
1	22	20	0.5
2	12	13	0.7
3	1	2	0.4
4	0	0	
5	0	0	

Table 6: Quality of surgical field in both groups.

There were no statistically significant differences between the two groups as regards to pain score value at 2 h postoperatively, p>0.05 (Table 7).

At 4 h, 6 h and 8 h postoperatively the pain score values were statistically significant less in group D when compared to group E. (P<0.05), however it was comparable between both groups at 12 h and 18 hours postoperatively p>0.05 (Table 7).

Time	Group D: N=35	Group E: N=35	P1
2 h	1.42 ± 0.56	1.52 ± 0.64	0.573
4 h	1.32 ± 1.65	3.35 ± 0.45	0.03
6 h	2.54 ± 0.72	4.52 ± 0.55	0.01
8 h	3.45 ± 0.35	4.85 ± 0.82	0.04
12 h	4.54 ± 0.64	5.62 ± 0.65	0.5
18 h	4.35 ± 0.73	4.42 ± 0.74	0.2
All data expressed as mean ± SD			

Table 7: Pain score value in both groups.

As regards to the time of first analgesic request we found that, the time was statistically significant less in group E when compared to group D it was 9.45 ± 2.65 h in group D while it was 4.55 ± 0.55 h in group E (P<0.05), the amount of tramadol consumption was statistically significant less in group (D) than group (E) (P<0.05) (Table 3).

There were no differences in the postoperative values of blood urea, serum creatinine, AST, and ALT when compared to the baseline values in both groups (Table 8).

Values	Time	Group D: N=35	Group E: N=35	P
Blood Urea (mg/dL)	Baseline preoperative	15.52 ± 4.45	14.45 ± 3.65	0.3
	Day one postoperative	14.25±4.42	15.35 ± 4.34	0.23
	Day two postoperative	13.45±4.65	14.32 ± 5.55	0.43
Creatinine (mg/dL)	Baseline preoperative	0.65 ± 0.12	0.62 ± 0.15	0.42
	Day one postoperative	0.62 ± 0.15	0.65 ± 0.22	0.22
	Day two postoperative	0.64 ± 0.22	0.62 ± 25	0.45
AST Unites	Baseline preoperative	15.25 ± 2.45	16.32 ± 3.55	0.34
	Day one postoperative	18.55 ± 3.42	18.52 ± 4.65	0.52
	Day two postoperative	16.45 ± 4.65	1855 ± 3.42	0.12
ALT Unites	Baseline preoperative	20.52 ± 4.45	19.55 ± 4.54	0.35
	Day one postoperative	19.54 ± 4.52	20.55 ± 5.65	0.23
	Day two postoperative	20.55 ± 5,62	20.5 ± 4.55	0.34
AST: Aspartate Amino Transferase; ALT: Alanine Amino Transferase. All data expressed as mean ± SD				

Table 8: Comparison of blood urea, serum creatinine, AST, ALT in both groups.

There was a significant reduction in volatile anaesthetic and fentanyl consumption in dexmedetomidine group compared to the esmolol group.

Total fentanyl consumption in esmolol group was 80.5 ± 12.6 µg and 30.45 ± 6.52 µg in dexmedetomidine group.

Total isoflurane concentration used in esmolol group was 1 ± 0.22% and in dexmedetomidine group it was 0.75 ± 0.52 % (Table 9).

None of the patients in either group developed bradycardia less than 60 beats per minute.

It was observed that hypotension in 3 patients in dexmedetomidine group required intervention with ephedrine and IV fluid bolus.

None of the patients in either group needs addition of nitroglycerine.

Types of surgery	Group D: N=35	Group E: N=35	p
FESS	21	22	
Rhinoplasty	2	3	
Septoplasty	7	6	
Unilateral Choanal atresia	5	4	
Total fentanyl consumption (μg)	30.45 ± 6.52	80.5 ± 12.6	0.02
Total isoflurane concentration (%)	0.75 ± 0.52 %	1 ± 0.22%	0.034
FESS: Functional Endoscopic Sinus Surgery			

Tables 9: Types of nasal surgery, total fentanyl consumption, total isoflurane concentration.

Discussion

Our study demonstrated that, both dexmedetomidine and esmolol were effective in optimizing the surgical condition for patients underwent nasal surgery under general anesthesia by reducing heart rate and blood pressure which minimizing surgical site bleeding, allows better visualization, decrease operative time with no reported adverse events. Also there were no significant changes in renal and liver function postoperatively.

The present study shows using dexmedetomidine or esmolol anesthesia, controlled hypotension could be achieved without using additional antihypertensive agents in all patients.

Dexmedetomidine was associated with prolonged postoperative analgesia, decrease opioid consumption, and less postoperative adverse events.

Induced hypotension was probably not used in children in the early years although it is safer in them because their circulation is not compromised by atherosclerosis.

Controlled hypotensive anesthesia was used in pediatric surgery since 1953. After that it became a popular technique in many pediatric surgical operations which associated with major bleeding include scoliosis surgery, vascular surgery, nasal surgery, middle ear surgery and neurosurgery.

Advances in the understanding of the physiology, pharmacology of induced hypotensive anesthesia, and the advances in the monitoring techniques, lead to the evolution and safety of the technique.

The desired level of hypotension depends on the age, condition, and position of the patient, and on the surgical requirement. In young children placed in the supine position, a systolic pressure of 55 or 60 mm Hg can be safely used to induce a dry surgical field [4].

With hypotension, the operating time for Harrington rod insertion was reduced from 3 to 1¼ h because blood loss was reduced from 3 to 4 units on average to one or less and the surgeons could see more clearly what they were doing [10].

The nasal surgery in pediatric patients carries a major challenge to both anesthesiologist and surgeon. The surgeon face small nostrils, narrow nasal passages, the anatomical landmark may not be clearly developed, and small, thin bony structure of nasal septum and paranasal structure.

The anesthesiologist has to produce condition which facilitate the surgery, avoid the serious complications, decrease the operative time, by minimize the intraoperative bleeding and allow better visualization, this can be achieved by controlled hypotensive anesthesia which is the key issue in the success of nasal surgery in pediatric age group under general anesthesia.

the main advantages of hypotensive anesthesia are decrease of blood loss, decrease blood transfusion, improve quality of surgical field, decrease in operation time, no significant changes in the vital organs functionality provided that patient selection and adequate monitoring are used.

The complications of hypotensive anesthesia are secondary hemorrhage, renal impairment, thromboembolic complications (cerebral, coronary), rebound hypertension, cardiac arrest, increased ICP, and impaired cognitive function.

Contraindications of hypotensive anesthesia are, cerebrovascular disease, cardiovascular diseases (MI, HT, and Aortic stenosis), renal dysfunction, increased ICP, pregnancy, severe pulmonary disease, and severe hypovolemia.

The risk hypotensive anesthesia is inadequate tissue perfusion of vital organs, when the patient is not appropriately selected or the MAP drops below the accepted limit.

The present study was in line with the following studies:

Amin et al., concluded that, both dexmedetomidine and esmolol are safe and effective in inducing controlled hypotension which decrease the surgical area bleeding score and provide ideal surgical condition in children undergoing cochlear implant surgery under general anesthesia [11]. Shams et al. reported that, both dexmedetomidine and esmolol were used in patients undergoing FESS and it was found to be safe agents for inducing controlled hypotension and effective in providing better surgical field. Dexmedetomidine has advantage as analgesic, sedative and decrease the anesthetic requirements [12].

Erbesler et al. compared the effects of esmolol and dexmedetomidine for the controlled hypotensive anesthesia and found that the groups were comparable as regards to hemodynamics, quality of surgical field and surgeon satisfaction. Dexmedetomidine was associated with a prolonged time of muscle relaxant, however esmolol was associated with higher costs [13].

Both esmolol and dexmedetomidine, was used in previous study and proved to be effective and safe method to reduce the intraoperative blood loss in patients undergoing scoliosis surgery [14].

Dexmedetomidine was evaluated in patients underwent FESS with either conscious sedation or local anesthesia and found to be effective in inducing dry surgical field with hemodynamic stability and reduce the postoperative analgesic use [15,16].

Dexmedetomidine is a highly specific and selective alpha-2-adrenergic agonist with sedative, anxiolytic, and organ protective effects. The clinical applications of dexmedetomidine in children include premedication, prevention of emergence delirium, as part of multimodal anesthetic regimen and sedation in the pediatric intensive care unit [17].

Dexmedetomidine is a highly specific α_2 agonist with anesthetic, analgesic, and sympatholytic properties [18-20]. The sympatholytic effect is associated with decreases in arterial blood pressure, heart rate, and noradrenaline secretion. So, dexmedetomidine can prevent perioperative rise in arterial blood pressure and heart rate [21,22].

The probable mechanism by which the dexmedetomidine reduce blood pressure is due to stimulation of peripheral alpha 2 adrenoceptors of vascular smooth muscle and inhibition of central sympathetic out flow this results in decrease in blood pressure and heart rate.

Dexmedetomidine was found to be a useful and effective adjuvant to minimize bleeding and induce dry surgical field in both ear and nasal surgery [23-28].

Tobias et al. found that, Dexmedetomidine was proved to be an effective agent used alone without need for beta blockers for controlled hypotensive anesthesia during anterior spinal fusion [29].

Ülger et al. concluded that dexmedetomidine was found to be better in maintaining hemodynamic stability, dry surgical field without reflex tachycardia or rebound hypertension. Liver and renal functions were not affected by dexmedetomidine [30].

Surgical bleeding can result from cut in capillary so; the amount of blood loss will depend on blood flow in the capillary bed. The blood loss results from the arterial injury depend on MABP. Venous blood loss will be dependent on venous return and venous tone [5].

Esmolol is an ultra-short acting intravenous cardioselective beta-antagonist. It has an extremely short elimination half-life (mean:9 minutes; range 4-16minutes) and a total body clearance approaching 3 times of cardiac output and 14 times of hepatic blood flow [6].

The hypotensive anesthesia induced with beta blocker results in increase in the sympathetic tone due to increase norepinephrine release, enhance endocrinal and metabolic responses, which leads to vasoconstriction of arterioles and precapillary sphincters that result from unopposed alpha-adrenergic effects. Beta blockers decrease CO and therefore decrease the blood flow to the tissue. So, beta blocker would be appropriate for decreasing the bleeding which result from capillary injury [31-35].

The time to first analgesic requirements was shorter in esmolol group and amount of analgesic requirements were less in dexmedetomidine group. Pain score was significantly better in dexmedetomidine group. Also, dexmedetomidine decreased the need for pain medication in the PACU.

In line with our result, El Saied et al. reported that dexmedetomidine infusion in pediatric patients allowed rapid recovery from anesthesia and reduced need for analgesic requirements in the postoperative period [36].

Moreover, Feld et al. [37] found that dexmedetomidine provided good postoperative analgesia and decreasing the need of morphine consumption postoperatively.

Also, Ibraheim et al. found that dexmedetomidine was significantly reduces fentanyl consumption when compared to the esmolol and control groups [38].

In addition, Unlugenc et al. found that dexmedetomidine (1 µg/kg) given 10 min before induction of anesthesia significantly decreases postoperative morphine requirements without effect on recovery time [39].

Additionally, dexmedetomidine significantly reduces the requirements for rescue sedation by 80% and analgesia by 50% in

postoperative patients for up to 24 h. Its sedative properties differ from other sedative drugs as patients being more easily arousal without respiratory depression [40].

Also, Gurbet et al. reported that, continuous dexmedetomidine infusion during abdominal surgery associated with effective postoperative analgesia, and decreases postoperative opioids consumption without increasing the adverse effects [41].

Moreover, Amin et al. concluded that, dexmedetomidine decrease postoperative opioid consumption in children undergoing cochlear implant surgery when compared to patients received esmolol [11].

Our study demonstrated that, both renal and liver functions were not affected by hypotensive anesthesia or drugs used for inducing controlled hypotension.

Our result in agreement with Ulger et al. who reported that, both liver and renal functions were not affected by dexmedetomidine [30].

Also Ozcan et al. reported that, there were no significant differences between AST, ALT, blood urea and creatinine values before surgery, and in postoperatively [29].

Our study found no significant difference between both groups as regard postoperative nausea and vomiting.

However, previous studies [42,43] reported that, the incidence of postoperative nausea and vomiting was less in children receiving dexmedetomidine in comparison with those receiving fentanyl during extracorporeal shock wave lithotripsy. This could explained by that fentanyl may the cause of increased in the incidence of PONV.

the present study has some limitations include the following: we didn't use control group because it is not ethically to expose the patients to unnecessary bleeding, the amount of blood loss not measured, subjective scale was used by surgeon to assess the quality of surgical field, and we did not measure the depth of anesthesia. Further study was needed to compare the dexmedetomidine with other agent used for controlled hypotensive anesthesia in children.

Conclusion

Our study demonstrated that both dexmedetomidine and esmolol are safe and effective agents for inducing controlled hypotension and both drugs are effective in optimizing surgical condition and induce dry surgical field allow better visualization, and reduce operative time in pediatric patients undergoing nasal surgery with no reported complications. Dexmedetomidine offers the advantage over esmolol it prolongs postoperative analgesia and decrease the opioid used postoperatively.

References

1. Maniglia AJ (1991) Fatal and other major complications of endoscopic sinus surgery. Laryngoscope 101: 349-354.

2. Lindop MJ (1975) Complications and morbidity of controlled hypotension. Br J Anaesth 47: 799-803.

3. Degoute CS, Ray MJ, Manchon M, Dubreuil C, Banssillon V (2001) Remifentanil and controlled hypotension; comparison with nitroprusside or esmolol during tympanoplasty. Can J Anaesth 48: 20-27.

4. Ragab SM, Hassanin MZ (2010) Optimizing the surgical field in pediatric functional endoscopic sinus surgery: A new evidence-based approach. Otolaryngol Head and Neck Surg 142: 48-54.

5. Degoute CS (2007) Controlled hypotension: a guide to drug choice. Drugs 67: 1053-1076.

6. Wiest D1 (1995) Esmolol. A review of its therapeutic efficacy and pharmacokinetic characteristics. Clin Pharmacokinet 28: 190-202.

7. Coughlan MG, Lee JG, Bosnjak ZJ, Schmeling WT, Kampine JP, et al. (1992) Direct coronary and cerebral vascular responses to dexmedetomidine. Significance of endogenous nitric oxide synthesis. Anesthesiology 77: 998-1006.

8. Fromme GA, MacKenzie RA, Gould AB Jr, Lund BA, Offord KP (1986) Controlled hypotension for orthognathic surgery. Anesth Analg 65: 683-686.

9. Merkel SI, Voepel-Lewis T, Shayevitz JR, Malviya S (1997) The FLACC: a behavioral scale for scoring postoperative pain in young children. Pediatr Nurs 23: 293-297.

10. Brown TC (2012) Early experiences of vasodilators and hypotensive anesthesia in children. Paediatr Anaesth 22: 720-722.

11. Amin SM, Elmawy MGE (2016) Optimizing surgical field during cochlear implant surgery in children: Dexmedetomidine versus Esmolol, Egypt J Anaesth.

12. Shams T, El Bahnasawe NS, Abu-Samra M, El-Masry R (2013) Induced hypotension for functional endoscopic sinus surgery: A comparative study of dexmedetomidine versus esmolol. Saudi J Anaesth 7: 175-180.

13. Erbesler ZA, Bakan N, Karaören GY, Erkmen MA (2013) A Comparison of the Effects of Esmolol and Dexmedetomidine on the Clinical Course and Cost for Controlled Hypotensive Anaesthesia. Turk J Anaesthesiol Reanim 41: 156-161.

14. Ibraheim OA, Abdulmonem A, Baaj J, Zahrani TA, Arlet V (2013) Esmolol versus dexmedetomidine in scoliosis surgery: study on intraoperative blood loss and hemodynamic changes. Middle East J Anaesthesiol 22: 27-33.

15. Guven DG, Demiraran Y, Sezen G, Kepek O, Iskender A (2011) Evaluation of outcomes in patients given dexmedetomidine in functional endoscopic sinus surgery. Ann Otol Rhinol Laryngol 120: 586-592.

16. Goksu S, Arik H, Demiryurek S, Mumbuc S, Oner U, et al. (2008) Effects of dexmedetomidine infusion in patients undergoing functional endoscopic sinus surgery under local anaesthesia. Eur J Anaesthiol 25: 22-28.

17. Yuen VM (2010) Dexmedetomidine: perioperative applications in children. Paediatr Anaesth 20: 256-264.

18. Bloor BC, Ward DS, Belleville JP, Maze M (1992) Effects of intravenous dexmedetomidine in humans. II. Hemodynamic changes. Anesthesiology 77: 1134-1142.

19. Belleville JP, Ward DS, Bloor BC, Maze M (1992) Effects of intravenous dexmedetomidine in humans. I. Sedation, ventilation, and metabolic rate. Anesthesiology 77: 1125-1133.

20. Aho M, Lehtinen AM, Erkola O, Kallio A, Korttila K (1991) The effect of intravenously administered dexmedetomidine on perioperative hemodynamics and isoflurane requirements in patients undergoing abdominal hysterectomy. Anesthesiology 74: 997-1002.

21. Flacke JW, Bloor BC, Flacke WE, Wong D, Dazza S, et al. (1987) Reduced narcotic requirement by clonidine with improved hemodynamic and adrenergic stability in patients undergoing coronary bypass surgery. Anesthesiology 67: 11-19.

22. Roizen MF (1988) Should we all have a sympathectomy at birth? Or at least preoperatively? Anesthesiology 68: 482-484.

23. Durmus M, But AK, Dogan Z, Yucel A, Miman MC, et al. (2007) Effect of dexmedetomidine on bleeding during tympanoplasty or septorhinoplasty. Eur J Anaesthiol 24: 447-453.

24. Dikmen B, Sahin F, Ornek D, Pala Y, Kilci O, et al. (2010) Dexmedetomidine for Controlled Hypotension In Middle Ear Surgery with Low-Flow Anesthesia. J Int Adv Otol 6: 331-336.

25. Nasreen F, Bano S, Khan RM, Hasan SA (2009) Dexmedetomidine used to provide hypotensive anesthesia during middle ear surgery. Indian J Otolaryngol Head Neck Surg 61: 205-207.

26. Chiruvella S, Donthu B, Venkata Siva J, Dora Babu S (2013) Controlled hypotensive anesthesia with dexmedetomidine for functional endoscopic sinus surgery: A randomized double blind study. J of Evolution of Med and Dent Sci 3: 9956-9563.

27. Lee J, Kim Y, Park C, Jeon Y, Kim D, et al. (2013) Comparison between dexmedetomidine and remifentanil for controlled hypotension and recovery in endoscopic sinus surgery. Ann Otol Rhinol Laryngol 122: 421-426.

28. Ozcan AA, Ozyurt Y, Saracoglu A, Erkal H, Suslu H, et al. (2012) Dexmedetomidine versus Remifentanil for Controlled Hypotensive Anesthesia in Functional Endoscopic Sinus Surgery. Turk J Anesth Reanim 40: 257-261.

29. Tobias JD, Berkenbosch JW (2002) Initial experience with dexmedetomidine in paediatric-aged patients. Paediatr Anaesth 12: 171-175.

30. Ulger MH, Demirbilek S, Köroglu A, Borazan H, Ersoy MO (2004) Controlled Hypotension with Dexmedetomidine for Middle Ear Surgery Inonu University Medical Faculty Journal 11: 237-241.

31. Dietrich GV, Heesen M, Boldt J, Hempelmann G (1996) Platelet function and adrenoceptors during and after induced hypotension using nitroprusside. Anesthesiology 85: 1334-1340.

32. Blau WS, Kafer ER, Anderson JA (1992) Esmolol is more effective than sodium nitroprusside in reducing blood loss during orthognathic surgery. Anesth Analg 75: 172-178.

33. Degoute CS, Dubreuil C, Ray MJ, Guitton J, Manchon M, et al. (1994) Effects of posture, hypotension and locally applied vasoconstriction on the middle ear microcirculation in anaesthetized humans. Eur J Appl Physiol Occup Physiol 69: 414-420.

34. Boezaart AP, Van der Merwe J, Coetzee A (1995) Comparison of sodium nitroprusside and esmolol-induced controlled hypotension for functional endoscopic sinus surgery. Can J Anaesth 42: 373-376.

35. Lim YJ, Kim CS, Bahk JH, Ham BM, Do SH (2003) Clinical trial of esmolol-induced controlled hypotension with or without acute normovolemic hemodilution in spinal surgery. Acta Anaesthesiol Scand 47: 74-78.

36. El Saied MH, Mohamed NN, Mohamed HM, Amin MI (2015) Dexmedetomidine versus fentanyl in anesthesia of cochlear implantation in pediatric patients. Egypt J Anaesth.

37. Feld JM, Hoffman WE, Stechert MM, Hoffman IW, Ananda RC (2006) Fentanyl or dexmedetomidine combined with desflurane for bariatric surgery. J Clin Anesth 18: 24-28.

38. Ibraheim OA, Abdulmonem A, Baaj J, Zahrani TA, Arlet V (2013) Esmolol versus dexmedetomidine in scoliosis surgery: study on intraoperative blood loss and hemodynamic changes. Middle East J Anaesthiol 22: 27-33.

39. Unlugenc H, Gunduz M, Guler T, Yagmur O, Isik G (2005) The effect of pre-anaesthetic administration of intravenous dexmedetomidine on postoperative pain in patients receiving patient-controlled morphine. Eur J Anaesthiol 22: 386-391.

40. Venn RM, Bradshaw CJ, Spencer R, Brealey D, Caudwell E, et al. (1999) Preliminary UK experience of dexmedetomidine, a novel agent for postoperative sedation in the intensive care unit. Anaesthesia 54: 1136-1142.

41. Gurbet A1, Basagan-Mogol E, Turker G, Ugun F, Kaya FN, et al. (2006) Intraoperative infusion of dexmedetomidine reduces perioperative analgesic requirements. Can J Anaesth 53: 646-652.

42. Ali A, El Ghoneimy M (2010) Dexmedetomidine versus fentanyl as adjuvant to propofol: comparative study in children undergoing extracorporeal shock wave lithotripsy. Euro J Anesthiol 27: 1058-1064.

43. Turgut N, Turkmen A, Gökkaya S, Altan A, Hatiboglu MA (2008) Dexmedetomidine based versus fentanyl-based total intravenous anesthesia for lumber laminectomy. Minerva Anesthesiol 74: 469-474.

14

Determination of the Effects of Sevoflurane Anesthesia in Different Maturing Stages of the Mouse Hippocampus by Transcriptome Analysis

Tomo Hayase*, **Shunsuke Tachibana and Michiaki Yamakage**

Department of Anesthesiology, Sapporo Medical University School of Medicine, Sapporo, Japan

***Corresponding author:** Tomo Hayase, Department of Anesthesiology, Sapporo Medical University School of Medicine, S 1, W 16, Chuo-ku, Sapporo 060-8543, Japan, E-mail: hayash@me.com

Abstract

Purpose: Postoperative cognitive dysfunction (POCD) is a serious complication after general anesthesia. POCD is more likely to occur in elderly patients, but the mechanism of POCD has not been fully elucidated. We hypothesized that the difference of mRNA expression profile in the brain depending on the maturing stage causes the difference in the effect of sevoflurane anesthesia. We investigated the mRNA expression profile of hippocampal cells in young mice and in aged mice under sevoflurane anesthesia using transcriptome analysis.

Methods: This study was conducted after approval from our institutional animal ethics committee, the Animal Research Center of Sapporo Medical University School of Medicine (project number: 12-033). Eight mice were assigned to two groups: a young group and an aged group. Each of the 4 mice in the two groups was anesthetized with 3.5% sevoflurane for 1 hour. Subsequently, mRNA was isolated from hippocampal cells and RNA sequencing was performed on an Illumina HiSeq 2500 platform. Mapping of the quality-controlled, filter paired-end reads to mouse genomes and quantification of the expression level of each gene were performed using R software.

Results: The *Lhx9* gene, which is thought to be associated with neuronal inflammation, was the most highly up-regulated gene in aged mice. The *Epyc* gene, which encodes a protein related to the phospholipase-C pathway and ERK signaling, was the most down-regulated gene in aged mice.

Conclusions: The findings suggest that sevoflurane anesthesia induces neuronal inflammation *via* a LIM-homeodomain family related gene in aged mice and causes POCD.

Keywords: Transcriptome analysis; Hippocampus; Postoperative cognitive dysfunction

Introduction

Postoperative cognitive dysfunction (POCD) is a frequent and serious complication after general anesthesia [1]. POCD is known to have a negative impact on the quality of life in affected patients [2]. Despite the high prevalence of POCD, the mechanism of POCD has not been fully elucidated. Recent studies have revealed that clinical risk factors of POCD are frontal cortex function, lifestyle, medication, and age [3-6]. General anesthesia might cause neuroinflammation in the developing brain [7], but it is difficult to determine cognitive changes caused by the anesthetic agent *per se*. POCD is usually transient, and it is difficult to establish clear diagnostic criteria for POCD [1,8]. Elucidation of the biological mechanism of POCD would be useful for improving the diagnosis and prevention of POCD. It is known that the requirement of volatile anesthetics is decreased with advance of age [9]. This suggests that volatile anesthetic agents cause different biological changes depending on the brain maturing stage.

We previously reported that exposure to sevoflurane changes mRNA profile in the juvenile mouse hippocampus by transcriptome analysis. In the juvenile mouse, the *Lhx9* gene was highly down-regulated by sevoflurane exposure, while the *Rtn4rl2* gene was highly up-regulated [10]. The *Lhx9* gene encodes a LIM-homeodomain factor,

which is essential for the development of thalamic neurons [11]. The *Rtn4rl2* gene encodes the Nogo receptor, which is involved in the adhesion of dendritic cells to myelin in the central nervous system [12]. These findings suggest that sevoflurane anesthesia induces neuroinflammation in juvenile mice, but data for aged mice have not been shown. Surgical stress induces systemic inflammation and increases levels of cytokines such as TNF-alpha. After transition of inflammatory cytokines to the blood-brain barrier, they activate glial cells, which cause neuroinflammation. Cholinergic neurons alter the activation of glial cells, but the alteration is affected by aging. Subsequently, the aging of cholinergic neurons is thought to be a potential biological mechanism of POCD and the reason why POCD is likely to occur in elderly patients [13].

Is general anesthesia itself harmful for the aged brain? [13] Is the anesthetic agent itself likely to cause neuroinflammation in the aged brain? Alternatively, the anesthetic agent might activate unknown pathways that lead to the occurrence of POCD. We hypothesized that the change in the mRNA expression profile in aged mice after sevoflurane exposure is different from that in juvenile mice, especially in the hippocampus, which integrates memory and cognitive function [14]. Recent progress in genomics has enable us to comprehensively analyze cellular modifications at the gene expression level using transcriptome analysis. The DNA microarray technique has uncovered various mechanisms of diseases; however, there has been no investigation of the association between POCD and the hippocampus by a transcriptome-wide association study.

In this study, the mRNA expression profiles of hippocampal cells in juvenile mice and in aged mice under sevoflurane anesthesia were investigated by using transcriptome analysis.

Materials and Methods

With approval from the Sapporo Medical University School of Medicine animal ethics committee (project number: 12-033) for this study, male C57/BL6 mice (8 weeks old, body weight of 20-25 g) were purchased from Japan SLC, Inc. (Hamamatsu, Japan) and housed at 22°C under controlled lighting (12:12-hour light/dark cycle) with food and water provided ad libitum. Eight male mice were assigned to two groups: a young group (8 weeks of age, n=4) and an aged group (35 weeks of age, n=4). In both groups, 3.5% sevoflurane (Maruishi Co., Ltd. Shizuoka, Japan) in 100% oxygen was provided to mice in a plastic chamber for 1 hour.

Then the mice were decapitated after being anesthetized with 3.5% sevoflurane. The brain of each mouse was immediately removed from the skull, frozen at -70°C with 2-methylbutane, and placed in a Petri dish containing ice-cold phosphate-buffered saline. The brain was cut along the longitudinal fissure of the cerebrum, and the regions posterior to the lambda were cut off using tissue matrices (Brain Matrices, EM Japan, Tokyo, Japan). Thereafter, the brain was placed with the cortex of the left hemisphere facing down and any non-cortical forebrain tissue was removed. Tissue blocks containing hippocampal cells were obtained using Brain Matrices (EM Japan). Meningeal tissue was removed from the hemisphere according to a previously described method [15]. Finally, dissected hippocampal cells were homogenized and lysed into six samples for each mouse using the RNeasy® Plus Micro Kit (Qiagen, Hilden, Germany) and QIAcube (Qiagen). Quality control for isolated RNA was performed using the Agilent 2200 TapeStation system (Agilent Technologies, Santa Clara, CA, USA). For samples to pass the initial quality control step, it was necessary to quantify >1 μg of sample and to have an equivalent RNA integrity number (eRIN) of ≥ 8. The eRIN determined by a 2500 Bioanalyzer Instruments (Agilent Technologies) has been reported to provide accurate information [16]. Isolated RNA was then pooled into two samples per group and labeled. A cDNA library was prepared using TruSeq® RNA Library Prep Kits (Illumina, Inc., San Diego, CA, USA) according to the manufacturer's instructions. RNA-seq was performed in the paired-end (101 cycles × 2) mode on an Illumina HiSeq 2500 platform (Illumina, Inc.).

Base call (.bcl) files for each cycle of sequencing were generated by Illumina Real Time Analysis software (Illumina, Inc.) and were analyzed primarily and de-multiplexed into a FASTQ (.fastq) file using Illumina's BCL2FASTQ conversion software (ver. 1.8.4, Illumina, Inc.). Raw paired-end RNA-seq reads in FASTQ formats were assessed for base call quality, cycle uniformity, and contamination using FastQC (http://www.bioinformatics.bbsrc.ad.uk/projects/fastqc/). Mapping of the quality control-filtered paired-end reads to mouse genomes and quantification of the expression level of each gene were performed using R software (ver. 3.1.1 with TCC package) [17,18]. The quality control-filtered paired-end reads were mapped to public mouse genome data published by UCSC (NCBI37/mm9, http://genomes.UCSC.edu/). Differential gene sets were filtered to remove those with fold changes <1.5 (up- or down-regulated) and with a false discovery rate-corrected P value of 0.05. Sample size was calculated with the following parameters: power ≥ 0.8, probability level <0.05, and anticipated effect size=14.

Results

All total RNA samples had a quality ≥ 1 μg and eRIN value ≥ 8. The average base calls after primary filtration were 41,778,221 base pairs, and the average mean quality score (Phred quality score) was 37.1. We investigated changes in expression levels of a total of 37,681 genes (Supplementary Table 1). A total of 7,716 genes were filtered because they showed little change in mRNA expression levels. Microarray plotting showed a total of 7,027 genes that were expressed differentially between the maturing stages. The *Lhx9* gene was the most highly up-regulated in aged mice (Table 1). The *Htr5b* gene, which encodes the serotonin receptor, the *Cbln3* gene, which encodes cerebellin 3 precursor protein, and the *Gabra6* gene, which encodes the gamma amino butyric acid type A (GABAA) receptor alpha 6 subunits, were highly up-regulated in aged mice (log2 ratios being 7.48, 7.33, and 6.27, respectively). The *Epyc* gene was the most down-regulated gene in aged mice (Table 2). The *Oprd1* gene, which encodes the delta opioid receptor, the *Drd1a* gene, which encodes dopamine receptor D1A, and the *Adora2a* gene, which encodes adenosine A2a receptor were highly down-regulated in aged mice (log2 ratios being 7.64, 5.54, and 5.52, respectively).

Gene name	Gene description	Log2 ratio
Lhx9	LIM homeobox protein 9	9.21
Pou4f1	POU domain, class 4, transcription factor 1	8.72
Htr5b	5-hydroxytryptamine (serotonin) receptor 5B	7.48
4631426E05Rik	RIKEN cDNA 4631426E05 gene	7.44
Cbln3	Cerebellin 3 precursor protein	7.33
Gpr151	G protein-coupled receptor 151	7.08
Irx3	Iroquois related homeobox 3 (Drosophila)	6.84
Umodl1	Uromodulin-like 1	6.72
Slc5a1	Solute carrier family 5 (sodium/glucose cotransporter), member 1	6.71

Irx2	Iroquois related homeobox 2 (Drosophila)	6.48
Iyd	Iodotyrosine deiodinase	6.41
Nrk	Nik related kinase	6.36
Hes3	Hairy and enhancer of split 3 (Drosophila)	6.35
Gabra6	Gamma-aminobutyric acid (GABA-A) receptor, subunit alpha 6	6.27
Bcl2l15	Bcl2-like 15	6.2
Gsbs	G substrate	6.13
Ntng1	Netrin G1	6.1
OTTMUSG00000003311	Predicted gene, OTTMUSG00000003311	5.97
Irx1	Iroquois related homeobox 1 (Drosophila)	5.96
Tyrp1	Tyrosinase-related protein 1	5.94
Lhfpl1	Lipoma HMGIC fusion partner-like 1	5.94
Gm941	Gene model 941, (NCBI)	5.89
Gtf2a1l	General transcription factor IIA, 1-like	5.88
Vsig8	V-set and immunoglobulin domain containing 8	5.69
Ldlrad2	Low density lipoprotein receptor A domain containing 2	5.64
Epb4.2	Erythrocyte protein band 4.2	5.61
Cnn1	Calponin 1	5.58
Epha1	Eph receptor A1	5.57
Tmem182	Transmembrane protein 182	5.56
4933436C20Rik	RIKEN cDNA 4933436C20 gene	5.53
Barhl2	BarH-like 2 (Drosophila)	5.52
EG667705	Predicted gene, EG667705	5.47
Avil	Advillin	5.4
Gpx2	Glutathione peroxidase 2	5.38
Aqp6	Aquaporin 6	5.38
Trim40	Tripartite motif-containing 40	5.33
Irx5	Iroquois related homeobox 5 (Drosophila)	5.31
Slc43a3	Solute carrier family 43, member 3	5.3
Wnt9b	Wingless-type MMTV integration site 9B	5.25
Ptprq	Protein tyrosine phosphatase, receptor type, Q	5.24
1700024G13Rik	RIKEN cDNA 1700024G13 gene	5.23
Slc17a6	Solute carrier family 17 (sodium-dependent inorganic phosphate cotransporter), member 6	5.14
Gabrr1	Gamma-aminobutyric acid (GABA-C) receptor, subunit rho 1	5.12
Adamts19	A disintegrin-like and metallopeptidase (reprolysin type) with thrombospondin type 1 motif, 19	5.12
Ramp3	Receptor (calcitonin) activity modifying protein 3	5.11

Neurog2	Neurogenin 2	5.09
Chrnb3	Cholinergic receptor, nicotinic, beta polypeptide 3	5.09
A530057A03Rik	RIKEN cDNA A530057A03 gene	5.08
Atp2a1	ATPase, Ca++ transporting, cardiac muscle, fast twitch 1	5.06
1810019J16Rik	RIKEN cDNA 1810019J16 gene	5.02
Rspo4	R-spondin family, member 4	5.01
Gucy2c	Guanylate cyclase 2c	5

Table 1: Genes those are highly up-regulated in aged mice.

Gene name	Gene description	Log2 ratio
Epyc	Epiphycan	-8.38
Oprd1	Opioid receptor, delta 1	-7.64
Sh3rf2	SH3 domain containing ring finger 2	-7.25
Clspn	Claspin homolog (Xenopus laevis)	-7.23
Dlx5	Distal-less homeobox 5	-6.89
Ovol2	Ovo-like 2 (Drosophila)	-6.86
Actn2	Actinin alpha 2	-6.43
Gm1337	Gene model 1337, (NCBI)	-6.3
3110039M20Rik	RIKEN cDNA 3110039M20 gene	-6.28
Cd4	CD4 antigen	-6.08
Krt9	Keratin 9	-5.99
Ankk1	Ankyrin repeat and kinase domain containing 1	-5.94
Nkx2-1	NK2 homeobox 1	-5.92
Bcl11b	B-cell leukemia/lymphoma 11B	-5.89
Nxph2	Neurexophilin 2	-5.86
Fgf3	Fibroblast growth factor 3	-5.64
Ucn3	Urocortin 3	-5.62
Drd1a	Dopamine receptor D1A	-5.54
Kcnv1	Potassium channel, subfamily V, member 1	-5.53
Tgm3	Transglutaminase 3, E polypeptide	-5.52
Adora2a	Adenosine A2a receptor	-5.52
Gucy2g	Guanylate cyclase 2g	-5.42
Hs3st2	Heparan sulfate (glucosamine) 3-O-sulfotransferase 2	-5.28
Gpr88	G-protein coupled receptor 88	-5.28
Rspo2	R-spondin 2 homolog (Xenopus laevis)	-5.27
Brs3	Bombesin-like receptor 3	-5.26

Indo	Indoleamine-pyrrole 2,3 dioxygenase	-5.25
Kcnj4	Potassium inwardly-rectifying channel, subfamily J, member 4	-5.22
Kcnh4	Potassium voltage-gated channel, subfamily H (eag-related), member 4	-5.21
Dlx6	Distal-less homeobox 6	-5.13
Tpsg1	Tryptase gamma 1	-5.11
Tbr1	T-box brain gene 1	-5.09
Arx	Aristaless related homeobox gene (Drosophila)	-5.09
Lhx6	LIM homeobox protein 6	-5.09
Ccdc88c	Coiled-coil domain containing 88C	-5.05
Serpina9	Serine (or cysteine) peptidase inhibitor, clade A (alpha-1 antiproteinase, antitrypsin), member 9	-5.03

Table 2: Genes that are highly down-regulated in aged mice.

Discussion

We first confirmed the quality of RNA samples for transcriptome analysis. The quality and amount of RNA samples are likely to vary depending on the type, state, and part of tissue, and it confirmation of the quality is an important requirement for transcriptome analysis [19]. Using a previously described method, we homogenized some of the hippocampal cells without any tissue fixation and freezing technique [15]. Consequently, we were able to obtain quality-controlled RNA samples in this study [20]. We investigated a total 37,681 genes using data published data by UCSC. A total of 18,814 genes showed very small average expression levels of mRNA, namely less than 1 count per sample, in the hippocampus of both juvenile and aged mice. In the remaining 18,867 genes, we found that a total of 7,027 genes were differentially expressed between the groups in this study. These data might support that the mRNA expression levels in hippocampus cells are different depending on the maturing stage and suggest mechanisms underlying the differences in efficacy of sevoflurane among maturing stages. Understandably, since a very large number of genes were expressed differently in the two groups, we could not identify the factor that critically alters the effect of sevoflurane in this study. Further study is needed to identify the factor that alters the effect of sevoflurane.

Next, we demonstrated that the *Lhx9* gene was the most up-regulated gene in aged mice. In our previous study, the *Lhx9* gene was found to be the most down-regulated gene in anesthetized juvenile mice, and we therefore could not determine whether the *Lhx9* gene was up-regulated in aged mice by sevoflurane *per se* [10]. However, the *Lhx9* gene showed divergent mRNA expression between juvenile and aged mice in the hippocampus. The *Lhx9* gene encodes a LIM-homeodomain factor that is essential for the development of gonads, spinal cord interneurons, and thalamic neurons [11,21,22]. In juvenile mice, sevoflurane might suppress brain development *via* LIM-homeodomain factors or compensate for the hyperexcitability of the thalamocortical network by suppressing LIM-homeodomain factors [23], while sevoflurane exposure might increase *Lhx9* gene expression or not change its expression. If it is assumed that expression of the *Lhx9* gene enhances neuroinflammation in the mouse hippocampus, sevoflurane might not induce neuroinflammation in aged mice or the neuroprotective mechanism might be vulnerable in aged mice. Expression of the *Lhx9* gene might contribute to the development of POCD, and this could be the focus of future research.

The *Htr5b* gene and the *Cbln3* gene were also highly up-regulated in aged mice in this study. Serotonin receptors encoded by the *Htr5b* gene are widely distributed in the central or peripheral nervous system and play a role in neurotransmission [24]. Serotonin antagonists are used as anti-emetic agents in chemotherapy induced emesis and postoperative nausea and vomiting. Our previous results also showed that serotonin receptor genes were not up-regulated by sevoflurane exposure in juvenile mice. These results might suggest that serotonin antagonists are more effective for postoperative nausea and vomiting in aged patients. The *Cbln3* gene is known as a protein-coding gene that accumulates at parallel fiber-Purkinje cell synapses, and the proteins provide an anatomical basis for a common signaling pathway regulating circuit development and synaptic plasticity in the cerebellum [25]. Assuming that the expression level of the *Cbln3* gene is increased because it acts protectively against neuroinflammation caused by sevoflurane, the juvenile brain might be more prone to neuroinflammation caused by sevoflurane. Therefore, further investigation is needed to determine whether the *Cbln3* gene has a protective effect in the hippocampus.

Notably, the *GABRA6* gene, which encodes GABAA receptor subunit alpha 6, was highly up-regulated in aged mice. The GABAA receptors increase tonic inhibition in somatostatin interneunons and alter circuit activity within the dentate gyrus [26]. GABAA receptors are also known to be a potential target of volatile anesthetics [27].

The *Epyc* gene was the most down-regulated gene in aged mice. The *Epyc* gene is located in the mapping interval of MYP3, which has been suggested to be a candidate gene for high myopia [28,29]. The EPYC protein is predominantly expressed in cartilage, and it is important for fibrillogenesis through the regulation of collagen fibrils [30,31]. It is unclear whether the *Epyc* gene is associated with the effect of sevoflurane. The *Oprd* gene, which encodes the delta-opioid receptor (OPRD), and the *Drd1a* gene, which encodes the dopamine receptor D1a, were also highly down-regulated in aged mice. The ghrelin, which is identified as the endogenous ligand for growth hormone secretagogue receptor 1 alpha, induces acute pain and increases OPRD-mRNA expression [32]. The serum growth hormone concentration in juvenile mice might be higher than that in aged mice and might cause the higher expression level of the *Oprd* gene in the brain. The methods used in this study might have been more harmful for juvenile mice than aged mice, or it is possible that juvenile mice are more likely to feel pain than aged mice. This result regarding the *Oprd* mRNA expressions suggest that juvenile mice should be treated without a painful sequence. Further investigation is needed to determine whether the treatment of mice affects the expression of the *Oprd* gene. The dopamine D1 receptor in the hippocampus is essential for the functional relationship between associative learning and synaptic strength at the CA3-CA1 synapse [33]. D1 receptor knock-out mice are known to have reduced spatial learning and fear learning. Sevoflurane *per se* might inhibit expression of the *Drd1a* gene in the hippocampus in aged mice and/or enhance expression of the *Drd1a* gene in juvenile mice. The juvenile mice showed more than 300 counts of *Drd1a*-mRNA per sample, while the aged mice showed less than 10 counts per sample in this study. Therefore, the difference between juvenile and aged mice in expression level of the *Drd1a* gene in the hippocampus suggests a difference in postoperative spatial cognitive function.

Interestingly, the *Adora2a* gene, which encodes adenosine A2a receptor, was also highly down-regulated in aged mice in this study. The adenosine modulation system mostly operates through inhibitory A1 receptors and facilitatory A2 receptors, and the adenosine receptors are mutually switching synaptic activities in the brain [34]. Brain insults up-regulate the adenosine A2a receptor through adaptive change of the brain, and adenosine A2a receptor bolsters neuronal plasticity. The *Adora2a* gene was reported to show an age-dependent decrease in the human hippocampus. In this study, the *Adora2a*-mRNA expression level was dramatically decreased in aged mice, whereas the published database showed that the mRNA expression level in the elderly human hippocampus was only half of that in the juvenile human [35]. This difference suggests that sevoflurane *per se* inhibits expression of the *Adora2a* gene in the hippocampus in aged mice, or the *Adora2a* gene expresses diversely among the animal species. The adenosine A2a receptor has been reported to be associated with caffeine-induced insomnia [36]. Down-regulation of the *Adora2a* gene might influence the excitation at emergence from general anesthesia and cause POCD in aged patients. Further study is needed to confirm the association between *Adora2a*-mRNA expression and POCD.

We could not determine whether the changes in mRNA expression levels of individual genes were caused by sevoflurane *per se* or other pathways. However, our results indicated that there was age-dependent variation in the mRNA expression profile. Although the molecular mechanisms of POCD after sevoflurane exposure were predicted in the present study, further experiments based on the regulation of individual genes are needed to confirm our speculations. Furthermore, we did not examine the behaviors of the animals that might suggest spatial learning, because the mRNA expression profile might change while recording their behavior. While our data cannot be directly extrapolated to humans, they might provide clues for the molecular mechanism of POCD. In addition, the sample size was small in this study, despite having been determined to obtain a power of ≥ 0.8, and we overlooked changes in the expression of genes that were expressed at low levels. Further studies with larger numbers of samples are needed to confirm the changes in genes that are expressed at low levels.

In conclusion, expression of the *Lhx9* gene, which is thought to be associated with neuronal inflammation, was the most highly up-regulated in aged mice. The *Epyc* gene, which encodes a protein related to the phospholipase-C pathway and ERK signaling, was the most down-regulated in aged mice. These findings may be useful for exploring the mechanisms of POCD and neuronal inflammation after general anesthesia.

Acknowledgements

This work was supported by a Grant-in-Aid for Young Scientists (B) (No.15K20050, 2015 – 2016, to T.H.) from the Ministry of Education, Culture, Sports, Science and Technology, Tokyo, Japan.

References

1. Rundshagen I (2014) Postoperative cognitive dysfunction. Dtsch Arztebl Int 111: 119-125.

2. Kastaun S, Gerriets T, Schwarz NP, Yeniguen M, Schoenburg M, et al. (2016) The Relevance of Postoperative Cognitive Decline in Daily Living: Results of a 1-Year Follow-up. J Cardiothorac Vasc Anesth 30: 297-303.

3. Kline RP, Pirraglia E, Cheng H, De Santi S, Li Y, et al. (2012) Surgery and brain atrophy in cognitively normal elderly subjects and subjects diagnosed with mild cognitive impairment. Anesthesiology 116: 603-612.

4. Zeki Al Hazzouri A, Haan MN, Kalbfleisch JD, Galea S, Lisabeth LD, et al. (2011) Life-Course Socioeconomic Position and Incidence of Dementia and Cognitive Impairment Without Dementia in Older Mexican Americans: Results From the Sacramento Area Latino Study on Aging. Am J Epidemiol 173: 1148-1158.

5. Feinkohl I, Winterer G, Spies CD, Pischon T (2017) Cognitive Reserve and the Risk of Postoperative Cognitive Dysfunction. Dtsch Arztebl Int 114: 110-117.

6. Wilder RT, Flick RP, Sprung J, Katusic SK, Barbaresi WJ, et al. (2009) Early exposure to anesthesia and learning disabilities in a population-based birth cohort. Anesthesiology 110: 796-804.

7. Shen X, Dong Y, Xu Z, Wang H, Miao C, et al. (2013) Selective anesthesia-induced neuroinflammation in developing mouse brain and cognitive impairment. Anesthesiology 118: 502-515.

8. Rasmussen LS, Larsen K, Houx P, Skovgaard LT, Hanning CD, et al. (2001) The assessment of postoperative cognitive function. Acta Anaesth Scand 45: 275-289.

9. Lerou JG (2004) Nomogram to estimate age-related MAC. Br J Anaesth 93: 288-291.

10. Hayase T, Tachibana S, Yamakage M (2016) Effect of sevoflurane anesthesia on the comprehensive mRNA expression profile of the mouse hippocampus. Med Gas Res 6: 70-76.

11. Failli V, Rogard M, Mattei MG, Vernier P, Rétaux S (2000) Lhx9 and Lhx9alpha LIM-homeodomain factors: genomic structure, expression patterns, chromosomal localization, and phylogenetic analysis. Genomics 64: 307-317.

12. McDonald CL, Steinbach K, Kern F, Schweigreiter R, Martin R, et al. (2011) Nogo receptor is involved in the adhesion of dendritic cells to myelin. J Neuroinflammation 8: 113.

13. Ramlawi B, Rudolph JL, Mieno S, Feng J, Boodhwani M, et al. (2006) C-Reactive protein and inflammatory response associated to neurocognitive decline following cardiac surgery. Surgery 140: 221-226.

14. Gol A, Kellaway P, Shapiro M, Hurst CM (1963) Studies of hippocampectomy in the monkey, baboon, and cat behavioral changes and a preliminary evaluation of cognitive function. Neulorogy 13: 1031-1041.

15. Beaudoin GM 3rd, Lee SH, Singh D, Yuan Y, Ng YG, et al. (2012) Culturing pyramidal neurons from the early postnatal mouse hippocampus and cortex. Nat Protoc 7: 1741-1754.

16. Fleige S, Pfaffl MW (2006) RNA integrity and the effect on the real-time qRT-PCR performance. Mol Aspects Med 27: 126-139.

17. Robinson MD, McCarthy DJ, Smyth GK (2010) edgeR: a Bioconductor package for differential expression analysis of digital gene expression data. Bioinformatics 26: 139-140.

18. Sun J, Nishiyama T, Shimizu K, Kadota K (2013) TCC: an R package for comparing tag count data with robust normalization strategies. BMC Bioinformatics 14: 219.

19. Gallego Romero I, Pai AA, Tung J, Gilad Y (2014) RNA-seq: impact of RNA degradation on transcript quantification. BMC Biol 12: 42.

20. Macmanes MD (2014) On the optimal trimming of high-throughput mRNA sequence data. Front Genet 5: 13.

21. Retaux S, Rogard M, Bach I, Failli V, Besson MJ (1999) Lhx9: a novel LIM-homeodomain gene expressed in the developing forebrain. J Neurosci 19: 783-793.

22. Birk OS, Casiano DE, Wassif CA, Cogliati T, Zhao L, et al. (2000) The LIM homeobox gene Lhx9 is essential for mouse gonad formation. Nature 403: 909-913.

23. DiGruccio MR, Joksimovic S, Joksovic PM, Lunardi N, Salajegheh R, et al. (2015) Hyperexcitability of rat thalamocortical networks after exposure to general anesthesia during brain development. J Neurosci 35: 1481-1492.

24. Thompson AJ, Lummis SC (2006) 5-HT3 receptors. Curr Pharm Des 12: 3615-3630.

25. Miura E, Matsuda K, Morgan JI, Yuzaki M, Watanabe M (2009) Cbln1 accumulates and colocalizes with Cbln3 and GluRdelta2 at parallel fiber-Purkinje cell synapses in the mouse cerebellum. Eur J Neurosci 29: 693-706.

26. Tong X, Peng Z, Zhang N, Cetina Y, Huang CS, et al. (2015) Ectopic Expression of α6 and δ GABAA Receptor Subunits in Hilar Somatostatin Neurons Increases Tonic Inhibition and Alters Network Activity in the Dentate Gyrus. J Neurosci 35: 16142-16158.

27. Wang X, Song ZG, Huang DX, Gao H, Wang Q, et al. (2016) A single nucleotide polymorphism in GABAA receptor isoforms is potentially responsible for isoflurane sensitivity in mice. Genet Mol Res 15.

28. Young TL, Ronan SM, Alvear AB, Wildenberg SC, Oetting WS, et al. (1998) A second locus for familial high myopia maps to chromosome 12q. Am J Hum Genet 63: 1419-1424.

29. Wang P, Li S, Xiao X, Guo X, Zhang Q (2009) An evaluation of OPTC and EPYC as candidate genes for high myopia. Mol Vis 15: 2045-2049.

30. Deere M, Dieguez JL, Yoon SJ, Hewett-Emmett D, de la Chapelle A, et al. (1999) Genomic characterization of human DSPG3. Genome Res 9: 449-456.

31. Kurita K, Shinomura T, Ujita M, Zako M, Kida D, et al. (1996) Occurrence of PG-Lb, a leucine-rich small chondroitin/dermatan sulphate proteoglycan in mammalian epiphyseal cartilage: molecular cloning and sequence analysis of the mouse cDNA. Biochem J 318: 909-914.

32. Liu FY, Zhang MM, Zeng P, Liu WW, Wang JL, et al. (2016) Study on the molecular mechanism of antinociception induced by ghrelin in acute pain in mice. Peptides 83: 1-7.

33. Ortiz O, Delgado-García JM, Espadas I, Bahí A, Trullas R, et al. (2010) Associative learning and CA3-CA1 synaptic plasticity are impaired in D1R null, Drd1a-/- mice and in hippocampal siRNA silenced Drd1a mice. J Neurosci 30: 12288-12300.

34. Cunha RA (2016) How does adenosine control neuronal dysfunction and neurodegeneration? J Neurochem 139: 1019-1055.

35. Kang HJ, Kawasawa YI, Cheng F, Zhu Y, Xu X, et al. (2011) Spatio-temporal transcriptome of the human brain. Nature 478: 483-489.

36. Byrne EM, Johnson J, McRae AF, Nyholt DR, Medland SE, et al. (2012) A genome-wide association study of caffeine-related sleep disturbance: confirmation of a role for a common variant in the adenosine receptor. Sleep 35: 967-975.

Dexamethasone as an Additive to Low Volume Interscalene Plexus Blockade: A Randomized Controlled Study

Andreas Liedler, Benedikt Sattler*, Ingo Zorn, Christian Fohringer, Sabine Ottenschlager, Herbert Steininger and Christoph Hormann

Department of Anesthesiology and Intensive Care Medicine, University Hospital St Polten, Austria

*Corresponding author: Benedikt Sattler, Department of Anesthesiology and Intensive Care Medicine, University Hospital St. Polten, Propst-Fuhrer-Straße 4, St Polten, Lower Austria, E-mail: benedikt.sattler@meduniwien.ac.at

Abstract

Background: Interscalene Blockade is widely used to ensure analgesia in surgery involving the shoulder. Both i.v. and perineural dexamethasone seem to be able to prolong the block duration and can therefore be used to reduce the use of analgesics.

However most of the studies focusing on dexamethasone as an additive use large volumes (20 ml) of local anesthetic agent.

Larger volumes may be associated with a higher rate of complications.

Therefore the hypothesis of this study is to prove whether dexamethasone is also able to prolong the pain free time when given together with a low volume (10 ml) of anesthetic agent.

Methods: The study was conducted as a prospective, double-blinded randomized trial. Patients with arthroscopic surgery of the shoulder were included in our study. The blockade was performed using ultrasound guidance to ensure a low rate of block failure. We used eight milligrams of dexamethasone (free of preservative) and ten millilitres of ropivacaine in a concentration of 0.75%. The primary endpoint was analgesic duration defined as the time between performance of the block and first analgesic request. The primary variable was analyzed using a log rank test. Secondary endpoints were the assessment of the pain at the surgical site ten hours after operation at rest and movement.

Results: 104 patients were included in our study. The ethics committee of Lower Austria approved the study and patients signed an informed consent in order to participate in our study. During the study five patients were excluded due to block failure. Using a log-rank test, we observed a prolongation of pain free time of 310 minutes.

The analysis of the NRS-score ten hours after surgery yielded a significant difference between the control and active group at rest. Unexpectedly the NRS – score at movement does not differ between the control and active group.

Conclusion: Dexamethasone used in a low volume plexus brachialis blockade is able to prolong the pain free time.

Keywords: Analgesia; Anaesthetics local; Brachial plexus; Dexamethasone; Postoperative; Regional

Introduction

The use of plexus blockades to reduce postoperative pain in shoulder surgery is very common [1]. Proper management of postoperative pain can reduce economic costs and allows earlier discharge of patients [2,3].

A single shot blockade does not last long enough to help patients over the first night after surgery without analgesics. Therefore continuous blockades have become more popular, but they have their limitations; like the potential risk of infections or catheter dislocation [4,5]. In our experience, management of such catheters in a daily setting is difficult and laborious. Regular checking is required to ensure proper functioning and analgesia. Furthermore, consistent with the literature, the rate of catheter dislocation is high. Prolongation of a peripheral block might provide sufficient analgesia in the first phase after surgery without the limitations of catheter application. A nerve block is also very efficient against pain induced hyperalgesia and pain related neuronal plasticity [6].

Many substances have been investigated to circumvent the problem of limited analgesia after single-shot blockade [7-11], among them the synthetic glucocorticoid dexamethasone. Dexamethasone has been shown to prolong the duration of an interscalene block [12-14].

However, most studies investigating dexamethasone used large volumes of local anesthetics at a low concentration [15-17].

We believe that the usage of lower volumes can decrease the incidence of adverse events. A lower volume does not spread as far as a high volume. Also the risk for systemic absorption is lower when using low volumes instead of high volumes.

Indeed, the incidence of phrenical nerve paresis and respiratory complications is reduced when using lower volumes [18,19]. Ultrasound guidance might further reduce the risk of adverse events [20]. Therefore one advantage of using lower volumes could lie in the lower rate of complications associated with interscalene plexus block.

Low volume blocks are well established for plexus block using the interscalene approach. We believe that low volume blocks are representing the current practice better than high volume blocks and therefore it is relevant to research the effects of dexamethasone on low volume blocks. Studies have proven that even volumes as low as 7 ml ensure proper plexus blockade.

Our hypothesis is that dexamethasone prolongs the analgesic effect of an interscalene plexus block when given with a low volume of local anesthetic agent.

Our primary endpoint was the analgesic duration defined as the time between performance of the block and first analgesic request.

Methods

The study was conducted as a prospective, controlled, randomized, double-blinded trial.

Participants

Participants (n=104) received either 8 mg dexamethasone (2 ml) with 10 ml (0.75%) ropivacaine (n=50) or 0.9% saline (2 ml) with 10 ml (0.75%) ropivacaine (n=49). The inclusion criteria for patients were the following: arthroscopy of the shoulder or repair of the rotatory cuff, Age>18 years and ASA I, II, III.

Exclusion criteria for patients included the following: patient is a fertile woman, opiates usage more than 30 mg oxycodon or equivalent a day, surgery involving bone structures, corticoid usage for more than 2 weeks in the past six months, Neuropathy or an injury of nerves in the upper limb, history of osteosynthesis or prosthesis. Fertile women were excluded from our study in order to spare expenses due to an otherwise needed pregnancy test.

The study protocol including off-label use of dexamethasone as an additive was approved by the Ethics committee of Lower Austria (GS4-EK-2/304-2013) and the local government and registered in the international registry for clinical trials (clinicaltrials.gov).

All participants were recruited at the University hospital of St. Polten, Austria and provided informed consent. We conducted a standardized anesthesia protocol. Patients received premedication of 3.5 to 7.5 mg midazolam.

The nerve block was performed either in a holding area or in the operating room. After the block was performed a general anesthesia was performed to optimize surgical conditions and to avoid patient's discomfort due to the beach chair position.

General anesthesia was performed using propofol 1.5 mg to 3 mg/kg, rocuronium 0.3 mg-0.5 mg/kg and fentanyl: 0.0075- 0.0125 mg/kg. After induction and airway management (endotracheal intubation), sevoflurane was used as maintenance anesthesia (MAC: 0.8-1).

The interscalene block was performed using ultrasound support with SonoSite Inc. M-Turbo devices. The probe used was an HFL38x (13-6 MhZ) linear probe. The tip of the needle was located at C6. Checking of local anesthetic spread over the anterior scalene muscle was not performed.

After performing nerve block, sensory discrimination between hot and cold and mobility of the shoulder was assessed. If the block failed the patient were excluded from the study. During surgery, vegetative reactions to incision were closely monitored. If any such reactions (increase of heart rate or blood pressure, sweating) occurred due to pain, the block was considered inefficient and the patient received additional analgesics (i.v.). If block failure occurred, the patient was excluded from the study.

Patients did not receive analgesics postoperatively unless demanded, ruling out bias due to use of analgesics. The time at which the patients demanded analgesia was documented. The primary endpoint was pain-free time after surgery, computed as the time point of request of drug be the patient subtracted by the time point of successful block.

Ten hours after nerve block, patients rated their pain at rest and movement on a numeric rating scale from zero to ten. This time point was chosen based on previous observations at our side concerning first analgesic request of patients. The standardized movement performed was abduction in the shoulder joint to a level of 45 degrees. Furthermore, possible side effects from the interscalene block were assessed. All variables were assessed by an anesthesiologist.

We decided to plan only one ward round, because further ward rounds would increase the overall overhead and the data they may be retrieve did not influence our primary endpoint. We tried to research a mean prolongation of the pain free time of two hours compared with the saline group considering a standard deviation of six hours.

Sample size was calculated using a standard deviation of 6 hours, a mean time of 10 hours prior to first analgesic request and a standardized effect size of 2 hours. The data needed to calculate the sample size was collected from observations of blocks performed prior to the trial and review of the data in literature [12,21].

The calculated sample size for our trial was 104 patients (assuming a block failure rate of 7%). The randomization sequence was created with the tool randomiser developed by the department of statistics at the University of Graz, Austria.

Patients were randomized at a block size of ten. Randomization lists were created by the dispensary of the hospital, making unblinding by the assessing anesthesiologist impossible. Randomization and production of the local anesthetics solution was performed by the dispensary, so all doctors and patients were unaware of the drug given. After inclusion the patient received an insurance contract and given an appointment for surgery.

The primary outcome was analyzed using the log rank test, with the assumption that the Kaplan-Meier curves would not intersect. Secondary outcome variables were analyzed using Mann-Whitney U test. Calculations were performed with SPSS [22]. Whiskers of box plots represents minimum and maximum NRS scores.

Results

Between March 2014 and April 2015, 104 patients were enrolled. Five patients were excluded due to failure of nerve block, resulting in an effective sample size of 99 patients (Figure 1). Table 1 provides baseline characteristics of the patients.

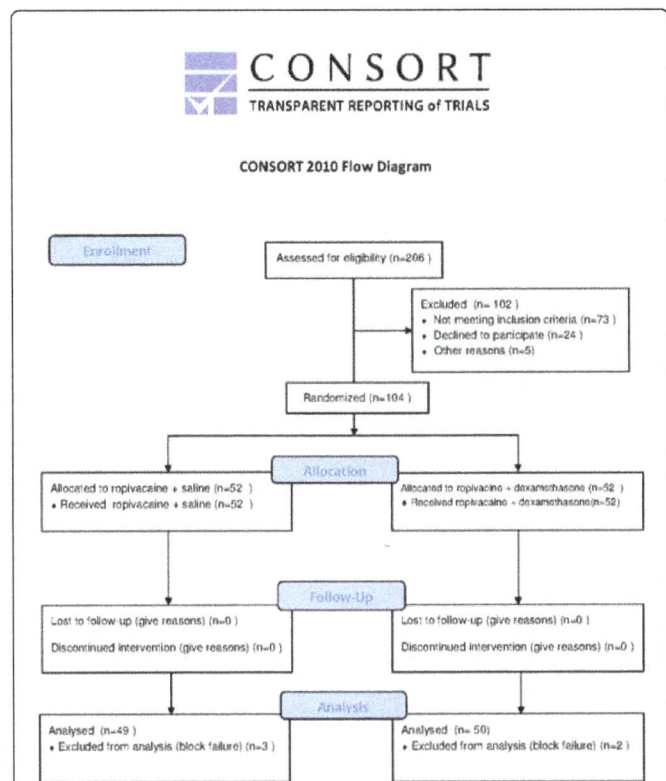

Figure 1: Patient flow through the study; provides an overview over the patient flow through our study. The figure adheres to the consort standard.

	Control (n=49)	Active Group (n=50)
Age mean (SD)	53.46 (SD:12.08)	49.7 (SD:15.53)
BMI mean (SD)	29.78 (SD:6.45)	27.06 (SD:4.38)
Sex (n)	Female:13, Male:36	Female:39, Male:11
Surgery duration (SD) minutes	75.94 (SD:44.83)	79.52 (SD:37.31)
ASA (n)	I:37,II:11,III:1	I:38,II:11,III:1
Type of surgical procedures performed (all athroscopical)		
Plain arthroscopy (n)	11	10
Arthroscopicrotatory cuff reconstruction (n)	18	22
Arthroscopic decompression (n)	18	13
Arthroscopic labrumrefixation (n)	2	5

Table 1: An overview about the descriptive data collected during the study.

Primary outcome

Mean pain-free time in the control group was 656.14 min with a standard error of 50.17 min. In contrast, in the active group, mean pain-free time was 966.80 min with a standard error of 60.30 min, resulting in a prolongation of pain-free time of 310.66 min by dexamethasone (p<0.001, Figure 2).

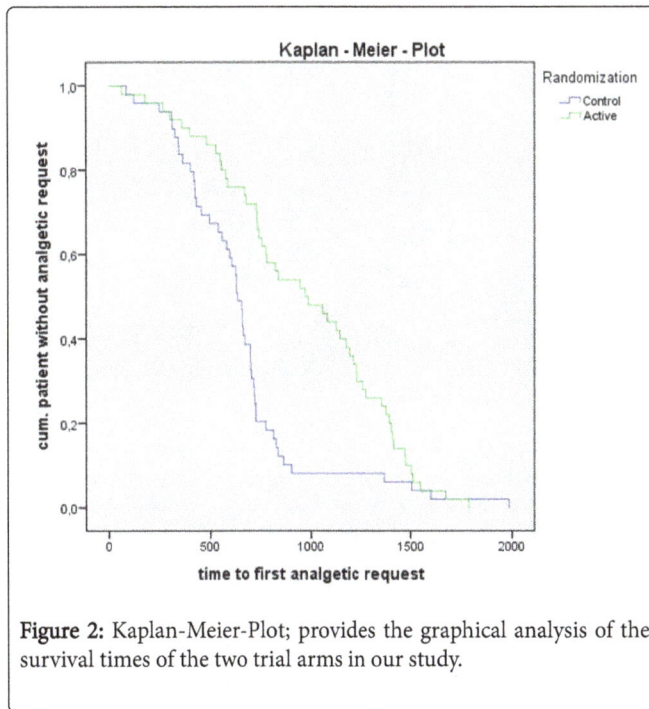

Figure 2: Kaplan-Meier-Plot; provides the graphical analysis of the survival times of the two trial arms in our study.

Therefore our trial showed that dexamethasone is able to prolong the pain-free time of the patients to around 310.66 minutes.

Post-hoc analyses were performed to assess the influence of gender, weight and age on primary outcome. We did not observe any correlations between these variables and pain-free time. Figure 2 shows the kaplan-meier plot for the control and the active group.

Secondary outcome

In the active group, the NRS score at rest after ten hours was significantly lower compared to the control group (p=0.016, Table 2 and Figure 3), whereas no difference of NRS score at movement was observed (p=0.451, Table 2 and Figure 4).

Group	NRS-Score-Type	Mean, minimum, maximum, range
Active	NRS at rest	1.88, 0, 8, 8
Active	NRS at movement	2.44, 0, 8, 8
Control	NRS at rest	2.98, 0,10,10
Control	NRS at movement	3.51, 0, 8, 8

Table 2: An overview about mean, minimum, maximum and range of the NRS-scores at rest and movement.

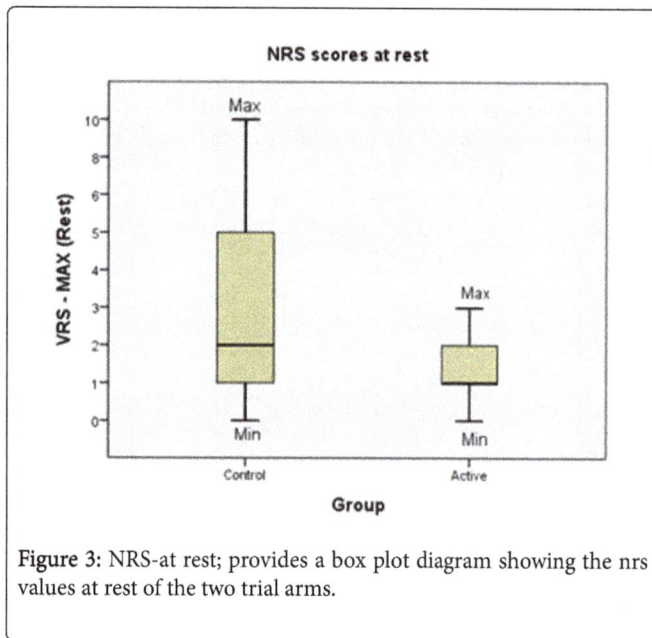

Figure 3: NRS-at rest; provides a box plot diagram showing the nrs values at rest of the two trial arms.

Concerning incidence of adverse events, no differences between groups were observed (Table 3).

Adverse Event	Active (n=50) or Control Group (n=49)	
Hoarseness	7 (14%)	9 (18%)
Horner Syndrom	11 (22%)	10 (20%)
Bezold-Jarisch-Reflex	0 (0%)	0 (0%)
Damage of nerves	0 (0%)	0 (0%)

Table 3: Shows the adverse events observed in the study population.

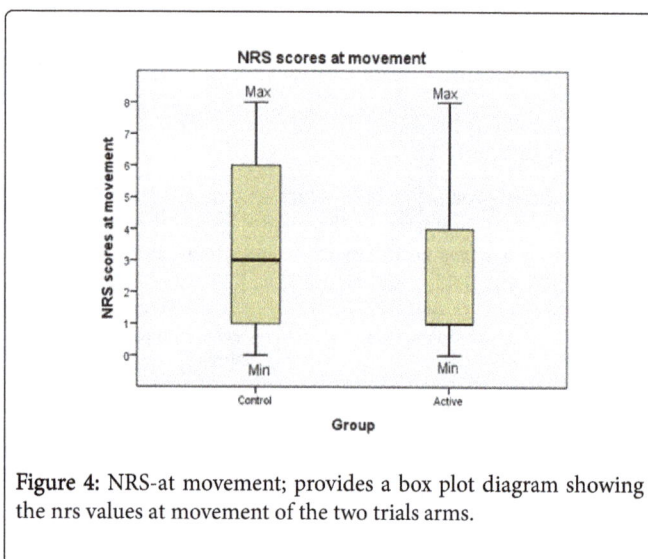

Figure 4: NRS-at movement; provides a box plot diagram showing the nrs values at movement of the two trials arms.

Discussion

In our study, dexamethasone used together with low-volume ropivacaine prolonged pain-free time compared to control.

The optimal dosage of dexamethasone as an analgesic additive is controversial. Liu et al. compared 1, 2, and 4 mg of dexamethasone given together with 30 ml bupivacaine (0.25%) [23]. In this study, no dose-dependent prolongation of pain-free time was observed. Woo et al. used a lower volume of ropivacain (12 ml) with 2.5, 5 mg or 7.5 mg dexamethasone and showed that there is a dose dependent prolongation of pain-free time [13].

The contradictor results might be due to the fact Liu performed a supraclavicular block and Woo a interscalene block. Another explanation might be that Woo used a low volume approach. The volume of local anesthetic could have an influence on the block enhancing capabilities of the additive. Another influence factor could be the use of different local anesthetic agents.

Using lower amounts of dexamethasone could be interesting, because only few data is available on adverse events originating from perineurally applied dexamethasone.

We overlooked different meta studies reporting on adverse events from dexamethasone. There was no case of nerval injury reported but long term adverse events with low frequency are possible. Also our trial does not discover any adverse events indicating potential damage to nerves due to the application of dexamethasone, but we only monitored the patients over a short time window of 24 hours. This window does not allow drawing conclusions about long term adverse events. The observation period in many of the studies researching dexamethasone as additive is too short to detect long term adverse events. A follow up after three to six months would be more appropriate to detect such adverse events.

Williams researched the effect of different additives in a rat model so the data cannot be extrapolated on humans [24].

Ropivacaine is more neurotoxic than dexamethasone and shows a time- and concentration-dependent effect [24]. High concentrations of ropivacaine, as used in this study, might increase the risk of neurotoxicity. However, we chose a high concentration to enhance duration and density of nerve block. Future studies to evaluate efficacy and safety of ropivacaine are warranted.

The incidence of phrenic nerve paralysis was not evaluated via ultrasound in our study. Although no patient experienced dyspnea after the procedure, this does not rule out nerve paralysis. Therefore, we cannot prove that a lower volume is associated with a decreased incidence of this side effect. However, current research indicates that lower volumes are associated with lower rates of phrenic nerve paralysis [18-20].

The effect of lower volumes on adverse events like hoarseness, Horner syndrome or vegetative disturbances is poorly described. In our study, the total rate of hoarseness was 16% which was lower compared to a study using 30 ml [23]. The incidence of Horner syndrome in our study was 21%, which was also lower. Furthermore, no difference in the occurrence of these adverse events between the active and control groups were observed. Our data therefore indicate that lower volumes may reduce side effects of interscalene plexus blockade. But when comparing two different studies precaution must be taken because different baseline characteristics and study methods can have an influence on the results.

We did not monitored vegetative disturbances as reaction to the block, because hemodynamic reactions to general anesthesia which was performed after nerve block could obscure the overall rate of side effects.

Despite randomization, sex, weight and age in the two groups was heterogeneously distributed. The difference in weight between active and control groups was significant. Weight might bias our results as the literature indicates that obese patients have a higher risk of block failure, probably due to difficulties locating the plexus, whereas relatively lower dosage of local anesthetics in relation to body weight does not appear to have an influence [25]. Ultrasound guidance helps to minimize risk of block failure in obese patients. In order to exclude a potential influence of these variables on our findings, we performed correlation analyses. This, however, did not yield any negative or positive correlations.

We could observe a significantly lower NRS (numerical rating scale) score ten hours after blockade in the dexamethasone group compared to control. However, the NRS score at movement did not differ between the groups. As early recovery of pain-free movement is of paramount importance post operatively, future studies might include additional time points of assessment during the first 24 h after surgery.

The ideal volume and concentration of local anesthetic agent for prolongation of the effect of dexamethasone remains elusive. Some studies favor a larger volume of local anesthetic over a higher concentration [26]. Another study implied that the higher volumes of ropivacaine not only enhance the effect of dexamethasone but also increase the effect of ropivacaine [27].

In conclusion, our study proved that dexamethasone (8 mg) used as an additive in a low volume (10 ml), high concentration (0.75%) single shot interscalene plexus blockade, is able to prolong the pain-free-time.

Acknowledgments

Author's contribution

A. L.: Patient recruitment, Study design and data collection

B. S.: Study design, Data analysis and writing up the first draft of the paper

C. F.: Patient recruitment and data collection

I. Z.: Patient recruitment and data collection

S. O.: Patient recruitment and data collection

H. S.: Patient recruitment and data collection

C. H.: Review and correction of the paper, Head of Department, Study design

Clinical Trials Number: NCT02178449

Declaration of Interests

The authors declared that there are no conflicts of interest.

Funding

The trials were funded solely by institutional aid. No external aid was contributed to the study.

References

1. Gonano C, Kettner SC, Ernstbrunner M, Schebesta K, Chiari A, et al. (2009) Comparison of economical aspects of interscalene brachial plexus blockade and general anaesthesia for arthroscopic shoulder surgery. Br J Anaesth 103: 428-433.

2. Hadzic A, Williams BA, Karaca PE, Hobeika P, Unis G, et al. (2005) For Outpatient Rotator Cuff Surgery, Nerve Block Anesthesia Provides Superior Same-day Recovery over General Anesthesia. Anesthesiology 102; 1001-1007.

3. Dolin SJ, Cashman JN, Bland JM (2002) Effectiveness of acute postoperative pain management: I. Evidence from published data. Br J Anaesth 89: 409-423.

4. Salviz E, Xu D, Frulla A, Kwofie K, Shastri U, et al. (2013) Continuous interscalene block in patients having outpatient rotator cuff repair surgery: a prospective randomised trial. Anesth Analg 117: 1485-1492.

5. Marhofer D, Marhofer P, Triffterer L, Leonhardt M, Weber M, et al. (2013) Dislocation rates of perineural catheters: a volunteer study. Br J Anaesth 111: 800-806.

6. Cervero F, Laird JMA (2007) One pain or many pains? A new look at pain mechanisms. New Physiol Sci 6: 268-273.

7. Fritsch G, Danninger T, Allerberger K, Tsodikov A, Felder TK, et al. (2014) Dexmedetomidine added to ropivacaine extends the duration of interscalene brachial plexus blocks for elective shoulder surgery when compared with ropivacaine alone: a single-center, prospective, triple-blind, randomised controlled trial. Reg Anesth Pain Med 39: 37-41.

8. Lee IO, Kim WK, Kong MH, Lee MK, Kim NS, et al. (2002) No enhancement of sensory and motor blockade by ketamine added to ropivacaine interscalene brachial plexus blockade. Acta Anaesthesiol Scand 46: 821-826.

9. Bailard N, Ortiz J, Flores A (2014) Additives to local anesthetics for peripheral nerve blocks: Evidence, limitations, and recommendations. American Journal of Health Systems Pharmacy 71: 373-378.

10. Lee AR, Yi HW, Chung IS, Ko JS, Ahn HJ, et al. (2012) Magnesium added to bupivacaine prolongs the duration of analgesia after interscalene nerve block. Can J Anaesth 59: 21-27.

11. Singelyn FJ, Dangoisse M, Bartholomee S, Gouverneur J (1992) Adding clonidine to mepivacaine prolongs the duration of anesthesia and analgesia after axillary brachial plexus block. Regional Anesthesia 17: 148-150.

12. Cummings KC 3rd, Napierkowski DE, Parra-Sanchez I, Kurz A, Dalton JE, et al. (2011) Effect of dexamethasone on the duration of interscalene nerve blocks with ropivacaine or bupivacaine. Br J Anaesth 107: 446-453.

13. Woo JH, Kim YJ, Kim DY, Cho S (2015) Dose-dependency of dexamethasone on the analgesic effect of interscalene block for arthroscopic shoulder surgery using ropivacaine 0.5%: A randomised controlled trial. Eur J Anaesthesiol 32: 650-655.

14. Tandoc MN, Fan L, Kolesnikov S, Kruglov A, Nader ND (2011) Adjuvant dexamethasone with bupivacaine prolongs the duration of interscalene block: a prospective randomized trial. J Anesth 25: 704-709.

15. Vieira PA, Pulai I, Tsao GC, Manikantan P, Keller B, et al. (2010) Dexamethasone with bupivacaine increases duration of analgesia in ultrasound-guided interscalene brachial plexus blockade. Eur J Anaesthesiol 27: 285-288.

16. Kumar S, Palaria U, Sinha AK, Punera DC, Pandey V (2014) Comparative evaluation of ropivacaine and ropivacaine with dexamethasone in supraclavicular brachial plexus block for postoperative analgesia. Anesth Essays Res 8: 202-208.

17. Jadon A, Dixit S, Kedia SK, Chakraborty S, Agrawal A, et al. (2015) Interscalene brachial plexus block for shoulder arthroscopic surgery: Prospective randomised controlled study of effects of 0.5% ropivacaine and 0.5% ropivacaine with dexamethasone. Indian J Anaesth 59:171-176.

18. Riazi S, Carmichael N, Awad I, Holtby RM, McCartney CJ (2008) Effect of local anaesthetic volume (20 vs 5 ml) on the efficacy and respiratory consequences of ultrasound-guided interscalene brachial plexus block. Br J Anaesth 101: 549-556.

19. Lee JH, Cho SH, Kim SH, Chae WS, Jin HC, et al. (2011) Ropivacaine for ultrasound-guided interscalene block: 5 mL provides similar analgesia but less phrenic nerve paralysis than 10 mL. Can J Anaesth 58: 1001-1006.

20. Gianesello L, Magherini M, Pavoni V, Horton A, Nella A, et al. (2014) The influence of interscalene block technique on adverse hemodynamic events. J Anesth 28: 407-412.

21. Desmet M, Braems H, Reynvoet M, Plasschaert S, Van Cauwelaert J, et al. (2013) I.V. and perineural dexamethasone are equivalent in increasing the analgesic duration of a single-shot interscalene block with ropivacaine for shoulder surgery: a prospective, randomised, placebo-controlled study. Br J Anaesth 111: 445-452.

22. Vandepitte C, Gautier P, Xu D, Salviz EA, Hadzic A (2013) Effective volume of ropivacaine 0.75 through a catheter required for interscalene brachial plexus blockade. Anesthesiology 118: 863-867.

23. Liu J, Richman KA, Grodofsky SR, Bhatt S, Huffman GR, et al. (2015) Elkassabany N. Is there a dose response of dexamethasone as adjuvant for supraclavicular brachial plexus nerve block? A prospective randomized double-blinded clinical study. J Clin Anesth 27 : 237-242.

24. Williams BA, Butt MT, Zeller JR, Coffee S, Pippi M (2015) Multimodal perineural analgesia with combined bupivacaine-clonidine-buprenorphine-dexamethasone: safe in vivo and chemically compatible in solution. Pain Med 16: 186-198.

25. Nielsen KC, Guller U, Steele SM, Klein SM, Greengrass RA, et al. (2005) Influence of obesity on surgical regional anesthesia in the ambulatory setting: an analysis of 9,038 blocks. Anesthesiology 102: 181-187.

26. Friedrickson M, Smith K, Biostat M, Wong A (2010) Importance of Volume and Concentration for Ropivacaine Interscalene Block in Prevent Recovery Room Pain and Minimising Motor Block after Shoulder Surgery. Anesthesiology 112: 1374-1381.

27. Fredrickson MJ, Abeysekera A, White R (2012) Randomized study of the effect of local anesthetic volume and concentration on the duration of peripheral nerve blockade. Reg Anesth Pain Med 37: 495-501.

Dexmedetomidine as an Adjuvant to Bupivacaine in Supraclavicular Brachial Plexus Block

Rajesh Meena*, Sandeep Loha, Arun Raj Pandey, Kavita Meena, Anil Kumar Paswan, Lalita Chaudhary and Shashi Prakash

Department of Anaesthesiology, BHU, India

*Corresponding author: Rajesh Meena, Assistant Professor, Department of Anaesthesiology, BHU campus, India, E-mail: drrajaiims86@gmail.com

Abstract

Background: Many drugs have been used as adjuvants to local anesthetic agents to prolong the duration of peripheral nerve blocks and decrease the time of onset.

In this study we assessed the effect of dexmedetomidine as an adjuvant to bupivacaine in supraclavicular brachial plexus block in terms of onset and duration of sensory and motor blockade, intraoperative sedation, postoperative analgesia, sedation and Complications /side effects if any.

Methods: 60 patients of age 18-70 yrs were divided into two equal groups for upper limb surgeries under supraclavicular brachial plexus block. Group BD was given 39 millilitres (ml) of 0.5% Bupivacaine+1 microgram/kg dexmedetomidine; Group BS was given 39 ml of bupivacine+1 ml of saline.

The following brachial plexus nerve block parameters were assessed hemodynamic parameters, onset and duration of sensory and motor blockade, Ramsay sedation score, verbal rating score, duration of analgesia, duration for rescue analgesia and number of analgesia given.

Results: The onset of sensory blockade was 2.54 minutes less in Group (BD) when compared to Group (BS). The onset of Motor Blockade is 3.26 minutes less in Group (BD) when compared to Group (BS).

The duration of sensory blockade is 195.65 minutes more in Group (BD) then Group (BS). The duration of Motor Blockade is 190.33 minutes more in Group (BD) when compared to Group (BS). The duration of Analgesia is 207.83 minutes more in Group (BD) when compared to Group (BS).

Ramsay sedation score in Gp (BD)continued to show slightly higher sedation scores at all times including postoperative period in comparison to Gp (BS) (P<0.01).

Conclusion: Dexmedetomidine is good adjuvant to local anesthestic agents, as its addition to bupivacaine was associated with prolonged sensory and motor blockade, mild sedation and prolonged analgesia.

Satisfactory hemodynamic stability without observed immediate post-operative side effects are other significant qualities related to it.

Keywords: Analgesia; Bupivacaine; Spuraclavicular brachial plexus block; Dexmedetomidine; Sedation

Introduction

An increasing demand for regional anesthesia from patients and surgeons both matches the fact that regional anesthesia can provide superior pain management and perhaps improves patient outcome.

Brachial plexus block is a popular and widely employed regional nerve block of the upper extremity. Various approaches to brachial plexus block have been described but supraclavicular approach is the easiest and most consistent method for anaesthesia and perioperative pain management in surgery below the shoulder joint.

Many drugs have been used as adjuvants to local anesthetic agents to prolong the duration of peripheral nerve blocks and decrease the time of onset.

Opioids, ketamine, dexamethasone, tramadol, Clonidine and few others drug have been reported to prolong the duration of anesthesia and analgesia during such blocks [1-3] all the adjuvants have some side effects and limitation on the basis of their mechanism of action.

The α2:α1 selectivity of dexmedetomidine is eight times that of clonidine and its high specificity for α2 subtype makes it a much more effective sedative and analgesic agent [4].

In this study we assessed the effect of dexmedetomidine as an adjuvant to bupivacaine in supraclavicular brachial plexus block in terms of (Figure 1):

- Onset and duration of sensory and motor blockade.
- Intraoperative sedation and postoperative analgesia and sedation.
- Complications /side effects if any

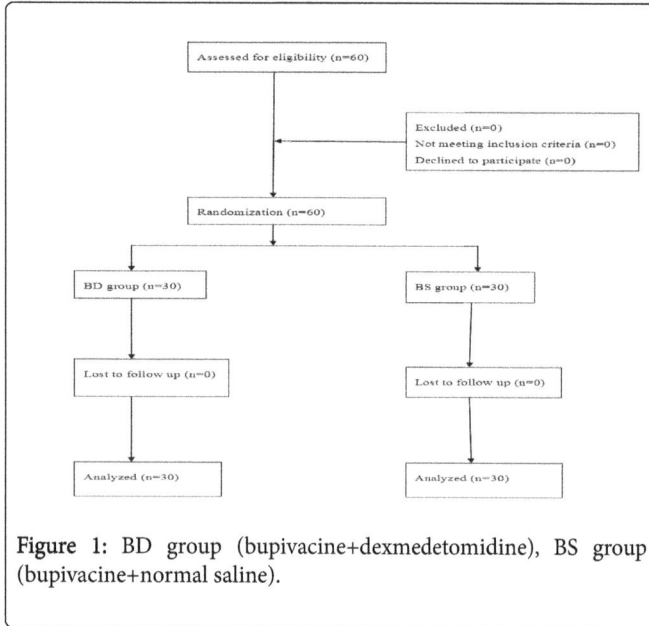

Figure 1: BD group (bupivacine+dexmedetomidine), BS group (bupivacine+normal saline).

Material and Method

This prospective, randomized, double blinded study was performed on 60 adult patients of age undergoing upper limb surgeries under supraclavicular brachial plexus block. Approval from local ethical committee was taken and written informed consent was obtained from patients. All patients were assessed for ASA physical status I and II.

Exclusion criteria

- ASA class III, IV and V
- Patient refusal for procedure
- Any bleeding disorder or patient on anticoagulants
- Neurological deficits involving brachial plexus
- Patients with allergy to local anaesthetics, dexmeditomidine.
- Local infection at the injection site
- Patients on any sedatives or antipsychotics
- Severe obesity/ Body mass index >35
- Hepatic impairment (CHILD B or higher)
- Renal impairment (creatinine >2 mg/dl)

Procedure

The patients were randomized by computer generated random number tables and divided into two equal groups:

- Group BS-(n=30) 39 millilitres (ml) of 0.5% Bupivacaine+1 ml saline
- Group BD-(n=30) 39 millilitres (ml) of 0.5% Bupivacaine+1 microgram (mcg)/kilogram (kg) Dexmedetomidine (dexem, by Themis, India) was given.

The drug solutions were prepared by an anesthesiologist not involved in the study. The anesthesiologist performing the block and observing the patient was blinded to the treatment group. Data collection was done by the same anesthesiologist who was unaware of the group allocation.

The patients undergoing surgical procedure were explained about the procedure. Intravenous cannulation with 18 G venflon was secured in the non-operating upper limb and inj. Midazolam 1 mg i.v and inj. ondansetron 4 mg i.v was given. ECG leads, O_2 saturation probe and NIBP cuff was attached. The patient was positioned supine with a roll under the shoulder to enhance neck extension and the head turned away from the side to be injected. The patients were administered brachial plexus block by supraclavicular route via the subclavian perivascular approach. Under all aseptic precautions, the injection site was identified to be 1 cm behind the midpoint of the clavicle, (where the pulsation of the subclavian artery was felt) and infiltrated with 1 ml of 2% lignocaine subcutaneously. A nerve stimulator (Neurostim LA II, Hugo Sachs Electronik, type 220/1 with 22G × 2" Pajunk needle) was used to locate the brachial plexus. The location endpoint was a distal motor response, that is, the movement of the fingers and the thumb with an output current of 0.5 mA. During injection of the drug solution, negative aspiration was done every 5 ml to avoid intravascular injection. Plexus block was considered successful when at least two out of the four nerve territories (ulnar, radial, median, and musculocutaneous) were effectively blocked for both sensory and motor block.

Onset of sensory time was defined as the time elapsed between the injection of drug and complete loss of cold perception of the arm, while motor blockade was defined as the time elapsed from injection of drug to complete motor block. Sedation of the patient was categorized using Ramsay Sedation Score.

Heart rate, NIBP, SpO_2, Respiratory rate was noted every 5 minutes (mins) during the first 15 mins, then every 15 mins throughout the surgery and first hour of postoperative period. Duration of sensory block (time elapsed between injection of drug and appearance of pain requiring analgesia) and duration of motor block (time elapsed between injection of drug and complete return of muscle power) was also recorded.

I.m Injection of Tramadol 150 mg was given as rescue analgesic when patients complained of pain which was assessed with visual analogue scale (VAS). Patients with VAS >3 (mild, annoying pain) received Inj. Tramadol 100 mg, IV for post op pain up to 12 hrs. When required.

Power of analysis

It was calculated according to duration of analgesia. With two sided type I error of 5% and study power at 80%, it was calculated that 25 patients were required in each group in order to detect difference of 35 min in the duration of analgesia between two groups.

Statistical analysis

The obtained data was analyzed using SPSS 16; descriptive data was compared and presented as Mean ± SD for continuous variables and as number and percentage for normal variable. The venous parameters studied during observation period were compared using student's 't' test or paired 't' test, for parametric variables and Chi-square test used for non-parametric variables.

The critical value of 'p' indicating the probability of significant difference was taken as <0.05 for comparison.

Results

The patients demographic data were recorded, observations were made perioperatively and postoperatively for changes in heart rate, blood pressure, oxygen saturation, sedation score, postoperative pain relief, onset of sensory and motor blockade, duration of sensory and motor blockade and duration of analgesia (Table 1).

As shown in Table 2, Base line heart rate was comparable in both groups (p>0.05). After 10 minutes of giving block there was decrease in heart rate ,which was more in Group (BD) compared to Group (BS) which is statistically significant (p<0.05).

	Group BD (n=30)	Group BS (n=30)
	Mean ± SD	Mean ± SD
Sex (M/F)	20/10	20/10
ASA I/II	21/9	22/8
Weight (Kg)	62.27 ± 7.70	63.60 ± 7.87
Height (Cm)	162.13 ± 7.56	162.13 ± 6.84
Age (yrs)	43.27 ± 12.81	43.7 ± 13.21

Table 1: Demographic and ASA characteristics.

Time interval	BD	BS	t-value	p-value
HR Baseline	74.57 ± 8.05	74.87 ± 8.95	-0.136	0.892
HR 5 min	75.70 ± 8.33	75.83 ± 8.27	-0.062	0.951
HR 10 min	75.00 ± 8.32	78.70 ± 8.02	-1.752	0.085
HR 15 min	71.23 ± 8.43	80.40 ± 6.81	-4.631	<0.001
HR 30 min	68.23 ± 7.09	80.40 ± 6.81	-6.776	<0.001
HR 45 min	66.77 ± 6.14	80.37 ± 6.82	-8.110	<0.001
HR 60 min	64.73 ± 2.71	79.67 ± 7.60	-10.130	<0.001
HR 75 min	65.23 ± 4.24	81.30 ± 6.75	-11.031	<0.001
HR 90 min	65.00 ± 3.69	80.70 ± 7.11	-10.725	<0.001
HR 120 min	64.97 ± 3.89	80.23 ± 6.95	-10.491	<0.001
HR 150 min	65.23 ± 4.24	81.30 ± 6.75	-11.031	<0.001
HR 180 min	66.77 ± 6.18	80.37 ± 6.72	-8.111	<0.001

Table 2: Comparison of Heart Rate (min) between both groups in perioperative and postoperative period.

As shown in Table 3 mean ± standard deviation of systolic blood pressure of patients in both groups were comparable at baseline (p>0.05), After giving the block there was fall in systolic blood pressure in both groups, but was not statistically significant until 15 minutes after giving block (p>0.05). After15 minutes till the end of surgery and also in the postoperative period ,there is more decrease in systolic blood pressure in Group (BD) compared to Group (BS), which is also statistically significant (p<0.05).

Time interval	BD	BS	t-value	p-value
SBP Baseline	125.40 ± 11.11	122.33 ± 10.99	1.074	0.287
SBP 5 min	125.47 ± 10.55	119.47 ± 6.53	2.647	0.010
SBP 10 min	117.20 ± 8.13	117.40 ± 5.63	-0.111	0.912
SBP 15 min	113.87 ± 7.51	118.60 ± 5.53	-2.776	0.007
SBP 30 min	114.00 ± 5.89	117.07 ± 5.50	-2.083	0.042
SBP 45 min	111.47 ± 5.53	118.87 ± 5.39	-5.243	<0.001
SBP 60 min	110.60 ± 6.06	118.47 ± 5.21	-5.388	<0.001
SBP 75 min	113.40 ± 5.63	119.00 ± 5.67	-3.835	<0.001
SBP 90 min	109.13 ± 5.29	119.07 ± 5.77	-6.946	<0.001
SBP 120 min	109.13 ± 6.69	118.33 ± 5.48	-5.820	<0.001
SBP 150 min	110.6 ± 5.99	118.57 ± 5.14	-5.384	<0.001
SBP 180 min	113.40 ± 5.60	119.00 ± 5.64	-3.835	<0.001

Table 3: Comparison of Systolic blood pressure (SBP) in mm Hg during perioperative and post-operative period among both groups.

As shown in Table 4 mean ± standard deviation of Diastolic blood pressure (DBP) of patients in both groups were comparable at baseline (p>0.05), After giving the block there was fall in Diastolic blood pressure (DBP) in BD group, It was statistically not significant until 10 minutes after giving block (p>0.05).

After 10 minutes till the end of surgery, there was fall in Diastolic blood pressure(DBP) in Group (BD) compared to Group (BS), which is statistically significant too (p<0.05).

During post-operative period, the diastolic blood pressure is constantly very close to base line in Group (BS). While in Group (BD), DBP continued to be low and stable which is statistically significant (p<0.05) (Figure 2).

Time interval	BD	BS	t-value	p-value
DBP Baseline	79.60 ± 6.15	80.67 ± 5.59	-0.702	0.485
DBP 5 min	78.87 ± 6.25	81.60 ± 4.99	-1.871	0.066
DBP 10 min	70.73 ± 3.98	80.60 ± 5.53	-7.923	<0.001
DBP 15 min	69.73 ± 4.25	81.60 ± 4.99	-9.904	<0.001

DBP 30 min	68.53 ± 3.67	80.60 ± 5.53	-9.946	<0.001
DBP 45 min	67.90 ± 3.68	82.00 ± 5.06	-12.335	<0.001
DBP 60 min	67.33 ± 3.75	81.60 ± 4.99	-12.508	<0.001
DBP 75 min	67.17 ± 4.13	80.60 ± 5.53	-10.645	<0.001
DBP 90 min	67.60 ± 4.14	81.60 ± 4.99	-11.821	<0.001
DBP 120 min	68.17 ± 3.36	80.60 ± 5.53	-10.511	<0.001
DBP 150 min	67.17 ± 4.13	81.60 ± 5.53	-11.60	<0.001
DBP 180 min	68.17 ± 3.36	80.60 ± 4.5	-11.52	<0.001

Table 4: Comparison of diastolic blood pressure (DBP) in mmHg during perioperative and post-operative period among both groups.

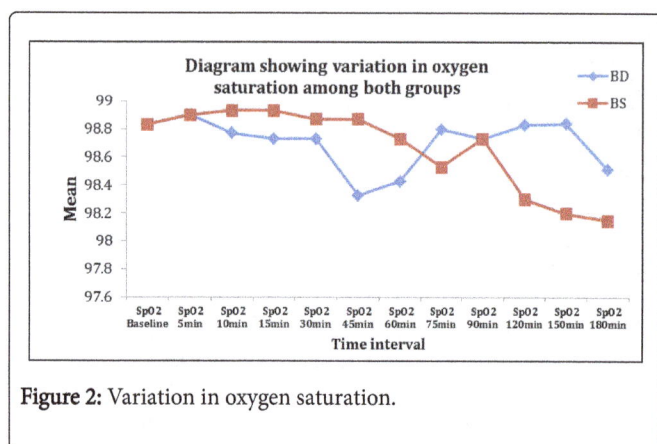

Figure 2: Variation in oxygen saturation.

As shown in Table 5 the mean ± standard deviation of Ramsay sedation scores (RSS) of patients in both groups were comparable at baseline and at 5, and 10 minutes. But after 15 minutes, the patients in Group (BD) continued to show slightly higher sedation scores at all times including postoperative period 150 and 180 minutes when compared with Group (BS) which was statistically significant too (p<0.01).

Time interval	BD	BS	t-value	p-value
RSS baseline	1.00 ±0 .000a	1.00 ± 0.000a	-	-
RSS 5 min	1.13 ± 0.346	1.43 ± 0.679	-2.157	0.035
RSS 10 min	1.43 ± 0.568	1.50 ± 0.682	-0.411	0.682
RSS 15 min	2.07 ± 0.640	1.50 ± 0.682	3.319	0.002
RSS 30 min	2.10 ± 0.607	1.50 ± 0.682	3.598	0.001
RSS 45 min	2.10 ± 0.607	1.50 ± 0.682	3.598	0.001
RSS 60 min	2.10 ± 0.607	1.57 ± 0.679	3.207	0.002
RSS 75 min	2.13 ± 0.571	1.50 ± 0.682	3.898	0.000
RSS 90 min	2.20 ± 0.484	1.43 ± 0.626	5.306	0.000
RSS 120 min	2.10 ± 0.607	1.50 ± 0.682	3.598	0.001
RSS 150 min	2.13 ± 0.571	1.50 ± 0.682	3.898	0.000

RSS 180 min	2.20 ± .484	1.43 ± .626	5.306	0.000

Table 5: Comparison of Ramsay sedation score (RSS) during perioperative and post operative period among both groups.

As shown in Table 6, The mean ± standard deviation of visual analogue scale (VAS) of patients in both groups during postoperative period shows better pain relief score in Group (BD) when compared to Group (BS),but it is not statistically significant(p<0.01). No patients in any group required rescue analgesic after 1st hour of surgery. Injection tramadol 100 mg intravenous was given for postoperative pain in both groups among patient having VAS>3.

Time interval	BD	BS	t-value	p-value
VAS Baseline 120 min	0.13 ± 0.346	0.20 ± 0.407	-0.684	0.497
VAS 125 min	0.13 ± 0.346	0.30 ± 0.466	-1.573	0.121
VAS 135 min	0.13 ± 0.346	0.33 ± 0.479	-1.853	0.069
VAS 150 min	0.67 ± 0.711	0.37 ± 0.556	1.820	0.074
VAS 180 min	0.83 ± 0.747	0.77 ± 0.728	0.350	0.727

Table 6: Visual analog score *vs.* group.

No. of analgesia required is less in group BD in comparison to BS and is also statistically significant (Figure 3).

As shown in Table 7, The mean ± standard deviation of the Onset of Sensory Blockade (OS) shows the time taken for onset of sensory blockade is less in Group (BD) when compared to Group (BS) and is statistically significant (p<0.01).

The onset of sensory blockade was 2.54 minutes less in Group (BD) when compared to Group (BS).

The mean ± standard deviation of the Onset of Motor Blockade (OM) shows the time taken for onset of motor blockade is less in Group (BD) when compared to Group (BS) and is statistically significant (p<0.01).

The onset of Motor Blockade is 3.26minutes less in Group (BD) when compared to Group (BS).

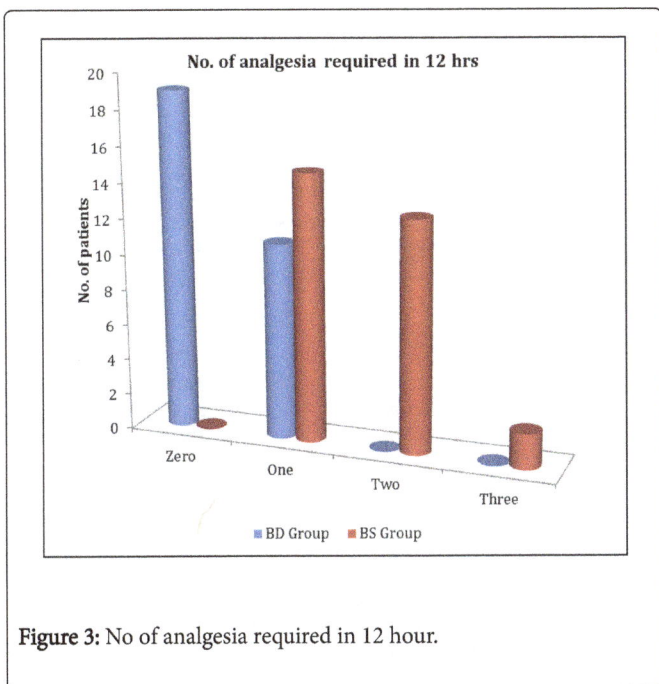

Figure 3: No of analgesia required in 12 hour.

Variables	BD	BS	t-value	p-value
Surgery time	72.83 ± 31.69	57.00 ± 26.11	2.112	0.039
Onset sensory block	8.83 ± 1.62	11.37 ± 1.56	-6.160	<0.001
Duration of sensory block	532.33 ± 85.32	336.67 ± 71.71	9.615	<0.001
Onset motor block	10.33 ± 1.60	13.07 ± 1.59	-6.615	<0.001
Duration of Motor block	486.67 ± 88.68	296.33 ± 75.28	8.962	<0.001
Duration of analgesia	569.00 ± 78.88	361.17 ± 71.22	10.710	<0.001

Table 7: Comparison of onset of Sensory Blockade (OS), Onset of Motor Blockade (OM), Duration of Sensory Blockade (DS), and Duration of Motor blockade (DM) and Duration of analgesia (DA) among both groups.

The mean ± standard deviation of the Duration of Sensory Blockade (DS) shows the duration of sensory blockade is more in Group (BD) when compared to Group (BS) and is statistically significant (p<0.01). The duration of sensory blockade is 195.65 minutes more in Group (BD) when compared to Group (BS).

The mean ± standard deviation of the Duration of Motor Blockade (DM) shows the duration of motor blockade is more in Group (BD) when compared to Group (BS) and is statistically significant (p<0.01). The duration of Motor Blockade is 190.33 minutes more in Group (BD) when compared to Group (BS).

The mean ± standard deviation of the Duration of Analgesia (DA) shows the duration of Analgesia is more in Group (BD) when compared to Group (BS) and is statistically significant (p<0.01). The duration of Analgesia is 207.83 minutes more in Group (BD) when compared to Group (BS).

Discussion

Anesthesiologists routinely use peripheral nerve blocks as an alternative or as an adjunct to general anesthesia, as well as for postoperative analgesia for a wide variety of procedures.

The selection of the optimal long-acting local anesthetic and its concentration for supraclavicular brachial plexus block has always been a debate. Bupivacaine, a local anaesthetic has faster onset and longer duration of action. Bupivacaine has been used with various adjuncts; more commonly with alpha-2 adrenergic receptors agonists. In this study we compared bupivacaine alone and bupivacaine with dexmedetomidine (an alpha-2 adrenergic receptor agonist).

In our study we found that heart rate was decreased from base line in the BD (bupivacaine + dexmedetomidine) group after 15 minutes (p<0.05) when compared to (BS) group (Table 2). Systolic blood pressure was decreased from base line in BD (bupivacaine +dexmedetomidine) group after 15 minutes and beyond in comparison to BS (bupivacaine) group (Table 3). Diastolic blood pressure was also decreased from base line after 15 minutes (p<0.05) in BD (bupivacaine + dexmedetomidine) group when compared to BS (bupivacaine) group (Table 4).

Marina Simeoforidou et al. suggested that spraclavicular block, possibly through extension of block to the ipsilateral stellate ganglion, alters the autonomic outflow to the central circulatory system and this influence depends on the block site [5]. Bradycardia and hypotension during surgery under brachial plexus block have been reported by many investigators; though most are transient, isolated and uncomplicated. Few cases with severe cardiovascular instability have occurred, including asystolic cardiac arrest. Ozalp et al. also noted that there was fall in heart rate and systolic blood pressure in their study on the analgesic efficacy of dexmedetomidine added to bupivacaine in patient controlled supraclavicular analgesia via the posterior approach [6].

Injection midazolam 1 mg was given to all patients and sedation was assessed using Ramsay sedation score (Table 5). There was no statistical significance in both groups until first 15 minutes after which patients in (BD) group showed RSS of 3 most of the times, with statistical significance of (p<0.05). Ozalp et al. [6] and Aliye Esmaoglu et al. [7] also observed that patients who received dexmedetomidine as adjuvant in brachial plexus block were sedated throughout the surgery. Though the exact mechanism of action is not known, centrally-acting alpha-2 agonists produce analgesia and sedation by inhibition of substance P release in the nociceptive pathway at the level of the dorsal root neuron and by activation of alpha-2 adrenoceptors in the locus coeruleus [8].

The onset of sensory and motor blockade was quick in group (BD) when compared with the group (BS) (p<0.05) (Table 7). Esmaoglu et al. [7] in his study on Dexmedetomidine added to Levobupivacaine in Axillary Brachial Plexus Block, observed that Sensory and motor block onset time were significantly shorter in group LD (levobupivacaine+ Dexmedetomidine) than in group L (levobupivacaine), and the difference was statistically significant (P<0.05) [8]. The onset of sensory blockade was 2.54 minutes less in Group (BD) when compared to Group (BS). The onset of motor Blockade was 2.66 minutes less in Group (BD) when compared to Group (BS).

In our study, the duration of sensory and motor blockade was prolonged in BD (bupivacaine + dexmedetomidine) group when compared to BS (bupivacaine) group (p<0.05) (Table 7). Duration of sensory blockade was prolonged by 195.66 minutes and motor blockade by 190.34 minutes. Esmaoglu et al. [7], Amar et al. [9] also found in their studies that administering perineural dexmedetomidine as part of a brachial plexus block resulted in a prolongation of motor block duration. The mechanism by which alpha-2 adrenergic receptor agonists produce analgesia and sedation is not fully understood but is likely to be multifactorial. Peripherally, alpha-2 agonists produce analgesia by reducing release of norepinephrine and causing alpha-2 receptor independent inhibitory effects on nerve fiber action potentials.

In this study, pain was assessed by visual analogue scale (VAS), and found that VAS score at 120, 125, 135, 150 and 180 minutes was less in group (BD) when compared to group (BS) (p<0.05) (Table 6) Duration of analgesia was prolonged by 207.8 minutes in group (BD). Esmaoglu et al. [7], Gandhi et al. [8] and Amar et al. [9] studies were analysed together and found out that there was increase in time to first analgesic request by 345 min (95% CI: 102.68, 587.23, P<0.005) or 70% when Dexmedetomidine was used as an adjunct to local anesthetics in various blocks when compared with local anesthetics alone.

No. of analgesia required in post-operative period was less in group BD when compared to group BS and also statistically significant (p<0.05) (Figure 3).

Oxygen saturation remained >95% at all times in groups, with no statistically significant difference between bupivacaine (BS) and bupivacaine+dexmedetomidine group (BD) (p>0.05). Respiratory rate of patients in both groups were comparable at baseline and at 5 minutes after the block (p>0.05). There was decrease in respiratory rate in Group (BD) after 10 min, which was statistically significant (p<0.05) (Figure 2) when compared with group (BS).

Summary and Conclusion

From this study we concluded that Dexmedetomidine is a good adjuvant to local anesthestic agents, as its addition to bupivacaine was associated with prolonged sensory and motor blockade, mild sedation and prolonged analgesia. Satisfactory hemodynamic stability without observed immediate post-operative side effects are other significant qualities related to it.

References

1. Yoginee SP, Rashmi B, Tushar P (2013) Efficacy of Dexmedetomidine as an adjuvant to 0.5% Ropivacaine in Supraclavicular Brachial Plexus Block for Postoperative Analgesia. Impact Factor 4: 2319-7064.

2. Duma A, Urbanek B, Sitzwohl C, Kreiger A, Zimpfer M, et al. (2005) Clonidine as an adjuvant to local anaesthetic axillary brachial plexus block: A randomized, controlled study. Br J Anaesth 94: 112-116.

3. Popping M, Elia N, Marret E, Wenk M, Tramèr MR (2009) Clonidine as an adjuvant to local anaesthetic for peripheral nerve and plexus blocks: A meta-analysis of randomized trials. Anesthesiology 111: 406-415.

4. Virtanen R, Savola JM, Saano V, Nyman L (1988) Characterisation of selectivity, specificity and potency of dexmedetomidine as an alpha 2-adrenoceptor agonist. Eur J Pharmacol 150: 9-14.

5. Marina S, George V, Eleni C, Metaxia B, Katerina T, et al. (2013) Effect of supraclavicular brachial plexus block on heart rate variability: Korean J Anesthesiol 64: 432-438.

6. Ozalp G, Tuncel G, Savli S, Celik A, Doger C, et al. (2006) The analgesic efficacy of dexmedetomidine added to ropivacaine in patient controlled supraclavicular analgesia via the posterior approach. Eur J Anaesthesiol 23: 220.

7. Esmaoglu A, Yegenoglu F, Akin A, Turk Y (2010) Dexmedetomidine Added to Levobupivacaine Prolongs Axillary Brachial Plexus Block. Anesth Analg 111: 1548-1551.

8. Rachana G, Alka S, Ila P (2012) Use of Dexmedetomidine along with Bupivacaine for brachial plexus block. Nat J Med Res 2: 67-69.

9. Ammar AS, Mahmoud KM (2012) Ultrasound-guided single injection infraclavicular brachial plexus block using bupivacaine alone or combined with dexmedetomidine for pain control in upper limb surgery: a prospective randomized controlled trial. Saudi JAnaesth 6: 109-114.

Dexmedetomidine *vs.* Magnesium Sulphate as an Adjuvant to Rocuronium Bromide, and Local Anaesthetic Mixture in Peribulbar Anaesthesia for Viteroretinal Surgery

Mona Mohamed Mogahed*, **Wessam Mohamed Nassar and Mohamed Ali Abdullah**

Faculty of Medicine, Tanta University, Egypt

*Corresponding author: Mona Mohamed Mogahed, Faculty of Medicine, Tanta University, Tanta, Egypt, E-mail: monamogahedfr@hotmail.com

Abstract

Background: A wide variety of additives have been used in a mixture with local anesthetics in PBA to fasten the onset, increase the potency and prolong the duration of the block to cover the long viteroretinalsurgeries. Dexmedetomidine, magnesium sulphateand rocuronium bromidehave been added to local anesthetics to achieve such goal.

Patients and methods: This randomized double-blind prospective study was carried out on 96 ASA I and II patients aged 40 to 65 years who were scheduled for elective vitreoretinal surgery in Tanta university. Patients were divided randomly allocated into three groups, 32 patients in each group. Group C received the combination of 3.5 ml bupivacaine 0.5%, 3.5 ml lidocaine 2%, 0.5 ml rocuronium bromide (5 mg) plus 0.5 ml Normal saline (0.9% NaCl), group D received the same local anesthetic rocuronium mixture supplemented plus with plus 0.5 ml Dexmedetomidine (5 Group M group received the same local anesthetic rocuronium mixture plus 0.5 ml $MgSO_4$ 5% (50 mg). the onset of corneal anesthesia, time to adequate condition to begin surgery, the score and duration of akinesia, number of patients requiring supplementary injection, IOP, sedation scores, intraoperative pain, patients and surgeon's satisfaction and incidence of complication were assessed.

Results: There was no statistical significance in the onset of corneal anesthesia between all groups with p value>0.05 (Group M 2.00 ± 0.70, Group M, 2.04 ± 0.77 and Group C 2.26 ± 0.62 min). However, the time adequate to start the surgery was significantly shorter (p<0.0001) in group M than in group D and group C (7.05 ± 1.54, 7.86 ± 1.61 and 8.63 ± 1.65 min respectively); also, it was significantly shorter in group D than group C. The duration of akinesia was significantly longer (p<0.0001) in group M compared with other groups (200.55 ± 7.55,180.11 ± 1.61 and 140.44 ± 13.04 min in group M, D and C respectively). IOP comparison was statistically insignificant between all groups with p value>0.05. No significant difference was noticed between the 3 groups regarding sedation score HR and MAP at all-time measures. As regards the akinesia score Mg group had the least akinesia score (p<0.0001) compared with the other groups in all measurement times. The VAS score and the need of supplemental dose were much higher in the control group. Patient satisfaction (p<0.0001) was best achieved in the D Group while surgeon satisfaction (p=0.01) was the best in M Group.

Conclusion: Adding Mg to local anesthetic mixture in peribulbar anesthesia resulted in a fast onset, long duration and better akinesia score while Dexmedetomidine supplementation offered more patient satisfaction.

Keywords: Peribulbar anaesthesia; Rocuronium; Dexmedetomedine; Magnesium

Introduction

Vitreoretinal surgery is a surgery involving the vitreous and retina, they are lengthy procedures and associated with significant pain [1], it has traditionally been performed under general anesthesia but local anesthesia has increased in popularity in recent years [2].

The retro bulbar can provide adequate anesthesia, akinesia and control of intraocular pressure as well as postoperative analgesia [3]. However, many complications are associated with this technique such as globe perforation, brain stem anesthesia and retro bulbar hemorrhage, which is the most frequent complication [4].

Many believe that the peribulbar block is a safer technique however, it has the disadvantage of a slow onset of orbital akinesia and to produce it a larger volume or repeated injections of anesthetic solution is required due to limited diffusion of local anesthetics (LA) [5]. This also increases the frequency of complications such as globe perforation and hemorrhage [4]. To prevent this and to increase tissue diffusion, hyaluronidase and other adjutants such as clonidine, epinephrine and alkalinization were used to improve peribulbar block [6-8].

Neuromuscular blocking drugs, such as vecuronium [9] and atracrurium [10], and rocuronium have also been added to the local anaesthetic mixture and have been shown to accelerate onset and improve the quality of peribulbar block [11].

Magnesium (Mg) has antinociceptive effects due to its antagonistic effect of NMDA receptors, and its analgesic effect is based on its inhibitory properties for calcium channels [12]. At the motor nerve terminal, $MgSO_4$ inhibits acetylcholine release, thus it enhances the effect, speeds the onset and increases the clinical duration of neuromuscular blocking agents [13].

Dexemedetomidine is a highly selective a2-adrenoreceptor agonist that has an a2 to a1 selectivity ratio of 1620:1 [14]. It enhances central and peripheral neural blockades when added to LAs as an adjuvant. It has been used as additives to local anaesthetics in peripheral nerve block, brachial plexus block [15] and peribulbar block. Dexmedetomidine may be used to improve the reliability and efficacy of regional anesthesia [16]. It is also a potent and effective drug for decreasing IOP in rabbits [17].

In several studies, systemic magnesium sulphate [13] was proved to speed the onset and prolong the duration of neuromuscular blockade while the effects of dexmedetomidine on neuromuscular blockade is still unclear.

Using dexmedetomidine, and magnesium sulphate as adjuvants to peribulbar anesthesia has been investigated in several studies [18-20], comparing their effects versus rocuronium in peribulbar anesthesia [19,21] has been studied as well. To our knowledge little was done to investigate the local effects of dexmedetomidine or magnesium on the muscle relaxant potentiated block.

Patient and Methods

The study was carried out on 96 patients, aging (40-65 y), (ASA I&II) of both sex presented for viteroretinal surgery under local anesthesia in Tanta University Hospital Ophthalmology department. The duration of the study was 3 months. After approval from institutional ethics committee an informed consent was taken from each patient. All data of the patients was confidential with secret codes and private file for each patient, all given data were used for the current medical research only.

Exclusion criteria

Patient with renal and liver diseases, Cardiovascular instability, orthopnea, History of allergy to local anesthetics, Patient with coagulopathies and impaired platelet functions, Parkinsonism, claustrophobia, difficulty in communication, patients with high myopia, staphylomas, Local infection at the site of the block and extraocular muscles or eyelid abnormalities were excluded

This study was conducted in a randomized, double blind and prospective manner. Any unexpected risks appeared during the course of the research were cleared to the participants and ethical committee on time.

All physicians, patients, nursing staff, and data collector were blinded to the patient group assignment. For all patients, full clinical examination and laboratory investigations as regards renal and hepatic functions as well as cardiovascular status were done.

Using a computer-generated randomization schedule and serially numbered, opaque, sealed envelopes, patients were randomly allocated to one of three study groups; 32 patients in each group.

Patients were randomly allocated to one of three study groups; 32 patients in each group:

Group 1 (C group) (n=32): Each patient received the combination of 3.5 ml bupivacaine 0.5%, 3.5 ml lidocaine 2%, 0.5 ml rocuronium bromide (5 mg) plus 0.5 ml Normal saline (0.9% NaCl).

Group 2 (D group) (n=32): Each patient received the combination of 3.5 ml bupivacaine 0.5%, 3.5 ml lidocaine 2%, 0.5 ml rocuronium bromide (5 mg) plus 0.5 ml Dexmedetomidine (50 μ).

Group 3 (M group): (n=32): Each patient received the combination of 3.5 ml bupivacaine 0.5%, 3.5 ml lidocaine 2%, 0.5 ml rocuronium bromide (5 mg) plus 0.5 ml $MgSO_4$ 5% (50 mg).

Prior to performance of the block, a blinded observer evaluated the patient's eyelid and ocular movement at the site of surgery. On arrival in the anesthetic room, Standard monitors were attached and oxygen was administered at 2l/min via nasal prongs and a peripheral IV cannula was inserted

Peribulbar anesthesia was performed, by the same anesthesiologist who was blinded to the local anesthetic drug used. An infratemporal transconjuctival injection of the study drug (4 ml) using a 25gauge, 25 mm needle was performed followed by gentle massage for 30 seconds to facilitate the spread of the local anesthetic mixture.
A second transconjuctival injection of the study drug (4 ml) was performed medial to the lacrimal caruncle.

Injection of the intended volume of the study drug was stopped when there was fullness of the orbit and/or drooping of the upper eyelid during injection. Gentle ocular massage was done, the eye pad was removed every 2 min to assess ocular movements and the orbicular muscle. Corneal anesthesia was also evaluated using a small cotton wool at the same time intervals. To assess ocular akinesia, patients were asked to look in four directions: Lateral, medial, superior, and inferior. Ocular movement in each direction was scored as 2 if it was normal, 1 if it was limited, and 0 if there was no directional movement (total score 0-8). The patient was then asked to forcefully close his/her eyes to assess the orbicularis muscle on a scale of 0-2 (0=complete akinesia, 1=partial movement, 2=pronounced movement).

Time to adequate condition to begin surgery (defined as the presence of corneal anesthesia together with ocular movement score ≤ 1 and eyelid squeezing score of 0) was recorded using a stopwatch. If adequate condition to begin surgery was not obtained 10 min after performing the block, supplemental injection with 2 ml of lidocaine 2% either inferotemporally or medially was administered based on the anesthesiologist's assessment. At the end of surgery, all patients were asked to rate their intraoperative pain using a visual analogue scale (VAS) 0 being no pain and 10 being the worst imaginable pain. All adverse events including the presence of diplopia and/or ptosis were recorded.

The following were recorded in the three groups

Patients characteristics including age, sex, and weight, and ASA status, axial length of the globe measured by echocardiography, type and duration of surgery.

1. Baseline HR and MAP.

2. Onset time of corneal anesthesia every 30 sec.

3. Time to adequate condition to begin surgery defined as the presence of corneal anesthesia together with ocular movement score ≤ 1 and eyelid squeezing score.

4. The score of akinesia in the 1, 3, 5 and 10 minutes after injection (score 0 total, score 1 relative, score 2 no akinesia).

5. Number of patients requiring supplementary injection.

6. The offset time of akinesia in the recovery unit.

7. HR and MAP every 5 min in the first 20 min then every 10 min till the end of the surgery.

8. Sedation levels were assessed with modified Ramsay sedation scale (1-Anxious and agitated or restless or both, 2-Cooperative, oriented, and tranquil, 3-Responds to commands only, 4-Brisk response to light glabellar tap or loud auditory stimulus, 5-No response to light glabellar tap or loud auditory stimulus) at every 10 min during surgery and every 30 min in first 2 h.

9. Intraocular pressure measured using a Schiotz tonometer 5 min before the injection of LA as a baseline 10 min after the injection of LA.

10. Intraoperative pain at the end of the surgery using a visual analogue scale (VAS).

11. The surgeon's and patient's satisfaction (both blinded to group assignment) were assessed using a satisfaction verbal rating scale from 0 (total dissatisfaction) to 10 (total satisfaction).

12. Incidence of complications: Complications during or after the block: Such as episodes of nausea or vomiting, occulocardiac reflex arrhythmia, convulsions, allergy, weakness, diplopia, ptosis and subconjunctival haemorrhage were recorded.

Statistical methods

Based on the previous study of nicholson et al. [18], which resulted in mean ocular movement score of 5 in group 1 and 7 in group 2, Initial sample size estimation showed that 41 patients should be included for detecting a clinically meaningful in ocular movement score of 2 (at least), with (α=0.05, two side, power of 90%).

However, to enable detection of potential variations and avoid potential errors, 45 patients will be included in each group. All analyses were performed on an intention to treat basis. Data were analyzed using Statistical Program for Social Science (SPSS) version 18.0. Quantitative data were expressed as mean± standard deviation (SD). Qualitative data were expressed as frequency and percentage.

The following tests were done

1. (X^2) test of significance was used in order to compare proportions between qualitative parameters.

2. One-way analysis of variance was used for intergroup comparisons as regards normally distributed.

3. Variables Probability (P-value).

a). P-value<0.05 was considered significant.

b). P-value<0.001 was considered as highly significant.

c). P-value>0.05 was considered insignificant.

Results

A total of 96 patients were randomly included in this study, all of them had performed viteroretinal surgeries under peribulbar anesthesia, all cases complete the surgeries under local anesthesia, none of them required general anesthesia (Table 1 and Figures 1-3).

		Group D	Group M	Group C	F or X_2	P value
Age (years)		58.1 ± 5.1	58.3 ± 4.3	59.2 ± 4.9	0.58	0.56
Sex	M	25 (55.5%)	23 (51.1%)	24 (53.3%)	0.178	0.914
	F	20 (44.4%)	22 (48.8%)	21 (46.6%)		
Duration (min)		128.1 ± 25.6	131.2 ± 20.9	124.6 ± 24.3	0.852	0.43

Table 1: Demographic data and duration of surgery.

Table 1 showed that both the demographic data regarding (age, sex) and duration of surgeries were statistically comparable in three groups.

	MAGNESIUM (n=45) Mean ± SD	DEXEMEDE (n=45) mean ± SD	CONTROL (n=45) mean ± SD	ANOVA	P value	Post hoc
Time for adequate conditions to start the surgery (min)	7.05 ± 1.54	7.86 ± 1.61	8.63 ± 1.65	9.26	<0.0001	P1 0.02* P2 0.000** P3 0.02 †
Onset time of corneal anesthesia (min)	2.00 ± 0.70	2.04 ± 0.77	2.26 ± 0.62	5.39*	0.06	-------
Offset time: (min)	200.55 ± 7.55	180.11 ± 1.61	140.44 ± 13.04	405.7	<0.0001	P1 0.000* P2 0.000** P3 0.000 *†
IOP pre: (mmhg)	11.00 ± 1.85	11.30 ± 2.16	11.00 ± 2.18	0.13	0.73	
IOP at 10 min (mmhg)	12.98 ± 2.78	12.41 ± 2.68	13.35 ± 3.12	1.23	0.29	

P<0.05 dex. group compared to magnesium group; **p<0.0001 control group compared to magnesium group; † P<0.05 dex. Group compared to magnesium group *† p<0.0001 dex group *versus* control group.

Table 2: comparison between the 3 groups regarding time for adequate conditions to start the surgery, Onset time of corneal anesthesia, Offset time, preoperative IOP and IOP at 10 min post-injection.

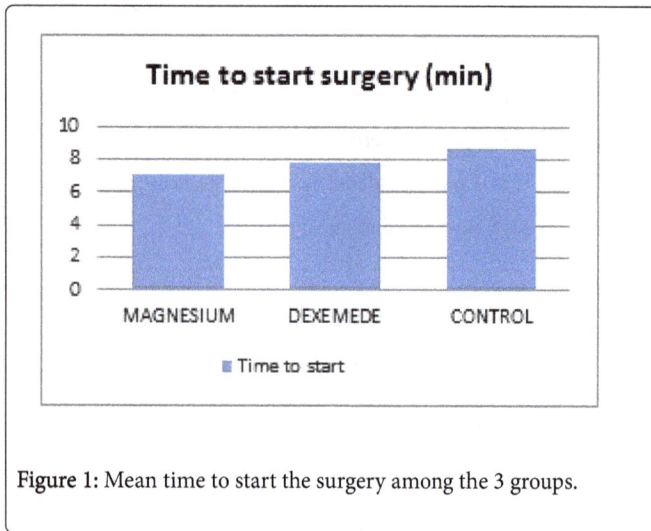

Figure 1: Mean time to start the surgery among the 3 groups.

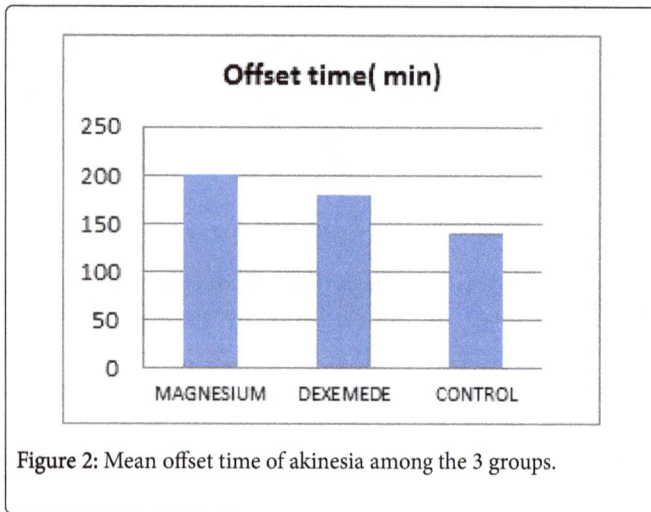

Figure 2: Mean offset time of akinesia among the 3 groups.

As shown in Table 2 the time of onset time of corneal anesthesia, showed no significant difference between the 3 groups. while the time for adequate conditions to start the surgery in Magnesium group was significantly the shortest among both dexmedetomidine and control groups, also, dexmedetomidine had significantly shorter time than control group. The Offset time of akinesia was significantly the longest in magnesium group than in dexmedetomidine and control groups with dexmedetomidine group had also a significantly longer offset than the control. As regards the IOP it was found that dexmedetomidine had the lowest values in 10 min IOP measurements but without statistical significance.

	MAGNESIUM (n=45) mean ± SD	DEXEMEDE (n=45) mean ± SD	CONTROL (n=45) mean ± SD	Kruskal Wallis test	P value
Sedation score 10 min	1.44 ± 0.50	1.53 ± 0.69	1.24 ± 0.43	5.17	0.07
Sedation score 30 min	1.55 ± 0.75	1.66 ± 0.85	1.28 ± 0.45	4.42	0.11
Sedation score 60 min	1.47 ± 0.58	1.64 ± 0.90	1.26 ± 0.44	3.56	0.16
Sedation score 120 min	1.40 ± 0.49	1.46 ± 0.62	1.22 ± 0.42	2.65	0.07

Table 3: comparison between the 3 groups regarding sedation score at different time measures.

Table 3 shows No significant difference between the 3 groups regarding sedation score at all-time measures.

	MAGNESIUM (n=45) mean ± SD	DEXEMEDE (n=45) mean ± SD	CONTROL (n=45) mean ± SD	Kruskal Wallis test	P value	Post hoc
1 min	5.93 ± 1.26	6.44 ± 1.23	7.24 ± 0.74	15.79	0.000†	P1 0.03* P2 0.000** P3 0.001***
3 min	3.33 ± 1.50	3.75 ± 1.36	5.97 ± 1.32	55.03	0.000†	P1 0.42 P2 0.000** P3 0.000***
5 min	1.71 ± 1.23	1.95 ± 1.29	3.95 ± 1.49	53.84	0.000†	P1 0.74 P2 0.000**

						P3 0.000***
						P1 0.33
						P2 0.001**
10 min	0.08 ± 0.41	0.28 ± 0.75	0.80 ± 1.15	15.35	0.000†	P3 0.04***
† P<0.0001* dex group compared to magnesium group; ** control group compared to magnesium group; *** control group compared to dex group.						

Table 4: Comparison between the 3 groups regarding Akinesia score at different time measure.

Table 4 shows that Magnesium group significantly had the least akinesia score at 1 min than both dexmedetomidine and control group (p<0.0001). The akinesia score between magnesium and dexmedetomidine group at 3, 5 and 10 min showed that magnesium had insignificantly lesser values than dexmedetomidine.

	MAGNESIUM (n=45)	DEXEMEDE (n=45)	CONTROL (n=45)	χ^2	P value
	No%	No%	No%		
No:	4395.6	4088.9	3168.9	13.19	0.001*
Yes:	24.4	511.1	1431.1		

Table 5: Comparison between the 3 groups regarding the need of supplementary injection.

Table 5 shows that control group had significantly (p<0.001) more need for supplementary injection than both Magnesium and dexmedetomidine group while it was insignificantly lesser in Magnesium group when compared with dexmedetomidine group.

Table 6 showed that Patient and surgeon satisfaction were significantly (<0.05) p lower in control group than both Magnesium and dexmedetomidine groups. To be noticed that patient satisfaction was best achieved in dexmedetomidine group while surgeon satisfaction had highest scores in magnesium group but this remark was of no significance between both groups.

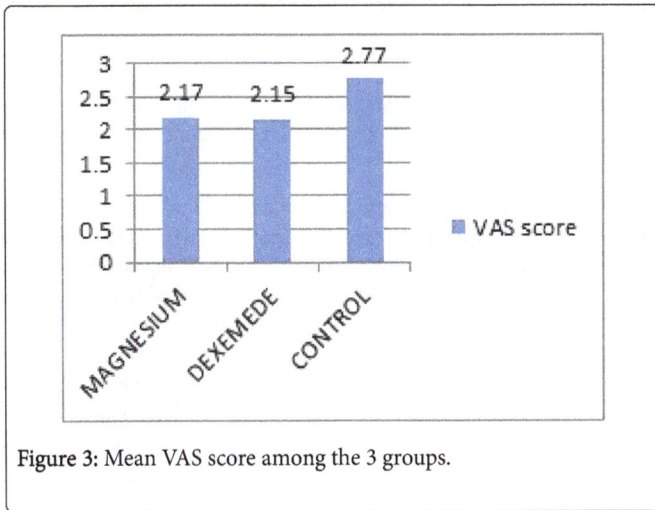

Figure 3: Mean VAS score among the 3 groups.

Intraoperative pain assessed by VAS score showed that control group has the highest score if compared with both Magnisum and dexemede group with a mean of (2.77 ± 0.87).

	MAGNESIUM (n=45) mean ± SD	DEXEMEDE (n=45) mean ± SD	CONTROL (n=45) mean ± SD	ANOVA	P value	Post hoc
Patient satisfaction	8.24 ± 1.17	8.57 ± 1.25	7.60 ± 1.05	8.24	0.000†	P1 0.47 P2 0.01** P3 0.000***
Surgeon satisfaction	8.62 ± 1.19	8.40 ± 1.23	7.97 ± 1.15	4.47	0.01*†	P1 0.37 P2 0.004** P3 0.04***
† P<0.0001, *† P<0.01, ** control group compared to magnesium group; *** control group compared to dex group.						

Table 6: Comparison between the 3 groups regarding patient and surgeon satisfaction.

Discussion

Using nondepolarizing muscle relaxants such as atracurium [10], vecuronium [9] and rocuronium [11], as adjuvants to local anesthetics in peribulbar anesthesia has been proved in several studies to improve the quality and the duration of the block.

In our study, we compared the effects of adding Dexmedetomidine or magnesium sulphate as an adjuvant to rocuronium bromide and local anesthetic mixture in peribulbar anesthesia for viteroretinal surgery.

Although performing viteroretinal surgeries under topical anesthesia has been tried in several studies [22-24]. Many ophthalmic surgeons prefer to operate on completely akinetic eyes. Iatrogenic complications, such as retinal tearing [25] or hemorrhage may occur due to sudden movement of the eye during the surgery.

The addition of neuromuscular blockers as adjuvants to the local anesthetic does not influence analgesia; however, they induce akinesia in extraocular muscles, but the mechanisms are still unclear. It may be due to local action in the motor neurons extraocular muscles or by interfering the muscle spindle activity resulting in lower muscle tone and spasm [26].

Our study investigated the effects of adding $MgSO_4$ or Dexmedetomidine to NDMRS in peribulbar blocks. Our study showed that the time taken to achieve suitable akinesia (score 0 or 1) to start surgery was significantly shorter in magnesium than dexemedetomine and control groups, also it was significantly shorter in dexemedetomine than in control group.

Similarly the akinesia score, $MgSO_4$ and DEX groups showed significant more akinesia when compared with the control group in all measurement times.

Also, $MGSO_4$ group had significantly more akinesia (lesser akinesia score) than DEX group in min 1 and insignificantly lesser score in 3, 5, 10 min. This could be explained by the local effects of $MgSO_4$ on the motor end plate While the duration of akinesia in magnesium group was statistically prolonged when compared with the other groups, and in the same manner Dexmedetomidine group akinesia lasted statistically longer time than in the control group.

Several studies were made on the effects of magnesium on nondepolarizing muscle relaxant. SinghS et al. [13] found pretreatment with $MgSO_4$ before non-depolarizing muscle relaxant, resulted in faster onset of neuromuscular block, needed for intubation of trachea. Also, it resulted in an intensified and prolonged neuromuscular blockade and delayed recovery. Similar results were obtained by Ghodraty MR et al. [27] who studied the effects of different doses of $MgSO_4$ on theproperties of neuromuscular blockade by cisatracurium during induction of anesthesia and found that the speed of onset and the intensity of muscle relaxation increased as higher doses of magnesium were used.

$MgSO_4$ by acting as a calcium channel blocker at presynaptic level reduces acetylcholine release at the motor endplate, which lowers the excitability of the muscle and the amplitude of endplate potential, resulting in the augmentation of a neuromuscular blockade by NDMRs [13]. However, A study done by Wang H et al. [28] found that this potentiation of NDMRs by magnesium can be in part due to a combined effect on adult muscle-type acetylcholine receptors.

According to our results, regarding the onset of corneal anesthesia, there were no statistically significant differences between all groups although it was insignificantly delayed in the control group. Meanwhile, regarding the duration of anesthesia, we found it was more prolonged in magnesium group than the other two groups and in Dexmedetomidine group than the control group.

This was quite similar to the results of the study done by Hamawy TY et al. [21] who studied the effects of Rocuronium *versus* magnesium as an adjuvant to local anesthetics in peribulbar block and found that magnesium sulfate did not show any benefit as regards the onset of the block.

A meta-analysis done by Morrison AP et al. [29] found that the addition of intrathecal magnesium to local anesthetic did not result in a significant delay on the onset nor prolonged duration of sensory blockade.

In contrary, Haghighi M et al. [30] who studied the effect of Magnesium Sulfate Axillary Plexus Blockade he found a delayed onset and prolonged duration of sensory block in magnesium group.

A metanaylsis done by Zhang et al. [31] studying the effect of different doses of intrathecal Dexmedetomidine on spinal anesthesia showed that Dexmedetomidine had a dose dependent effect on fastening the onset and prolonging the duration of sensory and motor blockade.

Abd El-Hamid AM et al. [32], addition of $MgSO_4$ to local anesthetic in peribulbar eye block produces predictable rapid onset of anesthesia without any side-effects, Dogru et al. [33] also found statistically decreased motor and sensory block onset times by the addition of magnesium to levobupivacaine for axillary brachial plexus block in chronic renal failure patients scheduled for arteriovenous fistula surgery.

Narang et al. [34] observed that the addition of magnesium sulfate as adjunct to lignocaine for total intravenous anesthesia for upper limb surgery hastened the onset of sensory and motor block and decreased tourniquet pain.

When magnesium was compared with clonidine as an adjunct for epidural bupivacaine, the onset of anesthesia was rapid, but the duration of analgesia was shorter in magnesium group in comparison to clonidine group [35]. Sedation was seen in the clonidine group. The author established that magnesium is predictable and safe adjunct to epidural bupivacaine. Abd El-Hamid [32] also found the longer duration of peribulbar block in the patients receiving clonidine with local anesthetic in comparison to the patients receiving magnesium.

Dexmedetomidine was used in several studies as an additive to local anesthetics producing variable effects on the onset and duration of sensory and motor blocks.

Eskandr AM et al. [36] studied the effects of adding Dexmedetomidine in subtenon block and found that it significantly fastened the onset of sensory and motor block, prolonged the duration of analgesia with little effects on duration of akinesia.

Similarly El-Ozairy et al. [37] studying the effects of adding different doses of Dexmedetomidine in peribulbar block in viteroretinal surgeries found that higher dose (50 μgm DEX group) was combined with significantly faster onset and prolonging duration of both sensory and motor blocks than all other groups while the smaller dose (50 μgm DEX group) was combined with significantly prolonged duration of both sensory and motor blocks than the control group with no significant effects on the onset of corneal anesthesia nor the akinesia of the globe.

Hafez M et al. [38] studying the effect of adding different doses of Dexmedetomidine to peribulbar block in 160 patients undergoing vitreoretinal surgeries found a shorter onset time of corneal anesthesia in all groups which was statically significant in higher doses (D20, D25) when compared with the control group , as regards the onset of akinesia none of the groups had a statistically significant effects when compared with control group while the duration of analgesia and akinesia were statistically prolonged only in the D25 Group when compared with the control group.

A metanaylsis done by Abdullah FW et al. [39] showed that using dexemedetomine in as an additive different (either in brachial plexus or neuraxially) blocks produced different effects. When used intrathecally, it statistically speeded the onset of sensory and motor blocks which this was not the case when used perineurally in the brachial plexus while time to 1st analgesic requirement and duration of motor block were statistically prolonged in both perineural and neuroaxial technique.

Memis D et al. [40] studying the effects of intravenous dexemedetomine on rocuronium requirements in sevoflurane anesthesia showed marked reduction in rocuronium doses and explained this by the hemodynamic effects of dexemedetomine which could affect the pharmacokinetics of rocuronium.

Dexmedetomidine is a selective alpha 2 adrenoreceptor agonist. It produces a dose dependent sedation and analgesia, recently, Dexmedetomidine has been used as adjuvant to LA drugs in peripheral nerve block and eye block [41] this action is mainly due to blocking the hyperpolarization-activated cation current [42].

A study done by Talke PO et al. [43] on the effects of Dexmedetomidine on the neuromuscular blockade the authors showed that dexmedetomidine resulted in a more decrease in the muscle force using mechanomyog-raphy. Although these changes were statistically significant, the investigators concluded that they were not clinically relevant. The mechanism by which α2-adregenic receptor agonist produces analgesia and sedation is not fully understood but is likely to be multifactorial. Peripherally, α2-agonist produces analgesia by reducing the release of norepinephrine and causing α2-receptor-independent inhibitor effect on nerve fiber action potential. Centrally, α2-agonists produce analgesia and sedation by inhibition of substance P release in the nociceptive pathway at the level of the dorsal root neuron and by activation of α2-adrenoreceptor in the locus coeruleus [44].

As regards, hemodynamics our results showed no statically significant changes in HR nor in MAP in different measurement times, this was quite different from Significant decrease in HR and MAP noticed in many studies, when dexmedetomidine was added to local anesthetics [45,46]. this could be explained by that dexemedtomidine in these studies was given either parentrally or neuroaxially resulting in a central action by decreasing the sympathetic outflow and norepinephrine release.
While our results were similar to Hafez M et al. [38] study who failed to find any statically significant effects of peribulbar dexemedtomidine on haemodymaics.

As regards IOP, our results showed non-significant reduction in IOP in DEX and when compared with the control group and magnesium group.

Also, Hafez M et al. [38] study found a significant reduction in IOP at 5 and 10 min after injection in higher dose (D25) group compared to the baseline in the same group and also with the control group, while he found nonsignificant reduction in IOP in the smaller dose group.

In Eskander AM et al. [35] study, a significant reduction in IOP in DEX group was found at the end of surgery when compared to preoperative values and also when compared with the control group.

In Abdelhamid et al. [32] study more significant reduction was noticed in the IOP when Dexemedetomidine is injected intravenously.

The effects of dexmedetomidine on IOP could be explained by its vasoconstrictive effects on cilliary body blood vessels resulting in a decrease in aqueous humour formation [47]. The combined effects of dexmedetomidine on improving aqueous humour drainage thereby decreasing sympthatic vasoconstriction of aqueous drainage system [48] could be another explanation.

Regarding the assessment of Pain, the VAS during surgery showed significant lower scores in DEX and $MgSO_4$ groups when compared with the control group with non-significant difference between DEX and $MgSO_4$ groups.

This is in contrary to Hafez et al. [38] who found no significant effect to Dexmedetomidine addition in different doses on VAS score when compared to the control group.

The need of supplementary injections was significantly higher in the control group.

The sedation score was significantly higher in dexmedetomidine group when compared with other groups this could be explained by the systemic absorption of dexmedetomidine exerting central sedation effects by α2 agonistic effects which is similar to other studies [33].

References

1. Fekrat S, Elsing SH, Raja SC, Campochiaro PA, Haller JA, et al. (2001) Eye pain after vitreoretinal surgery: a prospective study of 185 patients. Retina 21: 627-632.

2. Jaichandran V (2013) Ophthalmic regional anaesthesia: A review and update. Indian J Anaesth 57: 7-13.

3. Grizzard WS (1989) Ophthalmic anesthesia. Ophthalmol Annu 265-293.

4. Kumar CM (2006) Orbital regional anesthesia: complications and their prevention. Indian J Ophthalmol 54: 77.

5. Palte HD (2015) Ophthalmic regional blocks: management, challenges, and solutions. 8: 57-70.

6. Kallio H, Paloheimo M, Maunuksela EL (2000) Hyaluronidase as an adjuvant in bupivacaine-lidocaine mixture for retrobulbar/peribulbar block. Anesth Analg 91: 934-937.

7. Youssef MM, Girgis K, Soaida SM (2014) Clonidine versus fentanyl as adjuvants to bupivacaine in peribulbar anesthesia. Egypt J Anaesth 30: 267-272.

8. Zahl K, Jordan A, McCroarty J, Sorensen B, Gotta AW (1991) Peribulbar Anesthesia Effect of Bicarbonate on Mixtures of Lidocaine, Bupivacaine and Hyaluronidase with or without Epinephrine. Ophthalmology 98: 239-242.

9. Reah G, Bodenham AR, Braithwaite P, Esmond J, Menage MJ (1998) Peribulbar anaesthesia using a mixture of local anaesthetic and vecuronium. Anaesthesia 53: 551-554.

10. Godarzi M, Beyranvand S, Arbabi S, Sharoughi M, Mohtaram R, et al. (2011) Comparing the effect of using atracourium and cis-atracourium as adjuvant agents to the local anesthetic substance on peribulbar-induced akinesia. Acta Medica Iranica 49: 509-512.

11. Ghanem MT, Tawfeek MA (2016) Adding low dose rocuronium to local anesthetic mixture: Effect on quality of peribulbar blockade for vitreoretinal surgery. Egypt J Anaesth 32: 201-205.

12. Kogler J (2009) The analgesic effect of magnesium sulfate in patients undergoing thoracotomy. Acta Clin Croat 48: 19-26.

13. Singh S, Malviya D, Rai S, Yadav B, Kumar S, et al. (2014) Pre-treatment with Magnesium sulphate before non-depolarizing muscle relaxants: Effect on speed on onset, induction and recovery. Intern J Med Sci Public Health 3: 1238-1243.

14. Chetty S (2011) Dexmedetomidine for acute postoperative pain. SAJAA 17: 139-140.

15. Gandhi RR, Shah AA, Patel I (2012) Use of dexmedetomidine along with bupivacaine for brachial plexus block. Natl J M ed Res 2: 67-69.

16. Yoshitomi T, Kohjitani A, Maeda S, Higuchi H, Shimada M, et al. (2008) Dexmedetomidine enhances the local anesthetic action of lidocaine via an α-2A adrenoceptor. Anesth Analg 107: 96-101.

17. Vartiainen J, MacDonald E, Urtti A, Rouhiainen H, Virtanen R (1992) Dexmedetomidine-induced ocular hypotension in rabbits with normal or elevated intraocular pressures. Invest Ophthalmol Vis Sci 33.

18. Mohamed AZE, Genidy MM (2017) Magnesium sulphate versus dexmedetomidine as an adjuvant to local anesthetic mixture in peribulbar anesthesia. Egyptian J Anaesth.

19. Bakr RH, Abdelaziz HMM (2017) Rocuronium versus dexmedetomidine as an adjuvant to local anesthetics in peribulbar block: A double blind randomized placebo controlled study. Egyptian J Anaesth.

20. Sinha R, Sharma A, Ray B, Chandiran R, Chandralekha C, et al. (2016) Effect of addition of magnesium to local anesthetics for peribulbar block: A prospective randomized double-blind study. Saudi J Anaesth 10: 64-67.

21. Tamer YH, John NB (2013) Rocuronium versus magnesium as an adjuvant to local anesthetics in peribulbar block. Ain-Shams J Anesth 6: 317-321.

22. Nicholson G, Sutton B, Hall GM (2000) Comparison of 1% ropivacaine with 0.75% bupivacaine and 2% lidocaine for peribulbar anaesthesia. British J Anaesth 84: 89-91.

23. Celiker H, Karabas L, Sahin O (2014) A Comparison of Topical or Retrobulbar Anesthesia for 23-Gauge Posterior Vitrectomy. J Ophthalmol 237028.

24. Bahçecioglu H, Ünal M, Artunay Ö, Rasier R, Sarici A (2007) Posterior vitrectomy under topical anesthesia. J Ophthalmol 42: 272-277.

25. Dogramaci M, Lee EJK, Williamson TH (2012) The incidence and the risk factors for iatrogenic retinal breaks during pars plana vitrectomy. Eye (Lond) 26: 718-722.

26. Sztark F, Thiocoip M, Favarel Garrigues JF, Lassie P, Petitjean, et al. (1997) The use of 0.25% lidocaine with fentanyl and pancuronium for intravenous regional anaesthesia. Anaesth Analg 84: 777-779.

27. Ghodraty MR, Saif AA, Kholdebarin AR, Rokhtabnak F, Pournajafian AR, et al. (2012) The effects of magnesium sulfate on neuromuscular blockade by cisatracurium during induction of anesthesia. J Anesth 26: 858-863.

28. Wang H, Liang Q, Cheng L, Li X, Fu W, et al. (2011) Magnesium sulfate enhances non-depolarizing muscle relaxant vecuronium action at adult muscle-type nicotinic acetylcholine receptor in vitro. Acta Pharmacologica Sinica 32: 1454-1459.

29. Morrison AP, Hunter JM, Halpern SH, Banerjee A (2013) Effect of intrathecal magnesium in the presence or absence of local anaesthetic with and without lipophilic opioids: a systematic review and meta-analysis. British journal of anaesthesia 110: 702-712.

30. Haghighi M, Soleymanha M, Sedighinejad A (2015) The Effect of Magnesium Sulfate on Motor and Sensory Axillary Plexus Blockade. Anesthesiology and Pain Medicine 5: e21943.

31. Zhang Y, Shan Z, Kuang L, Xu Y, Xiu H, et al. (2016) Review Article The effect of different doses of intrathecal dexmedetomidine on spinal anesthesia: a meta-analysis. Int J Clin Exp Med 9: 18860-18867.

32. Abdelhamid AM, Mostafa A (2011) Evaluation of the effect of magnesium sulphate vs clonidine as adjunct to local anesthetic during peribulbar anesthesia . Ain Shams J Anesthe 4: 21-22.

33. Dogru K, Yildirim D, Ulgey A, Aksu R, Bicer C, et al. (2011) Adding magnesium to levobupivacaine for axillary brachial plexus block in arteriovenousfistule surgery. Bratisla vs kelekarskelisty 113: 607-609.

34. Narang S, Dali JS, Agarwal M, Garg R (2008) Evaluation of the efficacy of magnesium sulphate as an adjuvant to lignocaine for intravenous regional anesthesia for upper limb surgery. Anaesth IntensiveCare 36: 840-844.

35. Ghatak, T, Chandra G, Malik A, Singh D, Bhatia V K (2010) Evaluation of the effect of magnesium sulphate vs clonidine as adjunct to epidural bupivacaine. Indian J Anaesthe 54: 308.

36. Eskandr AM, Elbakry AEAA, Elmorsy OA (2014) Dexmedetomidine is an effective adjuvant to subtenon block in phacoemulsification cataract surgery. Egyptian J Anaesthe 30: 261-266.

37. El-Ozairy, Hala S, Ayman I, Tharwat (2014) Comparative study of the effect of adding two different doses of dexmedetomidine to levobupivacaine/hyaluronidase mixture on the peribulbar block in vitreoretinal surgery." Ain-Shams J Anaesthe 7: 393.

38. Hafez M, Fahim MR, Abdelhamid MHE, Youssef MHI, Salem AS (2016) The effect of adding dexmedetomidine to local anesthetic mixture for peribulbar block in vitreoretinal surgeries. Egyptian J Anaesthesia.

39. Abdallah FW, Brull R (2013) Facilitatory effects of perineural dexmedetomidine on neuraxial and peripheral nerve block: a systematic review and meta-analysis. Br J Anaesth.

40. Memiş D, Turan A, Karamanlıoğlu B, Şeker Ş, Pamukçu Z (2008) Dexmedetomidine reduces rocuronium dose requirement in sevoflurane anaesthesia. Current Anaesthesia & Critical Care 19: 169-174.

41. Abdelhamid A, Mahmoud A, Abdelhaq M, Yasin H, Bayoumi A (2016) Dexmedetomidine as an additive to local anesthetics compared with intravenous dexmedetomidine in peribulbar block for cataract surgery. Saudi J Anaesth 10: 50-54.

42. Brummett CM, Hong EK, Janda AM, Amodeo FS, Lydic R (2011) Perineural dexmedetomidine added to ropivacaine for sciatic nerve block in rats prolongs the duration of analgesia by blocking the hyperpolarization-activated cation current. Anesthe 115: 836-843.

43. Talke PO, Caldwell JE, Richardson CA, Kirkegaard-Nielsen H, Stafford M (1999) The effects of dexmedetomidine on neuromuscular blockade in human volunteers. Anesth Analg 88: 633-639.

44. Guo TZ, Jiang JY, Buttermann AE, Maze M (1996) Dexmedetomidine injection into the locus ceruleus produces antinociception. Anesthe 84: 873-881.

45. Magdy H, Mohsen M, Saleh M (2015) The effect of intrathecal compared with intravenous dexmedetomidine as an adjuvant to spinal bupivacaine anesthesia for cesarean section. Ain-Shams J Anaesth 8: 93.

46. Bajwa SJS, Bajwa SK, Kaur J, Singh G, Arora V, et al. (2011) Dexmedetomidine and clonidine in epidural anaesthesia: A comparative evaluation. Indian J Anaesth 55: 116.

47. Macri FJ, Cervario SJ (1978) Clonidine. Arch Ophthalmol 96: 2111-2113.

48. Vartianinen J, MacDonald E, Urtti A, Ronhiainen H, Virtanen R (1992) Dexmedetomidine induced ocular hypotension in rabbits with normal or elevated intraocular pressure. Invest Ophthalmol Vis Sci 33: 2019-2023.

Does the Type of Anesthesia for Caesarean Section Affect the Neonate? A Non-Randomized Observational Study Comparing Spinal versus General Anesthesia

Reena Nayar[1*], Jui Lagoo[1] and Chandra Kala[2]

[1]Department of Anesthesiology, St Johns Medical College Hospital, Bangalore, India

[2]Department of Pediatrics, St Johns Medical College, Bangalore, India

[*]**Corresponding author:** Reena Nayar, Professor, Department of Anesthesiology, St Johns Medical College Hospital, Sharjapur Road, Bangalore, Karnataka 560034, India, E-mail: anesthesia62@hotmail.com

Abstract

The influences on neonates due to choice of anesthesia for cesarean section deliveries, general versus spinal were the focus of this prospective non randomized observational study.

Aims and objectives: To study the effects of choice of obstetric anesthesia during Cesarean Section (General (GA) or spinal (SA): on mothers by assessing Mean arterial Blood pressure changes and Time to delivery from initiation of Anesthesia, & Uterine Incision: on neonates by assessing Apgar Scores and Umbilical cord blood parameters.

Material and methods: Two groups of 20 expectant mothers each, posted for elective caesarean sections ASA 1 & 2. Group A: SA Group B: GA. Informed consent, IERB approval, Results: The two groups were comparable in terms of age, weight, pre-operative mean arterial pressure and gravid status. The mean speed of surgery in minutes was significantly faster under General Anesthesia (8.65 to 17.6) when measured from induction of anesthesia to delivery time, and (1.65 to 2.4) when measured from uterine incision to delivery time. The upper limit of block of spinal anesthesia was variable, but mostly centered around T4, T6. The maximum values of Fluctuations in the Blood pressure in the two groups showed that the SA group had a drop in the mean arterial pressure up to 54 mmHg, while the GA group showed a rise in the mean arterial pressure up to 107 mmHg. The neonatal cord blood parameters across the two groups showed no significant differences in pH, PCO_2, HCO_3, and base excess. However umbilical cord venous blood oxygenation (35.86) and Oxygen saturation (58.71) were significantly better when delivery was under GA in comparison with SA (26.59 and 44.58).

Discussion: The benefits of a faster surgical time achieved under General anesthesia were not quantifiable as no difference in apgar score in the neonates of the two groups at 1 or 5 minute. The fluctuations in Blood pressure likewise did not translate to evidence of fetal hypoxia. The increased blood oxygenation as a consequence of controlled anesthesia was the only noteworthy finding in the cord blood analysis.

Conclusion: There were no statistically significant changes on the apgar score of neonates or their blood biochemistry, if the choice of anesthesia for cesarean section were general or spinal. Cord blood oxygenation was higher with general anesthesia.

Keywords: Anesthesia for caesarean section; Obstetric anesthesia; Effect on neonates; General anesthesia; Spinal anesthesia

Introduction

The choice of anesthesia for obstetric anesthesia has been traditionally influenced by patient and physician preferences.

Maternal safety, the absence of narcotic effects, avoidance of inhalant anesthesia, or intra venous drugs leading to an awake mother, who can initiate lactation early and with less pain due to post-operative residual analgesia and hence a better psychological outcome, are compelling arguments favouring use of regional anesthesia.

Epidural anesthesia or Spinal with epidural anesthesia is gradually becoming the preferred anesthesia choice in obstetric anesthesia. Spinal anesthesia is still a mainstay in Caesarean Section as it avoids a general anaesthetic with concomitant risks of failed intubation especially in anatomical abnormalities, and risks of ventilation in respiratory diseases. The mother is conscious and the partner is able to be present at the birth of the child. The post-operative analgesia from intrathecally administered opioids and non-steroidal anti-inflammatory drugs are also good. Ease of administration, improved needles which reduce the post puncture headache and faster onset time of anesthesia favour the use of spinal anesthesia

General Anesthesia with its superior control over ventilation, avoidance of hypotension seen with spinal anesthesia, speed of induction, and lack of awareness of the perioperative period is preferred in emergency situations and in selected elective procedures [1].

Apocryphal anecdotes attribute to Dr Walter Channing of Harvard in 1847 the first attempt to report on the effects of anesthesia on the neonate by crudely attempted to smell ether at the cut ends of the cords stating that there were negligible effects on the neonate! [2]. The influences on neonates due to anesthesia for cesarean section deliveries is usually not a factor in the choice, and it is maybe time to revisit this issue. Neonatal impact needs to be considered in the decision paradigm, especially as advances in anesthesia and monitoring have altered the reality of practice of obstetric anesthesia.

In our tertiary level referral hospital setting we conducted this pilot prospective non randomized observational study to look at this aspect of caesarean anesthesia.

Aims and Objectives

To study the effects of choice of obstetric anesthesia during Caesarean Section (General (GA) or spinal (SA)), on mothers by assessing

Mean arterial Blood pressure changes.

Time to delivery from initiation of Anesthesia & Uterine Incision

To study the effects of choice of obstetric anesthesia (GA *vs.* SA) in Neonates by assessing

i) Apgar Scores

ii) Umbilical cord blood parameters: such as: pH, PCO_2, PO_2, HCO_3, etc.

Materials and Methods

After obtaining Institutional Ethical Board clearance (IERB/RS/1/1/132/11) Intra mural funding for the study was obtained from the St Johns Hospital Research Society, (PO167).

Two groups of 20 expectant mothers each, posted for elective caesarean sections who were ASA 1 & 2 were included in the study. The choice of anesthesia was made after discussion with the patient and obstetrician. Inclusion in the two arms of the study was post hoc, and not randomized. Informed consent for the study was obtained from the mothers.

Patients undergoing emergency caesarean section due to maternal or fetal causes were excluded from this study. Epidural anesthesia and spinal with epidural is a feature of a parallel study hence not reported in this analysis.

Group A: Spinal anesthesia

Group B: General anesthesia

The anesthesia techniques in both followed standard institutional guidelines and no deviations were noted.

For general anesthesia after preoxygenation for 3 minutes, intravenous Rapid sequence induction with thiopentone sodium (5 mg/kg), succinyl choline (2 mg/kg), followed by intubation, and maintained with 50% oxygen, nitrous oxide and isoflurane mixture, and atracurium (0.3 mg/kg body weight initially, with bolus of 10 mg). After delivery, and clamping of the umbilical cord, oxytocin drip (20 units in 500 ml normal saline) and Fentanyl 2 mcg/kg was administered. Patients were reversed with neostigmine 50 mcg/kg and glycopyrrolate 10 mcg/kg and extubated.

For spinal anesthesia after preloading with normal saline, 10 ml/kg body weight, 2 ml of 0.5% hyperbaric bupivacine was introduce intrathecally at L 3-4 space, via a 25 gauge spinal needle. Oxygenation

at 5 litre/minute with mask was administered during the delivery. Vasopressors ephedrine (6 mg boluses) was given when Mean Arterial Pressure (MAP) dropped to less than 20% of the base line.

Documentation of maternal and fetal parameters, umbilical cord venous blood readings were done as per our standard institutional proforma. The blood pressure (NIBP automated) and heart rate was recorded every minute for the first five minutes, and thereafter at 5 minute intervals till completion of the procedure. Maternal factors such as Previous LSCS, Obesity (BMI), maternal age at delivery, week of pregnancy at time of delivery, smoking status in the mother, and birth weight in the neonate were identified as potential Confounders. Multivariate regression analysis, with adjusted odds ratio was calculated. The sample size in each arm was 20, as this was a pilot study to detect trends in our institution with current standardized protocols. Descriptive statistics were reported using mean and Standard Deviation for the continuous variables, and number and percentages for the categorical variables. Inferential statistics used Independent Sample T Test between the two groups for comparison of clinical and demographic parameters. P value less that 5% was considered as statistically significant and multivariate regression analysis for confounders using SPSS version 17.1.

Results

The two groups of expectant mothers chosen for the study were comparable in terms of age, weight, pre-operative mean arterial pressure and gravid status (Table 1).

Parameters		Spinal Anesthesia	General Anesthesia
Age in Years			
	Mean	28.35	26.55
	Standard Deviation	3.376	4.915(SED: 1.3)
	Range	22-34	20-35
Weight in Kg			
	Mean	61.5	53.25
	Standard Deviation	11.56	4.79 (SED: 2.79)
	Range	40-83	45-61
Mean arterial pressure (mm Hg)			
	Mean	84.95	86.7
	Standard Deviation	8.153	5.4
	Range	68-100	76-96
Gravid status			
	I	5	11
	II	10	4
	III	5	4
	IV	0	1

Table 1: Maternal Demographics.

Did the choice of anesthesia affect the surgical time?

Two parameters were studied to determine the influence of anesthesia on surgical time, the time from induction of anesthesia to delivery time, and the time from uterine incision to delivery time. (Table 2). The speed of surgery in our study was significantly faster under General Anesthesia (8.65 mins mean to 17.6 mins mean) when measured from induction of anesthesia to delivery time, and likewise (1.65 min to 2.4 min mean) when measured from uterine incision to delivery time.

Parameters		Spinal Anesthesia	General Anesthesia
Anesthesia to Delivery time in minutes			
	Mean	17.6	8.65
	Standard Deviation	4.99	4.46 (P value 0.0001)
Uterine Incision to Delivery Time			
	Mean	2.4	1.65
	Standard Deviation	1.31	0.87 (P value 0.041)

Table 2: Maternal Demographics.

Did the Level of block in Spinal Anesthesia alter the maximum fluctuation in Blood pressure?

The upper limit of block of spinal anesthesia was variable, but mostly centered around T4, T6. The drop in Blood pressure as an average from the base line did not appear to be related to the level of block (Table 3).

Level of Block	No of cases	Drop in BP (Avg) from Baseline
T2	1	60 mm
T4	6	58.2 mm
T6	10	53.5 mm
T8	3	57.0 mm

Table 3: Upper limit of spinal anesthesia block.

Did the fluctuations from the base line of mean blood pressure differ significantly between the two groups?

The maximum values of Fluctuations in the Blood pressure in the two groups during the course of the surgery were noted in both groups. The mean of these values showed that the Spinal anesthesia group as expected showed a drop in the mean arterial pressure up to 54 mm of Hg, while the General anesthesia group showed a gain in the mean arterial pressure up to 107 mm of Hg (Table 4).

Maximum fluctuation from Base line Mean Art Pressure	Spinal Anesthesia	General Anesthesia
Mean	54.6	107.45
Standard Deviation	8.623	5.482

Table 4: Maximum fluctuation from Base line Mean Art Pressure.

Did the choice of anesthesia have an effect on the neonates?

The neonatal apgar scores were normal both at one minute and 5 minutes in both groups studied, and there were consequently no significant differences across the two methods of anesthesia adopted for cesarean section (Table 5).

	Spinal Anesthesia	General Anesthesia
At one minute		
Mean	8	7.95
Standard Deviation	0.27	0.39
At 5 minutes		
Mean	9.1	9
Standard Deviation	0.304	0.4

Table 5: Neonatal Apgar scores.

Did the choice of anesthesia affect the Umbilical cord blood parameters?

The neonatal cord blood parameters across the two groups were biochemically similar. There were no significant differences noted in pH, pCO_2, HCO_3, and base excess across the two groups of neonates (Table 6).

	S.A	G.A
pH (Mean/S D)	7.32/.054	7.31/.049
pCO_2 (Mean/S D) mm/hg	43.73/7.21	45.75/8.41
HCO_3 (Mean/S D) mmol/L	22.16/2.9	22.78/2.83
Base Excess (Mean/ S D) mmmol/L	3.465/2.37	3.59/1.69

Table 6: Neonatal Biochemical parameters.

However umbilical cord blood oxygenation (35.86) and Oxygen saturation (58.71) were significantly better in the group delivered under general anesthesia in comparison with those values of the group delivered under spinal anesthesia (26.59 and 44.58) (Table 7).

	S.A	G.A
PO_2 in mm of Hg		
Mean	26.59	35.86
S.D	4.76	6.83 Significant difference P value (0.0001)
Oxygen Saturation percentage (SO_2)		
Mean	44.58	58.71

Table 7: Umbilical Cord blood oxygenation.

Analgesia in the spinal anesthesia group was maintained optimally in all patients without additional narcotics. In the post-operative period after general anesthesia, addition of narcotic medication, such as pethidine 5 mg/kg was used for analgesia hence a direct comparison was not made of this parameter.

Post section lactation and feeding initiation was earlier in the Spinal Anesthesia group (Mean 1.5 h with a SD of 15), compared to the General Anesthesia group (Mean of 4 h with an SD of 45).

Did use of vasopressors in the event of fall in the BP during Spinal anesthesia affect Neonatal cord blood parameters?

Fall in maternal BP (MAP<20% from baseline) necessitated the use of vasopressors in 7 out of 20 patients. However, no significant alteration in neonatal cord blood parameters were noted.

In summary the two Groups were comparable in the Maternal Parameters pre delivery. The GA group surgical time was much faster measured both as an Initiation of anesthesia to delivery and the Uterine Incision to delivery time. In the spinal anesthesia group the Level of anesthesia mainly at T6 but a variation of the highest level was noted. The neonatal outcomes too showed no variation across Apgar Scores, pH, HCO_3, Base Excess, Lactate and PCO_2. However in the General Anesthesia group PO_2 and SO_2 were higher.

Discussion

The choice of anesthetic most appropriate for a cesarean depends on many factors, such as the urgency of the situation, maternal medical condition etc. But as better understanding of materno fetal conditions, risks and benefits have evolved; obstetric anesthesia practice too has continuously evolved. Given that the principal purpose of a caesarean section is to deliver a baby in as good or better condition than when the decision to operate is taken, it appears logical to examine critically the influence of the choice of anesthesia on the neonatal outcome [3].

This aspect has been studied earlier with equivocal results [4-7]; however, given the availability of newer anesthetic agents and more rigid protocols; the current study was an attempt to look at this aspect of obstetric anesthesia in our institutional setting.

In the present study, using comparable groups we noted that surgical time, as estimated from induction to delivery, and uterine incision to delivery was significantly reduced in the General anesthesia group.

Krishnan et al. in their study concluded that delivery should be completed within 6-8 minutes after GA induction to prevent neonatal resp depression due to inhalant gas [6]. Evans et al. while noting the incidence of respiratory depression in children born of a general anesthesia attributed it to the effect of nitrous oxide crossing the placenta in case of a delay in delivery [3]. Kamat et al. noted a lowering of Apgar score in prolonged delivery time [5].

In our study the mean time from Initiation of anesthesia to delivery was 8.6 mins in the G.A group but no significant changes in Apgar score were noted when compared to the SA group with a mean time of 17.6 mins.

This finding is similar to what was noted by authors earlier [5,6]. The precise significance of this negative correlation can be questioned, given the lack of adverse effects on the neonate even if there were a surgical delay given controlled conditions in modern operation suites.

The role of Oxygenation of the mother during Cesarean Section was also studied earlier, and it was noted that fetal hypoxia improved when 65% oxygen was given to mothers [7]. The lateral decubitus position was reportedly beneficial for fetal oxygenation [8].

In our study, we noted significantly higher PO_2, (35.86 mmHg) and SO_2 values (58.71 %) in GA cases, who received 50% oxygen and were delivered in left lateral position as a routine. However, as neither group had any significant alteration in Apgar scores, the significance of these findings must remain equivocal. It has been suggested that other neurobehavioural scoring systems may be more relevant than conventional Apgar Scoring in this regard [9].

The concern that hypotension the most common side effect of spinal anesthesis especially if untreated can lead to fetal acidosis because of diminished uteroplacental blood flow. Was highlighted as Fetal Acidosis is a risk for adverse neonatal outcome [10]. A pH<7 associated with neurologic and other organ damage. Some morbidity may be seen between pH=7-7 [1]. However, this has never been established in studies. In a study of 238 cases of cesarean sections, it was reported that significant neonatal acidosis, and lowered oxygenation were noted in neonates born of mothers receiving spinal anesthesia, though without evident effect on fetal wellbeing [11].

In our study too, we did not note any significant acidosis in blood gas analysis, in the group of neonates, who were delivered receiving Spinal Anesthesia even though there was significant maternal hypotension in that group.

The use of vasopressors to correct significant drop in blood pressure during spinal anesthesia did not cause significant alteration in cord blood parameters. This finding was similar to results from an earlier retrospective database analysis comparing cord blood parameters when phenylephrine was used instead of ephedrine [12].

Analysis of Ischaemic modified albumin (IMA) in cord blood as an early marker for ischemic events has been used to explore subtle alterations in blood oxygenations [13].

On the basis of our study no clear advice for a change in protocols was made in our institution. We note that though Spinal Anesthesia leads to a significant drop in BP, no significant fetal acidosis develops. However the oxygenation of the neonate is significantly better with General Anesthesia. Hence case individualisation was still recommended on the basis of the study. There were no alterations in umbilical cord blood values across the group in this limited sample, hence no further conclusions were drawn.

Larger patient numbers, inclusion of Epidural and spinal with epidural anesthesia cases, Emergency cases, study of IMA and other ischemia markers and a longer term follow up of neonates to validate these observations are aspects being reviewed at our centre for further prospective analysis.

References

1. McCallum RH (2013) Anesthesia for Cesarean delivery. Shnider and Levinsons-Anesthesia for Obstetrics (5thedn) Wolters Kluwer /Lippincott Williams& Wilkins, Philadelphia. Chapter 12: 174.

2. Campbell D, Sam Vincente M (2013) Placental transfer of drugs. Shnider and Levinsons-Anesthesia for Obstetrics (5thedn) Wolters Kluwer / Lippincott Williams& Wilkins, Philadelphia 3: 46.

3. Evans CM, MurphyJF, Gray OP, Rosen M (1989) Epidural versus General Anesthesia for Elective Cesarean Section, Effect on Apgar Score and acid-base status of the newborn. Anaesthesia 44: 778-782.

4. Ong BY, Cohen MM, Palahniuk RJ (1989) Anesthesia for Cesarean section-Effects on Neonates. Anesth Analg 68: 270-275.

5. Kamat SK, Shah MV, Chaudhary LS, Pandya S, Bhatt MM (1991) Effect of induction delivery and uterine delivery on apgar scoring of the newborn. J Postgrad Med 37: 125-127.

6. Krishnan L, Gunasekaran N, Bhaskaranand N (1995) Neonatal Effects of Anesthesia for Caesarean Section. Indian J Pediatr 62:109-113.

7. Zagorxycki MT (1984) General Anesthesia in Caeserean Section: Effect on Mother and Neonate. Obsteric Gynecol Survey 39: 134-137.

8. Hodgson CA, Wanchob TD (1994) A comparison of Spinal and general anesthesia for elective cesarean section: effect on neonatal condition at birth. Int J Obstet Anesth 3: 25-30.

9. BeckmannM, Calderbank S (2012) Mode of anesthetic for category 1 ceasarean sections and neonatal outcomes. Aust NZ J Obstet Gynaecol 52: 316-320.

10. Saini CK, DeySK, Chaturvedi P, Tikle AC (1992) Effect of General and Spinal Anesthesia on Neuro Behavioural Response in Cesarean Babies, Indian Pediatrics 29: 621-626.

11. Peropoulous F, Siristatidis C, Salamalekis E, Creatsas G (2003) Spinal and Epidural versus general anesthesia for elective cesarean section at terk: effect on the acid base status of the mother and newborn. J Mat Fetal Neonatal Med 13: 260-266.

12. Strouch ZY, Dakik CG, White WD, Habid AS (2015) Anesthetic technique for cesarean delivery and neonatal acid-base status. A retrospective database analysis. Int J Obst Anaesth 24: 22-29.

13. Omur D, Hacivelioglu SO, Oguzalp H, Uyan B, Kiraz HA, et al. (2013) The effect of anaesthesia technique on maternal and cord blood ischaemia-modified albumin levels during caesarean section: A randomized controlled study. J Int Med Res 41: 1111-1119.

Effect of Different Doses of Dexmedetomidine on Stress Response and Emergence Agitation after Laparoscopic Cholecystectomy: Randomized Controlled Double-Blind Study

Mohamed F Mostafa[1*], **Ragaa Herdan**[1], **Mohammed Yahia Farrag Aly**[2] and **Azza Abo Elfadle**[3]

[1]Department of Anesthesia, Faculty of Medicine, Assiut University, Egypt

[2]Department of Surgery, Faculty of Medicine, Assiut University, Egypt

[3]Department of Clinical Pathology, Assiut University Hospital, Assiut, Egypt

*Corresponding author: Mohamed F Mostafa, Lecturer of Anesthesia and Intensive Care, Faculty of Medicine, Assiut University, Assiut, Egypt, E-mail: mo7_fathy@yahoo.com

Abstract

Background: Emergence agitation (EA) may develops during recovery from general anesthesia. It causes confusion, disorientation, and unpredictable behaviours. Surgical stress response activates the sympathetic nervous system and increase the release of catabolic hormones leading to prolonged hospital stay.

Objectives: We designed this study to assess the effect of different doses of intra-operative dexmedetomidine infusion on surgical stress response, emergence agitation and postoperative outcome.

Study design: A controlled double-blind study was conducted using a computer-generated randomization scheme.

Setting: The study was conducted in Assiut University Hospitals, Assiut, Egypt.

Methods: 90 patients scheduled for laparoscopic cholecystectomy were randomly assigned into three equal groups to receive intraoperative dexmedetomidine infusion over 20 minutes before end of surgery. Group I received 1 µg/kg, group II received 0.75 µg/kg and group III received 0.5 µg/kg.

Results: We found that dexmedetomidine (0.5, 0.75 or 1 µg/kg) can decrease the incidence of EA when infused 20 minutes before skin closure in laparoscopic cholecystectomy in adults. Lower agitation scores, pain scores, cortisol and glucose levels were observed during the first 2 hours postoperatively with no serious complications.

Limitations: First, we think a larger number of patients may be needed to detect better comparison between different doses of dexmedetomidine in preventing EA and monitor possible complications. Second, we did not take in mind any other preoperative predisposing factors that may affect the incidence of EA especially anxiety or smoking. Finally, we did not use any monitoring for depth of anesthesia which has an important factor in the incidence of emergence agitation.

Conclusion: We conclude that low doses of dexmedetomidine infusion (0.5 µg/kg) over 20 minutes before skin closure are effective as higher doses (0.75 and 1 µg/kg) to decrease stress response and incidence of emergence agitation in laparoscopic cholecystectomy in adults with less adverse effects.

Keywords: Dexmedetomidine; Stress; Emergence agitation; Laparoscopic cholecystectomy

Introduction

Emergence agitation (EA) may develop during recovery from general anesthesia. It causes confusion, disorientation, and unpredictable behaviors [1]. It is more common in children than adults [2]. Serious complications may occur as a result of agitation such as bleeding, self extubation, removal of catheters, hypoxia or even aspiration [3]. The exact etiology and sequence of EA in adults are not well-cleared yet [4].

Tissue injuries during surgeries can lead to stress response [5]. Surgical stress response activates the sympathetic nervous system and increases the release of catabolic hormones. Changes in heart rate, blood pressure and cortisol levels also may occur [6]. Prolonged hospital stay may be the result of all these events [7].

The highly selective alpha-2 receptor agonist; Dexmedetomidine; has many anti-stress, sedative and analgesic actions [8]. It decreases surgical stress response and leads to better stable hemodynamic properties [9]. Dexmedetomidine decreases the postoperative supplemental analgesic requirements and pain intensity. Information about dexmedetomidine and EA is limited especially in adult patients [10].

Objectives

We designed this study to assess the effect of different doses of intraoperative dexmedetomidine infusion on the surgical stress response and general anesthesia. Also, we evaluated the effect of these doses on the post-anesthetic emergence agitation, quality of recovery after surgery, postoperative analgesic requirements and complications.

Methods

Eligibility

This study was carried out after approval from our Faculty Ethical Committee (ref. no. IRB00008718). Clinical trials registration was approved under this number NCT02917018. All patients were informed with complete information about the anesthesia and analgesia techniques that would be provided to them. A written informed consent was obtained from each patient before entry in this study.

Sample size calculation

It is based on the pilot study, where the incidence of surgical stress response in laparoscopies is found to be more than 70% and intervention that can cause 25% reduction in this incidence will be interesting. With a power of 90% and type I error of 5%, 27 patients were required to be in each group (α=0.05 and β=90%), but to avoid possible loss of samples (dropouts) during the study, the number of patients in each group is increased to 30.

Study design

A controlled double-blind study was conducted on 90 patients scheduled for elective laparoscopic cholecystectomy. They were randomly allocated using a computer-generated randomization program into three equal groups to receive intraoperative infusion of dexmedetomidine (Precedex, 100 µg/ml, Hospira, Inc., Rocky Mount, IL, USA). Access to the randomization codes was only available to one anesthesiologist. Group I received 1 µg/kg, group II received 0.75 µg/kg and group III received 0.5 µg/kg diluted to 50 ml NaCl 0.9% by syringe pump over 20 minutes before end of surgery. The study drugs and randomization were prepared by the second anesthesiologist while drug administration and observations were done by the first anesthesiologist.

Inclusion criteria

ASA I-II, Age 20 to 60 years, both sex and Laparoscopic cholecystectomy under general anesthesia

Exclusion criteria

Any cardiac disease, diabetes, reactive upper airway disease, known allergies to dexmedetomidine, cognitive disorders, renal insufficiency or hepatic dysfunction. Chronic use of analgesics, cortisone or drugs known to interact with dexmedetomidine.

Preoperative assessment and preparation: The day prior to surgery, all patients underwent pre-anesthetic check-up including detailed history, general & systemic examination and weight measurement.

Anesthetic technique

With no premedication, all patients received pre-oxygenation by O_2 100% for 3-5 minutes and intravenous access was secured. NaCl 0.9% 4 ml/kg/h were infused intraoperatively. General anesthesia was induced by fentanyl 1 µg/kg, propofol 2 mg/kg and nimbex (cisatracurium) 0.15 mg/kg. Endotracheal intubation then was inserted using oral ETT of appropriate size under direct laryngoscopy and secured at the angle of the mouth. Sevoflurane inhalational anesthetic (2-4 %) in 100% oxygen and nimbex 0.03 mg/kg were used for maintenance of anesthesia. The lungs were mechanically ventilated to keep intra-operative EtCO$_2$ between 35-40 mmHg.

Intraoperative monitoring: Routine monitors including ECG, non-invasive blood pressure, pulse oximetry and EtCO$_2$ were recorded every 5 minutes during the intraoperative 20 minutes of the study drug administration. Bradycadia (heart rate<60 beat/minute) was treated with IV atropine 0.5 mg. Hypotension (mean arterial blood pressure<60 mmHg) was treated with IV ephedrine 5 mg increments. Durations of anesthesia, sevoflurane % and duration of surgery were recorded.

At the end of surgery and stoppage of sevoflurane inhalation, neostigmine 0.04 mg/kg and atropine 0.02 mg/kg were used for muscle relaxant reversal (Time 0 in the emergence process), patients were extubated and transferred to the PACU for recovery and monitoring.

Assessment in PACU: Routine monitoring was continued during staying in the PACU. During emergence, the level of agitation was evaluated using the Ricker Sedation-Agitation Scale "RSAS" [11]. The maximum level of agitation was recorded for each patient at time 0, 5, 10, 20, 30, 60, 90 and 120 minutes.

Emergence agitation was defined when RSAS $\geq$ 5. Dangerous agitation was defined when RSAS=7 and it was treated with fentanyl 1 µg/kg.

Duration of stay in PACU was recorded. Criteria for discharge from PACU were applied according to the modified Aldrete scoring system. A score $\geq$ 9 was required for discharge [12].

Postoperative analgesia: The 10 points Visual Analogue Scale (VAS) for pain measurement was used to assess the severity of postoperative pain. Score 0 indicated no pain and score 10 indicated severe pain. If VAS $\geq$ 4, rescue analgesia was indicated. Perfalgan (perfalgan_, paracetamol 1000 mg. UPSA laboratories, France) infusion was used as supplemental analgesia. The first dose and the total amount in 24 hours of perfalgan were recorded. Patient's satisfaction was also recorded at the end of the first 24 hours postoperatively.

Blood sampling: All blood samples (2 ml each sample) were venous and obtained from peripheral vessels (antecubital vein) away from the limb infused with fluids. Samples were withdrawn 20 minutes pre-operatively, 20 minutes after skin incision, just after skin closure and 2 hours after end of surgery. The blood samples were centrifuged at 3500 $\times$ g for at least 10 minutes and then serum samples were collected for cortisol level analysis. Blood glucose levels were also recorded at the same times.

Statistical analysis

Statistical analysis was conducted with SPSS version 20 (SPSS Inc., Chicago, IL, USA) for Windows. Quantitative data were compared using One-way ANOVA and Student's t-test. Qualitative data were analyzed using the Chi-square test. P-values <0.05 were considered statistically significant.

Results

90 patients were enrolled in our study and randomly allocated into 3 equal groups of 30 patients each. There was no statistically significant difference with respect to Patients' characteristics (age, sex, weight, BMI, duration of anesthesia, duration of surgery and time to extubation) between the three study groups (Table 1).

Variable		Group I (n=30)	Group II (n=30)	Group III (n=30)	P value
Age (years)		32.71 ± 13.30	36.31 ± 11.18	33.56 ± 13.19	NS
Sex					
	Male	11	16	13	NS
	Female	19	14	17	
Weight (kg)		65.18 ± 10.77	65.72 ± 11.09	63.64 ± 10.95	NS
BMI		23.89 ± 3.20	24.28 ± 3.10	23.55 ± 3.41	NS
Duration of Anesthesia (minutes)		80.22 ± 19.95	78.91 ± 20.86	80.50 ± 20.16	NS
Duration of Surgery (minutes)		71.15 ± 20.37	69.82 ± 21.09	70.44 ± 20.71	NS
Time to extubation after end of surgery (minutes)		9.11 ± 2.77	8.97 ± 3.10	8.90 ± 3.09	NS
Data were expressed as mean ± SD and numbers.					

Table 1: Patients' characteristics of the three study groups.

There was no statistically significant difference between the three study groups during the whole intraoperative and 2 hours postoperative periods regarding heart rate, mean arterial blood pressure, oxygen saturation or $EtCO_2$.

We noted slight insignificant reduction in heart rate and mean arterial blood pressure than the pre-infusion readings.

Emergence agitation scoring (RSAS)

We noted decrease incidence of agitation in our patients. It occurred only in 3 (10%) cases in the group I, in 3 cases (10%) in group II and in 5 cases (16.7%) in group III. The RSAS was 4.03 ± 1.49 in group I, 4.11 ± 1.35 in group II and 4.42 ± 1.05 in group III.

There was no statistically significant difference between the three study groups as regarding the incidence or the scoring of emergence agitation in the recovery room (Table 2).

Pain scoring

Patients in the three study groups recorded low VAS pain scores through the postoperative 2 hours in the recovery room. VAS was 3.79 ± 1.93 in group I, 3.64 ± 2.01 in group II and 3.75 ± 2.12 in group III. There was no statistically significant difference between the three study groups as regarding VAS pain scoring (Table 2).

Patients in group I stayed in the PACU for 42.32 ± 7.15 minutes while patients in group II stayed in PACU for 40.58 ± 8.03 minutes and patients in group III stayed in PACU for 43.19 ± 7.10 minutes with no statistically significant difference between the three groups (Table 2).

Variable	Group I (n=30)	Group II (n=30)	Group III (n=30)	P value
Incidence of agitation in PACU (no.)	3 (10%)	3 (10%)	5 (16.7%)	0.098
RSAS	4.03 ± 1.49	4.11 ± 1.35	4.42 ± 1.05	0.127
VAS	3.79 ± 1.93	3.64 ± 2.01	3.75 ± 2.21	0.108
Duration of stay in PACU (minutes)	42.32 ± 7.15	40.58 ± 8.03	43.19 ± 7.10	0.116
Data were expressed as no. percentages, mean ± SD.				

Table 2: Postoperative Emergence Agitation and Pain Scoring.

Supplemental analgesia

12 (40%) patients in group I required supplemental analgesia during the first 24 hours postoperatively while 15 (50%) patients in group II and 14 (46.7%) patients in group III required supplemental analgesia with no statistically significant difference between the three groups (Table 3). Regarding the time of 1st analgesic requirement and the total amount of supplemental analgesia, there were no statistically significant differences between the three groups (Table 3). 21 patients in group I, 20 patients in group II and 17 patients in group III were satisfied with the results of our study (Table 3).

Regarding serum cortisol and blood glucose levels, there were no statistically significant differences between the three study groups (Tables 4,5). These levels were increased after surgical skin incision and decreased at the end of surgery with drug infusion indicating the effect of dexmedetomidine in decreasing stress response related to surgery.

Variable	Group I (n=30)	Group II (n=30)	Group III (n=30)	P value
No. of patients need analgesia	12 (40%)	15 (50%)	14 (46.7%)	NS
Time of first analgesia (hours)	4.17 ± 1.12	4.90 ± 1.33	4.51 ± 1.62	NS
Total amount of Perfulgan in first 24 hours (grams)	28.31 ± 3.65	29.82 ± 3.99	29.79 ± 4.03	NS
Patients' Satisfaction				
Yes	21 (70%)	20 (66.7)	17 (56.7)	NS
No	9 (30%)	10 (33)	13 (43.3)	

Data were expressed as numbers, percentages, mean ± SD.

Table 3: Supplemental Analgesia and Patients' Satisfaction.

Variable	Group I (n=30)	Group II (n=30)	Group III (n=30)	P value
20 minutes preoperatively	92.57 ± 4.32	90.88 ± 4.91	89.96 ± 5.20	0.184
20 minutes after skin incision	232.13 ± 17.65	235.29 ± 19.14	234.66 ± 19.61	0.093
Just after skin closure	190.83 ± 14.77	193.25 ± 15.39	190.12 ± 15.01	0.101
2 hours after end of surgery	188.45 ± 11.27	190.76 ± 14.50	191.02 ± 11.16	0.237

Data were expressed as mean ± SD.

Table 4: Serum cortisol level changes in the three study groups.

Variable	Group I (n=30)	Group II (n=30)	Group III (n=30)	P value
20 minutes preoperatively	88.36 ± 6.71	90.84 ± 7.52	91.90 ± 7.81	0.085
20 minutes after skin incision	127.58±27.46	130.13±28.70	128.67 ± 28.59	0.104
Just after skin closure	120.33 ± 11.96	121.00 ± 11.58	121.51 ± 11.30	0.099
2 hours after end of surgery	121.64 ± 15.32	120.54 ± 16.06	120.72 ± 16.13	0.113

Data were expressed as mean ± SD.

Table 5: Blood glucose level changes in the three study groups.

There were no serious complications noted throughout the whole conduct of our study. Few cases of nausea, vomiting, headache, hypotension or bradycardia were recorded and treated promptly (Table 6).

Variable	Group I (n=30)	Group II (n=30)	Group III (n=30)	P value
Nausea & Vomiting	6 (20%)	7 (23.3%)	6 (20%)	NS
Bradycardia	1 (3.3%)	0 (0%)	0 (0%)	NS
Hypotension	2 (6.7%)	0 (0%)	0 (0%)	NS
Headache	4 (13.3%)	5 (16.7%)	2 (6.7%)	NS

Data were expressed as numbers, percentages.

Table 6: Postoperative complications in the three study groups.

Discussion

Emergence agitation (EA) can be defined as a transient condition of agitation, may occur during recovery from general anesthesia. Surgical stress response may have a role in EA pathogenesis [13]. Surgeries closed to diaphragm usually decrease the vital capacity, movement of the diaphragm and respiratory functions especially in PACU [14]. Many contributing factors can affect the incidence of EA and a lot of studies tried to discover these factors [15].

We found that dexmedetomidine (0.5, 0.75 or 1 μg/kg) can decrease the incidence of EA when infused 20 minutes before skin closure in laparoscopic cholecystectomy in adults. Lower pain scores were recorded during the first 2 hours postoperatively then supplemental analgesics were prescribed when needed.

Dexmedetomidine has anxiolytic, analgesic and sympatholytic effects through activation of α2 receptors in CNS, decreasing the neuronal activities and enhancing the vagal activities [16]. The α2 agonists have a clear role on CVS as they inhibit the release of catecholamines by vasoconstrictive effect augmentation [17].

Emergence from general anesthesia is equal to the stress of laryngoscopy. The effect of sudden decrease of anesthetic depth and rapid increase in catecholamines levels may lead to serious complications. Dexmedetomidine leads to a smooth transition from sudden cessation of anesthesia and the recovery [18].

One study concluded the intraoperative infusion of dexmedetomidine (0.4 μg/kg/hr) until extubation can decrease the incidence of EA after nasal surgeries in adults without increasing complications or delaying extubation [19]. Another study found dexmedetomidine can reduce EA after anesthesia in adults by about 46% [20].

Some investigators evaluated the effect of dexmedetomidine (0.1 or 0.3 μg/kg) on EA. They found the better results with the 0.3 μg/kg dose [21]. It has anesthetic-sparing, anxiolytics and analgesic effect with no respiratory depressant effect [22].

When dexmedetomidine was administered 0.3 or 0.5 μ/kg post-induction in the pre-school children, reduced incidence and severity of emergence agitation after sevoflurane anesthesia were observed. No delayed recovery or hemodynamic instability was associated with the smaller dose [23].

According to our observations, we did not find any serious hemodynamic changes throughout our study period. One case of slight bradycardia and two cases of hypotension were found insignificantly and easily corrected. Cortisol and glucose levels showed increased readings after start the operative maneuver then these levels decreased at the end of drug infusion and end of surgery.

Some studies showed the higher doses (0.5 or 1 µg/kg) of dexmedetomidine can decrease the incidence of EA after sevoflurane inhalation but can affect the hemodynamics of the patients [24]. Another study used different doses of dexmedetomidine (0.1-10 µg/kg/h) but there was a higher incidence of hypotension and bradycardia especially in large doses [25].

Use of dexmedetomidine 0.4 µg/kg as a bolus injection within 30 minutes after general anesthesia induction can stabilize the patient's heart rate and blood pressure during emergence after thyroid gland surgery and also decreases awakening and extubation times [26].

We used smaller doses of dexmedetomidine infusion to avoid rapid changes in hemodynamics. Stress response in anesthetized patients can lead to autonomic or endocrine disturbance. Hemodynamic changes are usually unpredictable [27]. Cortisol level is widely used as the marker of surgical stress response [28]. A dose-dependent decrease in heart rate and arterial blood pressure occurred with dexmedetomidine, and decrease of sympathetic nervous activity was observed through the recorded levels of norepinephrine in plasma [29].

A previous research reported that dexmedetomidine use can significantly reduce the circulating catecholamines and also can decrease the blood pressure and the heart rate [30]. Another researcher found the pretreatment with dexmedetomidine 1 µg/kg attenuated (but did not totally abolish) the cardiovascular and stress response responses to laryngoscopy and tracheal intubation after induction of general anesthesia [31].

Conclusions

We conclude that low doses of dexmedetomidine infusion (0.5 µg/kg) over 20 minutes before skin closure are effective as higher doses (0.75 and 1 µg/kg) to decrease stress response and incidence of emergence agitation in laparoscopic cholecystectomy in adults with less adverse effects.

Limitations

First, we think a larger number of patients may be needed to detect better comparison between different doses of dexmedetomidine in preventing EA and monitor possible complications. Second, we did not take in mind any other preoperative predisposing factors or premedication that may affect the incidence of EA especially anxiety or smoking. Finally, we did not use any monitoring for depth of anesthesia which has an important factor in the incidence of emergence agitation.

Acknowledgement

Clinical Trials Number: NCT02917018

References

1. Vlajkovic GP, Sindjelic RP (2007) Emergence delirium in children: many questions, few answers. Anesth Analg 104: 84-91.

2. Kim YS, Chae YK, Choi YS, Min JH, Ahn SW, et al. (2012) A comparative study of emergence agitation between sevoflurane and propofol anesthesia in adults after closed reduction of nasal bone fracture. Korean J Anesthesiol 63: 48-53.

3. Lepousé C, Lautner CA, Liu L, Gomis P, Leon A (2006) Emergence delirium in adults in the post-anaesthesia care unit. Br J Anaesth 96: 747-753.

4. O'Brien D (2002) Acute postoperative delirium: definitions, incidence, recognition, and interventions. J Perianesth Nurs 17: 384-392.

5. Huiku M, Uutela K, van Gils M, Korhonen I, Kymäläinen M, et al. (2007) Assessment of surgical stress during general anaesthesia. Br J Anaesth 98: 447-455.

6. Gulec H, Cakan T, Yaman H, Kilinc AS, Basar H (2012) Comparison of hemodynamic and metabolic stress responses caused by endo¬tracheal tube and Pro-seal laryngeal mask airway in laparoscopic cholecystectomy. J Res Med Sci 17: 148-153.

7. Agarwal A, Ranjan R, Dhiraaj S, Lakra A, Kumar M, et al. (2005) Acupressure for prevention of pre-operative anxiety: a pro¬spective, randomized, placebo controlled study. Anaesthesia 60: 978-981.

8. Gerlach AT, Dasta JF (2007) Dexmedetomidine: an updated review. Ann Pharmacother 41: 245-252.

9. Parikh DA, Kolli SN, Karnik HS, Lele SS, Tendolkar BA (2013) A prospective randomized double-blind study comparing dexmedetomidine vs. combination of midazolam-fentanyl for tympanoplasty surgery under monitored anesthesia care. J Anaesthesiol Clin Pharmacol 29: 173-178.

10. Blaudszun G, Lysakowski C, Elia N, Tramer MR (2012) Effect of perioperative systemic alpha2 agonists on postoperative morphine consumption and pain intensity: systematic review and meta-analysis of randomized controlled trials. Anesthesiology 116: 1312-1322.

11. Riker RR, Picard JT, Fraser GL (1999) Prospective evaluation of the Sedation-Agitation Scale for adult critically ill patients. Crit Care Med 27: 1325-1329.

12. Aldrete JA (1995) The post-anesthesia recovery score revisited. J Clin Anesth 7: 89-91.

13. Neufeld KJ, Leoutsakos JM, Sieber FE, Wanamaker BL, Gibson Chambers JJ, et al. (2013) Outcomes of early delirium diagnosis after general anesthesia in the elderly. Anesth Analg 117: 471-478.

14. Kawamura H, Yokota R, Homma S, Kondo Y (2010) Comparison of respiratory function recovery in the early phase after laparoscopy assisted gastrectomy and open gastrectomy. Surg Endosc 24: 2739-2742.

15. Kim HJ, Kim DK, Sohn TS, Lee JH, Lee GH (2015) A laparoscopic gastrectomy approach decreases the incidence and severity of emergence agitation after sevoflurane anesthesia. J Anesth 29: 223-228.

16. Gerlach AT, Dasta JF (2007) Dexmedetomidine: an updated review. Ann Pharmacother 41: 245-252.

17. Bekker A, Sturaitis MK (2005) Dexmedetomidine for neurological surgery. Neurosurgery 57: 1-10.

18. Guler G, Akin A, Tosun Z, Eskitasoglu E (2005) During the extubation the effect of dexmedetomidine on cardiovascular changes and quality of extubation in the old patients undergoing cataract surgery. Turkish J Anaesthesia 33: 18-21.

19. Hina K, Khawer M, Mohammad SM (2015) Effect of Dexmedetomidine on Emergence Agitation after Nasal Surgeries. Indian Journal of Clinical Anesthesia 2: 126-130.

20. Patel A, Davidson M, Tran MC, Quraishi H, Schoenberg C, et al. (2010) Dexmedetomidine infusion for analgesia and prevention of emergence agitation in children with obstructive sleep apnea syndrome undergoing tonsillectomy and adenoidectomy. Anesth Analg 111: 1004-1010.

21. Ibacache ME, Munoz HR, Brandes V, Morales AL (2004) Single-Dose Dexmedetomidine reduce agitation after sevoflurane anesthesia in children. Anesth Analg 98: 60-63.

22. Keith A, Sergio D, Paula M, Marc A, Wisemandle W, et al. (2010) Monitored anesthesia care with dexmedetomidine: a prospective, randomized, double-blind, multicenter trial. Anesth Analg 110: 47-56.

23. El-Gohary MM, Rizk SN (2011) Dexmedetomidine for Emergence Agitation after Sevoflurane Anesthesia in Preschool Children Undergoing Day Case Surgery: Comparative Dose-Ranging Study. Med. J. Cairo Univ 79: 17-23.

24. Jsik B, Arslan M, tunga AD, Kurtipek O (2006) Dexmedetomidine decreases emergence agitation in pediatric patients after sevoflurane anesthesia without surgery. Paediatr Anaesth 16: 748-753.

25. Feld JM, Hoffman WE, Stechert MM, Hoffman IW, Ananda RC (2006) Fentanyl or dexmedetomidine combined with desflurane for bariatric surgery. J Clin Anesth 18: 24-28.

26. Zhao XC, Tong DY, Long B, Wu XY (2014) Effects of different doses of dexmedetomidine on the recovery quality from general anesthesia undergoing thyroidectomy. Zhonghua Weizhongbing Jijiu Yixue 26: 239-243.

27. Bajwa SJ, Kaur J, Singh A, Parmar S, Singh G (2012) Attenuation of pressor response and dose sparing of opioids and anaesthetics with pre-operative Dexmedetomidine. Indian J Anaesth 56: 123-128.

28. Ram E, Vishne TH, Weinstein T, Beilin B, Dreznik Z (2005) General anesthesia for surgery influences melatonin and cortisol levels. World J Surg 29: 826-829.

29. Sagar G, Vigya G, Krishnaprabha R, Mahesh B (2014) Comparison of Dexmedetomidine with Fentanyl in Attenuation of Pressor Response during Laryngoscopy and Intubation. IOSR Journal of Pharmacy 4: 28-38.

30. Khan ZP, Ferguson CN, Jones RM (1999) alpha-2 and imidazoline receptor agonists. Their pharmacology and therapeutic role. Anaesthesia 54: 146-165.

31. Mondal S, Mondal H, Sarkar R, Rahaman M (2014) Comparison of dexmedetomidine and clonidine for attenuation of sympathoadrenal responses and anesthetic requirements to laryngoscopy and endotracheal intubation. Int J Basic Clin Pharmacol 3: 501-506.

Effect of Heparin Flush in Blood Drawn from Arterial Line on Activated Clotting Time and Thromboelastogram

Amit Lehavi*, Vitaliy Borissovski, Avishay Zisser and Yeshayahu (Shai) Katz

Department of Anesthesiology, Rambam Healthcare Campus, Haifa, Israel

*Corresponding author:** Lehavi A, Department of Anesthesiology, Rambam Healthcare Campus, Haifa, Israel, E-mail: amit.lehavi@gmail.com

Abstract

The usage of low dose heparin as an additive to normal saline is a very acceptable medical practice for the maintenance of arterial line. However, heparin potentially may affect the exactness of coagulation studies carried out on blood sampled from a heparin flushed arterial line. This prospective, comparative observational study was designed to evaluate the effect of blood sampling through a heparin flushed arterial catheter on the validity of common and advanced coagulation tests including activated clotting time (ACT) and thromboelastogram (TEG). Whereas heparin flush did not affect international normalized ratio (INR) and activated partial thromboplastin time (aPTT), it significantly prolonged ACT together with the R-time and K-time components of TEG. This advocated being cautious when measuring ACT and some TEG parameters from a heparin flushed arterial line in a clinical setting.

Abbreviations

INR: International Normalized Ratio; aPTT: Activated Partial Thromboplastin Time; ACT: Activated Clotting Time; TEG: Thromboelastogram; R: Reaction time (time from the start of a sample run until the first significant levels of detectable clot formation); K: Time from the measurement of R until a fixed level of clot firmness is reached; MA: Maximal Amplitude; CPB: Cardiopulmonary Bypass

Introduction

An arterial catheter is commonly inserted to allow a direct line access to the arterial tree of the vascular system for many indications including continuous accurate measurement of blood pressure and blood sampling for chemistry, gas and the coagulation status. The usage of a low dose heparin as an additive to normal saline is a very acceptable medical practice for the maintenance of arterial line. Whereas heparin does not affect the exactness of blood gas and chemistry tests, it may have a significant impact on the quality of the coagulation status examination, being involved in the blood clotting cascade. Although past publications had found that clotting studies carried out on blood sampled from an arterial line correlate well with those obtained from a venipuncture, except for some effect on activated partial thromboplastin time (aPTT) [1], more recent observation challenged these findings [2]. A literature search revealed very few articles comparing activated clotting time (ACT) sampled from an arterial heparin-flushed line with venous heparin-free line [3,4] and only one which mentions Thromboelastogram (TEG) in the context of reliance on clotting profile assessment and heparinized arterial line [2]. Since our hypothesis is the presence of even very low dose heparin may have a significant effect on more sensitive clotting measurements, and as the accurate assessment of blood clotting is crucial for patient safety, this prospective, comparative observational study was designed to evaluate the effect of blood sampling through a heparin flushed arterial catheter on the validity of common and advanced coagulation tests, including ACT and TEG.

Methods

The study was designed as a prospective, comparative observational study, and performed in the Cardiothoracic Anesthesia Unit of the Department of Anesthesiology in Rambam Healthcare Campus in Haifa, Israel A tertiary, university affiliated teaching hospital.

Following approval from the hospital's ethics committee and obtaining written informed consent, patients scheduled for elective cardiac or thoracic surgery requiring invasive blood pressure monitoring were enrolled to the study. Patients with known coagulation disorders were excluded from the study. The age, height, weight and European system for cardiac operative risk evaluation (EuroSCORE) risk assessment grading were recorded, as well as pre-operative hemoglobin concentration, platelet count, aPTT and international normalized ratio (INR) studies.

Aiming to evaluate the differences in coagulation studies in patients with near normal coagulation system, all blood samples were withdrawn prior to the commencement of surgery, and prior to administration of high dose heparin for cardiopulmonary bypass (CPB).

An 18G arterial catheter (BD Venflon, BD, Becton Drive, Franklin Lakes, NJ, USA) was inserted into a radial artery. Following the arterial line insertion, the catheter was flushed with 10 ml of the heparin containing solution and then connected to a flushing system (Art-Line, BioMetrix, Kiryat Mada, Jerusalem, Israel) containing a standard flush solution constituted of heparin 2 units/ml, sodium chloride 0.9%, 1.9 microgram/ml citric acid, and 8.7 microgram/sodium phosphate (Teva Pharmaceutical Industries LTD, Israel). The flushing system had been operated for at least 30 minutes prior to connecting to the patient.

Once a peripheral venous catheter or a second large bore peripheral venous catheter were installed, a blood sample was drawn and marked as "Venous blood", In parallel, 10 ml dead space blood [1,2] was aspirated from the catheter and discarded, immediately followed by another blood sample marked as "Arterial blood". Both the "Venous blood" and the "Arterial blood" samples were processed for coagulation tests in the same fashion using the same measurement equipment.

Activated clotting time (ACT) measuring the time of formation of a stable clot in activated blood , aPTT quantifying the intrinsic coagulation pathway, and international normalized ratio (INR) quantifying the extrinsic coagulation pathway, as well as Thromboelastographic values (R,K, Alpha Angel and MA) were measured. Blood for INR and aPTT studies was sent in a sodium citrate containing glass vial (Vaacuette®,Greiner Bio One International GmbH, Frickenhausen, Germany) to the hospital laboratory, and tests were performed using an automated equipment (Sysmex CA-1500, Siemens AG, Erlangen, Germany). Normal INR and aPTT ranges in our institution laboratory were 0.8-1.2 and 30-50 seconds, respectively.

ACT was determined using an ACT-II Coagulation timer (Medtronics Inc., Minneapolis, USA) using a HR-ACT kit in a temperature of 37°C. Two separate blood vials were used for each test, and their average was regarded as the ACT final value.

Thromboelastography was performed using a TEG® 5000 Thrombelastograph® Hemostasis Analyzer System (Haemoscope, Niles, IL, USA) Using citrated whole blood as per standard manufacturer operating instructions.

Sample size was calculated using retrospective patient chart review. All the variables were recorded on a computerized spreadsheet and assigned to each study subject by name and identification number. Data was evaluated by statistical package for the social sciences (SPSS) software, version 17 (SPSS Inc. Chicago, IL, USA). Descriptive statistic studies, including mean and standard deviation ware used. A paired T-Test was used to determine statistical significance. Normal distribution was assessed by both Back-of-the-envelope test and Kullback–Leibler divergences.

Results

Thirty six patients were enrolled to the study between 11 March 2010 and 8 August 2013 (20 males and 16 females). The average age was 68 ± 11 years, the average height 163 ± 11 cm and the average weight 73 ± 15 kg.

In pre-operative blood tests performed one to three days prior to the operation, the average hemoglobin concentration was 12.5 ± 19 g/dL, average platelet count 206 ± 65 X 109/L, average INR 1 ± 0.1 and average aPTT 28 ± 5 seconds.

Average INR of Arterial blood was the same as for venous blood. Similarly, aPTT for Arterial blood was 29 ± 5 seconds - prolonged by one second compared with venous blood ($P<0.01$).

Average ACT of Arterial blood sampled was 10 seconds [8.1%, ($P<0.01$)] longer compared with Venous blood.

Average R, defined as R-time (reaction time)- the time from the start of a sample run until the first significant levels of detectable clot formation (amplitude=2 mm in the TEG tracing) for Arterial blood was 1.2 second longer [12%, ($P<0.01$)] compared with Venous blood, Similar effect was found with average K, defined as K-time - the time from the measurement of R until a fixed level of clot firmness is reached (amplitude=20 mm in the TEG tracing), namely 0.3 second [16%, (P=0.03] prolongation for Arterial blood compared with venous blood. Neither Average TEG angle alpha (the kinetics of clot development of blood) nor average TEG MA [maximum amplitude a measurement of maximum strength or stiffness (maximum shear modulus) of the developed clot] showed insignificant difference between Arterial and Venous blood (Table 1).

Coagulation study	Venous blood	Arterial blood	Normal values	P*
INR	1.1 ± 0.1	1.1 ± 0.1	0.8-1.2	0.12
aPTT (Seconds)	28 ± 4	29 ± 5	25-35	<0.01
ACT (seconds)	122 ± 16	132 ± 14	80-160	<0.01
TEG R (seconds)	6.6 ± 2.1	7.8 ± 2.1	4-8	<0.01
TEG K (seconds)	1.9 ± 0.7	2.2 ± 0.8	1-4	0.03
Alpha Angle (degrees)	67 ± 7	69 ± 7	47-74	0.06
TEG MA (mm)	65 ± 7	65 ± 8	55-73	0.63

Table 1: Effect of blood sampled from venous blood or from Arterial line flushed with heparin on coagulation studies (Arterial blood).

Discussion

There is a heated debate in the literature if there is any real need to use heparin for arterial line maintenance. On the one hand, some studies present unequivocally approach that no significant difference in duration of patency exists between intravascular catheters flushed with saline or with a heparinized solution [5-7]. This position has important practical implications with regards to avoidance of exposure to heparin-associated risks [8] including inadvertent flow of extra fluid volume and unintended overdose from a pressurized bag of heparin solution together with additional costs associated with the use of a

unique solution and a potential for heparin induced thrombocytopenia (HIT) [9-11]. Yet, others encourage heparin usage because of longer duration of patency compared with saline, and do not fear either the higher costs, overdose or the not proven risk of HIT [11,12].

Indeed, there are recommendations to aspirate from the intravascular indwelled catheter a dead space volume of at least 5 mL comprising of flushing solution and blood, discard it and then redraw a certain volume of blood necessary to conduct the necessary test on it [13]. This action provides the operator with a sense of assurance that the tested sample is free of any contamination. With respect to INR and aPTT, our findings coincide with the literature [2,14]. However, apparently according to our study this feeling is baseless when it comes to more specific measurements which in our case are the advanced coagulation test of ACT and some TEG parameters. The differences, despite being small, may raises critical questions pertaining to the use of heparin flush in arterial line and the reliability of clotting functions tests which are nowadays more available, accessible and widespread as a means of monitoring and managing of many situations including heart, vascular, and transplantation surgery, major trauma, severe bleeding and more. Prolonged ACT may indicate a deficiency in coagulation factors, thrombocytopenia and aprotinin use [15-17]. Inasmuch R, the point at which most traditional coagulation assays reach their end-points is prolonged by anticoagulants and factor deficiencies and K, a measure of the speed to reach a certain level of clot strength and is prolonged by anticoagulants may be affected by heparin flush.

Conclusion

Due to the small sample size and limited clinical settings, we refrain from taking a position pro or against the use of heparin flush versus saline for arterial line maintenance, but suggest to be cautious when measurements such as ACT and some TEG parameters in a clinical setting has a potential to become affected by heparin contamination. Despite the relatively low clinical significance, it may be wise to compare blood samples drawn from a single site when evaluating coagulation changes over time.

References

1. Lew JK, Hutchinson R, Lin ES (1991) Intra-arterial blood sampling for clotting studies. Effects of heparin contamination. Anaesthesia 46: 719-721.

2. Alzetani A, Vohra HA, Patel RL (2004) Can we rely on arterial line sampling in performing activated plasma thromboplastin time after cardiac surgery? Eur J Anaesthesiol 21: 384-388.

3. Zisman E, Rozenberg B, Katz Y, Ziser A (1997) A comparison between arterial- and venous-sampled activated clotting time measurements. Isr J Med Sci 33: 786-788.

4. Leyvi G, Zhuravlev I, Inyang A, Vinluan J, Ramachandran S, et al. (2004) Arterial versus venous sampling for activated coagulation time measurements during cardiac surgery: a comparative study. J Cardiothorac Vasc Anesth18: 573-580.

5. Kulkarni M, Elsner C, Ouellet D, Zeldin R (1994) Heparinized saline versus normal saline in maintaining patency of the radial artery catheter. Can J Surg 37: 37-42.

6. Peterson FY, Kirchhoff KT (1991) Analysis of the research about heparinized versus nonheparinized intravascular lines. Heart and lung 20: 631-640.

7. Lapum JL (2006) Patency of arterial catheters with heparinized solutions versus non-heparinized solutions: a review of the literature. Canadian journal of cardiovascular nursing. Journal canadien en soins infirmiers cardio-vasculaires 16: 64-70.

8. Del Cotillo M, Grane N, Llavore M, Quintana S (2008) Heparinized solution vs. saline solution in the maintenance of arterial catheters: a double blind randomized clinical trial. Intensive care Med 34: 339-343.

9. Goode CJ, Titler M, Rakel B, Ones DS, Kleiber C, et al. (1991) A meta-analysis of effects of heparin flush and saline flush: quality and cost implications. Nurs Res 40: 324-330.

10. Walenga JM, Bick RL (1998) Heparin-induced thrombocytopenia, paradoxical thromboembolism, and other side effects of heparin therapy. Med Clin North Am 82: 635-658.

11. Kordzadeh A, Austin T, Panayiotopoulos Y (2014) Efficacy of normal saline in the maintenance of the arterial lines in comparison to heparin flush: a comprehensive review of the literature. J Vasc Access 15: 123-127.

12. Kumar M, Vandermeer B, Bassler D, Mansoor N (2013) Low-dose heparin use and the patency of peripheral IV catheters in children: a systematic review. Pediatrics 131: e864-872.

13. Reinhardt AC, Tonneson AS, Bracey A, Goodnough SK (1987) Minimum discard volume from arterial catheters to obtain coagulation studies free of heparin effect. Heart Lung 16: 699-705.

14. Cicala RS, Cannon K, Larson JS, Fabian TC (1988) Evaluation of coagulation studies from heparinized arterial lines with use of Lab-Site high-pressure tubing. Heart Lung 17: 662-666.

15. Ammar T, Fisher CF, Sarier K, Coller BS (1996) The effects of thrombocytopenia on the activated coagulation time. Anesth Analg 83: 1185-1188.

16. Wallock M, Arentzen C, Perkins J (1995) Factor XII deficiency and cardiopulmonary bypass. Perfusion 10: 13-16.

17. Sievert A, McCall M, Blackwell M, Bradley S (2003) Use of aprotinin during cardiopulmonary bypass in a patient with protein C deficiency. J Extra Corpor Technol 35: 39-43.

Effects of Types of Anesthesia on Neurobehavioral Response and Apgar Score in Neonates Delivered with Cesarean Section in Dilla University Referral Hospital

Semagn Mekonnen[1*] **and Kokeb Desta**[2]

[1]*Department of Anesthesiology, Dilla University, Dilla, Ethiopia*

[2]*Department of Anesthesiology, Debre Birhan University, Debre Birhan, Ethiopia*

*****Corresponding author:** Semagn Mekonnen, Department of Anesthesiology, Dilla University, Dilla, Ethiopia, E-mail: semmek17@gmail.com

Abstract

Background: Neonatal outcomes are affected by types of anesthesia and perioperative patient cares. Studies showed that neonatal neurobehavioral response and Apgar score were better in mothers who gave birth under spinal anesthesia than general anesthesia. But studies were inadequate locally and this study compared neonatal neurobehavioral response and Apgar score in mothers who undergo caesarean section.

Objective: The main objective of the study was to compare Neonatal neurobehavioral response and Apgar score in neonates delivered with caesarean section under spinal *vs.* General anesthesia.

Methods and materials: After approval from institutional review Board (IRB) of Dilla University, we studied 200 consecutive babies delivered with caesarean section under spinal and General Anesthesia from ASA I&II term pregnant mother in Dilla University Teaching and referral Hospital. Prospective effectiveness study design was employed. Mothers were randomly allocated in two equal groups 60 patients each by lottery method after informed consent.

Result: There was a significant mean difference between the two groups on mean Intraoperative systolic blood pressure. More women who received spinal anesthesia had lower intraoperative systolic blood pressure as compared to women who received general anesthesia (P<0.05). Neonatal Neurologic Adaptive capacity score at 15 minutes were better in spinal as compared to General Anesthesia. There were significant association between types of Anesthesia with the majority of the tests in 15 minute and 2 hrs period. But Neonatal Neurologic Adaptive capacity score at 24 hrs didn't show significant Association.

Conclusion: Spinal Anesthesia is associated with good neonatal outcomes even in emergency caesarean section with non-touching rapid sequence spinal anesthesia technique. General anesthesia should be preserved for cases contra indicated with spinal anesthesia.

Keywords: Apgar score; Neurologic adaptive capacity score; Anesthesia; Neonate

Introduction

Caesarean section is a procedure where by a baby is delivered through an incision on the abdominal wall and intact uterus of the mother under General or Spinal Anesthesia. It is usually life-saving and reserves the health of the mother and her baby [1,2].

General anaesthesia refers to the loss of ability to perceive pain associated with loss of consciousness produced by intravenous or inhalation anesthetic agents. For caesarean section, this involves the use of thiopentone for induction, tracheal intubation facilitated by suxamethonium, positive-pressure ventilation of the lungs with pre-oxygen plus a volatile agent, and a muscle relaxant [1].

Regional anaesthesia (spinal) refers to the use of local anaesthetic solutions to produce circumscribed areas of loss of sensation. This type of regional anaesthesia used for caesarean section involves the infiltration of a local anaesthetic agent directly into the subarachnoid space [1].

General and Regional Anesthesia for caesarean section are not ideal as each has benefits and risk to foetus. But the aim of clinician is to select the method which is harmless and most comfortable for the mother, least depressant to the new born [2].

Spinal anesthesia affects neonates either by decreasing uteroplacental perfusion secondary to sympathetic blocked induced hypotension or intratecally administered Opioids with local anesthetics that depress the respiratory center and end up with asphyxia and acidosis [3].

The outcome of Neonates delivered by Caesarean section is depending on preoperative maternal and neonatal condition, intraoperative management and postoperative care. Effective neonatal resuscitation with qualified resuscitator and adequate equipment must be provided and the Apgar score in the first minute and fifth minute and arterial oxygen saturation with pulse oximeter (89-94%) will signify adequate resuscitation minimal or no respiratory depression [4].

Incidence of Neonatal Mortality

The assessment of anaesthesia-related mortality has been employed since so many years back and defined as death of patients under, or following anesthesia within twenty four hours under the care of anesthetist [5].

Unlike other studies conducted in different parts of the world [2,4,6-27] incidence of neonatal death was reported only in one study, there were four deaths in general anesthesia and zero in spinal anesthesia [28].

Determinants of Neonatal Morbidity

Anesthesia related morbidity is any complication that could occur in patients under or following anesthesia under the care of anesthetist within twenty four hours and they are related with preoperative patient condition, intraoperative management and postoperative care [5].

Neonatal Neurobehavioral Response

Apgar sore assess the need for neonatal resuscitation and intraoperative anesthetic drugs effects are not easily appreciated [28]. As a result, the anesthesiologist and neonatologist discover new methods of assessment besides Apgar score. The neurologic and Adaptive capacity score is the one being employed because of its simplicity and feasibility.

According to a study conducted in America, the neonatal neurologic and Adaptive capacity score was much lower in babies delivered under general anesthesia than spinal anesthesia [7]. But a study conducted in Thailand showed Neonatal Adaptive Capacity Score in babies born either Spinal or general anesthesia had no significant difference [25].

Neonatal Intensive Care Unit (NICU) Admission and Hospital Stay

The factors contributing for long duration of hospital stay and NICU admission varies with preoperative maternal and neonatal condition, types of anesthesia administered intraoperative management and postoperative care.

According to an observational study conducted in Pakistan, babies delivered under general anesthesia had long duration of hospital stay and required neonatal Intensive care Unit Admission [22].

A study conducted in Turkey showed that neonatal ICU admission had no significant difference in mothers who received either spinal or general anesthesia [10].

According to another study conducted in Italy, rates of neonatal admission and need for oxygen ventilation were higher in babies delivered under general anesthesia. But the overall neonatal outcomes were not significant [24].

Apgar Score

The immediate neonatal outcome is usually measured with a tool called Apgar score in the first minute and fifth minutes after delivery.

According to different literatures, the first and fifth Apgar scores were better in neonates delivered under spinal anesthesia as compared to general anesthesia [4,6,8,10,12,14,16-19,21-25]. However, in other studies the fifth minute Apgar score didn't show significant different between the groups [2,11,13,15].

A study conducted in Ethiopia showed that neonatal outcomes were affected by uterine incision to delivery time. Neonates delivered in uterine incision to baby out less than three minute had better Apgar score [6].

During review of the literature, we found out many clinical trials and observational studies comparing neonatal outcomes delivered with caesarean section. However, still there are controversies on selection of types of anesthesia and effects of each on neonatal outcomes. Besides, there are no studies in Ethiopia comparing neonatal outcomes delivered with caesarean section in clinical trial or prospective observational study.

Apgar score is employed to confirm the need for resuscitation of the baby. However, Apgar score doesn't confirm effects of maternal preoperative and intraoperative administered drugs on neonatal neurologic effects. Anesthesiologists and pediatricians used different techniques to assess neurobehavioral response of neonates delivered with caesarean section. Neurologic and Adaptive capacity score is the recent techniques employed by Anesthesiologists. There were many clinical trials and observational studies conducted to assess the Apgar score of neonates delivered with caesarean section [4,6,8,10,12,14,17-25]. These studies showed that babies delivered under spinal anesthesia had better outcomes as compared to general anesthesia. Though studies conducted on effects of types of anesthesia to Neurobehavioral response of neonates were scarce worldwide, they showed that babies delivered under General anesthesia had low neurobehavioral response than Spinal anesthesia groups [2,7,13,16].

Methods and Materials

After approval from institutional review Board (IRB) of Dilla University, we studied 200 consecutive babies delivered with cesarean section under spinal and General Anesthesia from ASA I&II term pregnant mother in Dilla University Teaching and referral Hospital. Prospective effectiveness study design was employed. Mothers were randomly allocated in two equal groups 60 patients each by lottery method after informed consent. Mothers with spinal Anesthesia group was preloaded with 1-1.5 litres of crystalloids before spinal Anesthesia and Spinal Anesthesia was given with 2-2.5 ml of 0.5% bupivacaine in sitting position with strict aseptic technique. General Anesthesia was induced with rapid sequence induction with 3.5 mg/kg of thiopental and 1-2 mg/kg succinylcholine. General Anesthesia was maintained with 1-1.5 v% halothane, 0.1 mg/kg of vecronium and 1.5-2 mg/kg of Pethidine.

Data collection method and measurement of variables

Data were collected using a pre-tested structured questionnaire. The trained data collectors managed the data in intraoperative and postoperative period who were not responsible for the anesthetic management for that particular subject.

Preoperatively, the socio-demographic characteristics, ASA status, preoperative hematocrit and blood pressure were taken. Intraoperatively, the maternal blood pressure was taken every three minutes until delivery of the baby and the induction to delivery time also recorded. Just after delivery, the first and the fifth minute Apgar scores were recorded. The Apgar score was assessed with a standard table format which contains five parameters (Table 1) [10].

Sign	0	1	2
Appearance	Blue and pale	Body pink, extremities blue	Completely pink
Pulse rate	Absent	Bellow 100	Above 100
Grimace	No response	Grimace	Cry
Activity	No movement	Some flexion of extremities	Active movement
Respiration	Absent	Shallow and irregular	Deep and regular, strong cry

Table 1: Apgar scoring table.

Postoperatively, the baby was sent to ward along with his/her mother and the neurobehavioral response of the baby was assessed with Neonatal neurologic and Adaptive capacity score at 15 minutes, 2 and 24 hrs. The Neonatal Neurologic and Adaptive capacity score contains five assessment areas i.e. adaptive capacity, Active tone, Passive tone, primary reflexes and general neurologic status. Each criterion was given a score of 0 for absent or abnormal, 1 for slightly abnormal and 2 for normal and the maximum score will be 40 (Table 2) [26].

		0	1	2	Total score
Adaptive Capacity	Response to sound	Absent	Mild	Vigorous	
	Habituation to sound	Absent	7-12 stimuli	<6 stimuli	
	Response to light	Absent	Mild		
	Habituation to light	absent	7-12 stimuli	<6 stimuli	
	Consolability	Absent	Difficult	Easy	
Total					
Passive tone	Scarf sign	Encircles the neck	Elbow slightly passes midline	Elbow dose not reach midline	
	Recoil of elbow	Absent	Slow and weak	Brisky and reproducible	
	Popliteal angle	>110°	100-110°	<90°	
	Recoil of lower limb	Absent	Slow and weak	Brisky and reproducible	
Total					
Active tone	Active contraction of neck flexor	Absent/abnormal	Difficult	Good, head is maintained in the axis of the body	
	Active contraction of neck extensor	Absent or abnormal	Difficult	Good, head is maintained in the axis of the body	
	Palmar grasp	Absent	Weak	Excellent: reproducible	
	Response to traction (following Palmar grasp	Absent	Lifts part of the body weight	Lifts all body weight	
	Supporting reaction (upright position)	Absent	Incomplete transitory	Strong; lifts all body weight	
Total					
Primary reflexes	Automatic walking	Absent	Difficult to obtain	Perfect ; reproducible	
	Moro reflex	Absent	Weak; incomplete	Perfect	
	Sucking	Absent	Weak	Perfect : synchronous with swallowing	
Total					
General Assessment	Alertness	Coma	Lethargy	Normal	
	Crying	Absent	Weak	Normal	
	Motor activity	Absent /excessive	Weak	Normal	

Total			
Grand total			

Table 2: NACS scoring table.

Data processing and analysis

Chi square test and odds ratio were used to determine the association between hypothesized independent and dependent variables. Finally, multivariate analysis was used to control possible confounders and identify independent predictor of Neurobehavioral response and Apgar score.

Results

A total of 200 Neonates delivered with caesarean section from a term pregnant women were followed perioperatively for twenty and the response rate of the participants were hundred percent.

Socio-demographic characteristics

Data on maternal age, weight, height, Body Mass Index, and neonatal weight were summarized in Table 3.

Variables	Spinal anesthesia (n=100)	General anesthesia (n=100)	P value
Age (year)	23.21 ± 50	22.61 ± 5	0.414
Weight (Kg)	66.22 ± 12	63.5 ± 10	0.115
Height (cm)	162.02 ± 6.7	162.78 ± 4.5	0.351
BMI (kg/m^2)	23.21 ± 5.4	22.61 ± 4.8	0.414
Neonatal weight (g)	3556.2 ± 596	3295.9 ± 455	0.422
Data were stated as mean ± SD, BMI: Body Mass Index.			

Table 3: Socio-demographic Characteristics.

Maternal preoperative Characteristics

Data on maternal preoperative hematocrit, previous cesarean section and qualification of the anesthetist who provided anesthesia were shown in Table 4.

Variables	Spinal anesthesia (n=100)	General anesthesia (n=100)	P value
Preoperative SBP	122.10 ± 9.13	122.05 ± 14	0.798
PHCT	39.22 ± 4.77	38.39 ± 3.9	0.18
Previous C/S	24/100	15/100	0.108
Data were described as mean ± SD and number. SBP: systolic Blood Pressure. PHCT: preoperative Hematocrit.			

Table 4: preoperative maternal characteristics.

Intraoperative maternal characteristics

There was a significant mean difference between the two groups on mean Intraoperative systolic blood pressure. More women who received spinal anesthesia had lower intraoperative systolic blood pressure as compared to women who received general anesthesia (P<0.05). Severe reduction in blood pressure decreased placental perfusion which results in fetal acidosis and asphyxia. However, neonates delivered from spinal anesthesia with lower blood pressure and Normal blood pressure didn't show any difference (Table 5).

Variables	Spinal anesthesia (n=100)	General anesthesia (n=100)	P value
Base line	122.10 ± 9.13	122.05 ± 14	0.798
3rd minute	117.60 ± 12.23	119.53 ± 14	0.301
6th minute	102.20 ± 11.59	114.35 ± 19.78	0.000*
9th minute	97.8 ± 11.69	111.40 ± 19.12	0.000*
12th minute	100.32 ± 9.44	122.55 ± 14.95	0.000*
15th minute	103 ± 20.72	115.95 ± 12.06	0.000*
PACU entry	116.65 ± 14.98	117.19 ± 10.40	0.768

*Significant at P<0.05; Data were described as mean ± SD, PACU: Post Anesthetic Care Unit.

Table 5: intraoperative maternal systolic blood Pressure (mmHg).

Neonatal characteristics

There was no neonatal death in this study. The number of neonates required resuscitation was higher in general anesthesia, 24/100 and 14/10 respectively. But the mean difference was not significant (P>0.071) (Figure 1).

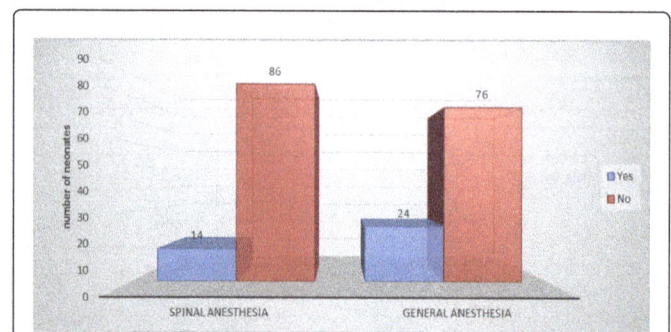

Figure 1: need of resuscitation.

Apgar score

There were significant mean difference on the mean first and fifth minute Apgar score (P<0.05). The Apgar score of neonates in the first minute less than seven was lower in general Anesthesia as compared to spinal anesthesia. Thirty one neonates from hundred had lower first minute Apgar score less than seven in General Anesthesia when compared to spinal Anesthesia groups which was only eleven neonates from hundred with lower first minute Apgar score less than seven (Table 6).

Variables	Spinal anesthesia (n=100)	General anesthesia (n=100)	P value
First minute Apgar	7.57 ± 0.96	7.13 ± 1.22	0.005*
Fifth minute Apgar	8.7 ± 0.67	8.34 ± 0.95	0.002*
Apgar score <7	11/100	31/100	0.001*
Apgar score >7	89/100	69/100	0.001*
Neonatal Psao$_2$	91.63 ± 4.43	91.52	0.24
Hospitalization	2.99 ± 0.86	3.05 ± 0.93	0.637

*Significant at P<0.05; Data were expressed as mean ± SD and number. PACU: Post Anesthetic Care Unit, Psao$_2$: percutaneous arterial oxygen saturation.

Table 6: Apgar score, neonatal oxygen saturation and duration of Hospitalization.

Neurologic adaptive capacity score

Neonates delivered under General and spinal Anesthesia was assessed with Neurologic Adaptive Capacity score to determine the effect of Anesthetic drug on neonatal immediate outcomes in 15 minute, 2 hrs and 24 hrs.

Neonates delivered under spinal anesthesia had highest score in 15 minutes when compared to babies delivered under General Anesthesia. There were significant association between types of anesthesia with the majority of the tests especially in 15 minute and 2 hrs period. However, there was no significant difference in 24 hrs assessment (Table 7).

Parameters	15 minutes			2 hrs			24 hrs		
	SA	GA	P value	SA	GA	P value	SA	GA	P value
Adaptive Capacity									
Response to sound	63	37	0.000**	74	56	0.008*	99	97	0.312
Habituation to sound	65	40	0.001**	76	57	0.006*	99	97	0.508
Response to light	73	54	0.020*	84	66	0.013*	99	97	0.508
Habituation to light	81	64	0.026*	88	72	0.018*	100	97	0.218
Consolability	57	53	0.045*	66	65	0.126	100	97	0.218
Passive tone									
Scarf sign	52	34	0.026*	64	53	0.127	100	96	0.13
Recoil of elbow	56	50	0.421	66	64	0.397	100	97	0.218
Popliteal angle	62	49	0.104	71	62	0.224	100	96	0.13
Recoil of lower limb	67	47	0.005*	79	61	0.010*	99	97	0.508
Active									
Neck flexion	66	38	0.000**	78	55	0.002*	100	97	0.246
Neck extension	64	35	0.000**	76	54	0.004*	100	97	0.246
Palmar grasp	73	59	0.076*	83	70	0.071	99	97	0.508
Palmar traction	45	29	0.026*	58	49	0.315	99	96	0.359
Supporting reaction	43	23	0.002**	57	46	0.088	99	96	0.359
Primary reflexes									
Automatic walking	44	26	0.028*	58	48	0.44	99	96	0.359
Moro reflex	59	38	0.008*	72	57	0.082	99	98	0.561
Suckling	72	65	0.287	82	74	0.172	99	98	0.561
General assessment									

Alertness	95	88	0.076	97	91	0.074	100	99	0.316
Crying	94	88	0.138	96	92	0.234	100	99	0.316
Motor activity	91	81	0.048[*]	94	87	0.091	100	98	0.155

[*]significant (0.001<P<0.05), [**] very significant (p<0.001) , GA: General Anesthesia, SA: spinal Anesthesia, P: p-value

Table 7: Number of Neonates who scored highest score in each item of Neurologic Adaptive Capacity Score after caesarean section under spinal and general Anesthesia, Dilla University Referral Hospital, Ethiopia, 2016.

Determinants of neonatal Apgar scores

To determine the predictor of lower Apgar score, bivariate and Multivariate logistic regression was conducted and the results was described below (Table 8).

Neonates born under General Anesthesia were more likely to have higher figures of Apgar score less than seven when compared to spinal anesthesia, (AOR=0.275, 95% CI=[0.129, 0.285]).

Neonates born with greater than three minutes from uterine incision to baby out were half times more likely to be asphyxiated (AOR=0.453, 95% CI= [0.224, 0.917]) as compared to babies born with less than three minutes from uterine incision to baby out.

Variables	Apgar Score at first minute		COR, 95% CI	AOR, 95% CI
	<7 N (%)	>7 N (%)		
Neonatal weight (kg)				
<3	19 (33.33)	38 (66.67)	0.383 (0.183, 0.779)[*]	0.383 (0.183, 0.779)[*]
>3	23 (16.08)	120 (83.92)	1	1
Type of anesthesia				
General	31 (31)	69 (69)	0.275 (0.129, 0.285)[*]	0.275 (0.129, 0.285)[*]
Spinal	11 (11)	89 (89)	1	1
Total fluid Requirement (ml)				
<1500	16 (38.09)	26 (61.91)	1	1
>1500	41 (25.95)	117 (65.05)	0.569 (0.278, 1.17)	0.569 (0.278, 1.17)
Time from skin incision To uterine incision (min)				
<3	32 (76.19)	10 (23.81)	1	1
>3	73 (46.20)	85 (53.80)	3.73 (1.72, 8.09)[*]	0.268 (0.124, 0.583)[*]
Time from uterine incision To baby out (min)				
<3	27 (64.29)	15 (35.71)	1	1
>3	71 (44.94)	87 (55.06)	2.206 (1.09, 4.46)[*]	0.453 (0.224, 0.917)[*]

[*]Significant at P<0.05, results were expressed in number and percent. COR: Crude Odd Ratio; AOR: Adjusted Odd Ratio; CI: Confidence Interval.

Table 8: Determinates of first minute Apgar score (n=200).

Discussion

The mean Apgar score at first minute was lower in neonates delivered under general Anesthesia when compared to spinal Anesthesia groups. This study is in line with many studies conducted elsewhere [2,10,11,13,17,18,20,21,24]. However, the mean fifth minute Apgar score didn't show significant mean difference in these studies.

But a study conducted other areas showed a significant mean difference at first and fifth minute [6,12,23,25].

In this study Neonatal Neurologic Adaptive Capacity Score in the 15 minute and 2 hrs time were higher in neonates delivered under spinal Anesthesia when compared to General Anesthesia. This study finding is in line with a study conducted in America [7]. However, the 24 hrs Neurologic Adaptive capacity score didn't show significant different. This significant difference in the first couple of hours might be due to lipid soluble intravenous drugs passing through the placenta and depress the neonate for some time. But a study conducted in Thailand didn't show significant difference between the groups on Neonatal neurologic Adaptive Capacity score [25].

A systemic review and meta-analysis on effects of types of anesthesia on maternal and neonatal outcomes also showed that neonatal Neurologic Adaptive Capacity Score didn't significant different (P>0.4) [2].

Neonatal resuscitation and intensive care Admission is higher in babies delivered under general Anesthesia as compared to Spinal Anesthesia but there was no significant mean difference (p>0.071). This study finding is in line with a study conducted in Turkey in which neonatal Intensive care Admission was 5 *vs.* 6 for spinal and general anesthesia respectively [10].

Another study in Turkey also showed that respiratory support didn't show any significant association (P>1) [22].

A study conducted in America showed that immediate neonatal intensive care Admission didn't have any significant difference. However, a study conducted in Pakistan showed that there were higher number of neonatal Admission in general anesthesia when compared to spinal Anesthesia, [28] *vs.* 6 respectively, P<0.001. These discrepancies might be due to longer induction delivery time with potent lipid soluble intravenous agents and/or more emergency cases with fetal distress in the sample of a study conducted in Pakistan.

Greater induction to delivery time is associated with low Apgar score. This study is in line with a study conducted in Gondar University.

Conclusion

The findings in this study revealed that the mean first minute and fifth minute Apgar score is much better in babies delivered under spinal Anesthesia when compared to general Anesthesia.

Apgar score less than seven at first minute was better in neonates delivered under spinal anesthesia. Neonatal Apgar score had a significant association with induction delivery time.

Neonatal Neurologic Adaptive Capacity Score was higher in neonates delivered under Spinal Anesthesia in 15 minute and 2 hrs when compared to General Anesthesia.

The neonatal respiratory support and Neonatal Intensive care Admission didn't show any significant difference between the groups.

Overall, spinal Anesthesia is associated with minimal neonatal outcomes even in emergency caesarean section with non-touching rapid sequence spinal anesthesia technique. General anesthesia should be preserved for cases contra indicated with spinal anesthesia.

Competing Interest

All authors declare that they have no conflict of interest associated with the publication of this manuscript.

Authors' Contribution

Semagn Mekonnen conceived and designed the study and collected data in the field, performed analysis, interpretation of data, and draft the manuscript. Kokeb Desta involved in the design, analysis, and interpretation of data and the critical review of the manuscript.

Acknowledgments

This study was funded by Dilla University who covered all the financial and material support for the research. We also want to acknowledge the participants for being volunteer and patient throughout the follow up.

References

1. Barash PG, Cullen BF, Stoelting RK, Calahan MK, Stock MC (2009) Handbook of clinical anesthesia. (6th edn) P: 697-702.

2. Afolabi BB, Lesi FE, Merah NA (2006) Regional versus general anesthesia for caesarean section. cochrane database of systematic reviews 18: CD004350.

3. Chattopadhyay S, Das A, Pahari S (2014) Fetomaternal outcome in severe preeclamptic women undergoing emergency cesarean section under either general or spinal anesthesia. Journal of Pregnancy 2014: Article ID 325098: 10 pages.

4. Haller G, Anaesthetist C, Clergue F (2011) Best Practice & Research Clinical Anaesthesiology Morbidity in anaesthesia⊠: Today and tomorrow. Best Pract Res Clin Anaesthesiol 25: 123-132.

5. Saygı AI, Ozdamar O, Gun I, Emirkadı H, Mungen E, et al. (2015) Comparison of maternal and fetal outcomes among patients undergoing cesarean section under general and spinal anesthesia⊠: a randomized clinical trial. sao paulo med j 133: 227-234.

6. Imtiaz A, Mustafa S, Haq N, Ali S, Imtiaz k (2009) Effect of spinal and general anaesthesia over apgar score in neonates born after elective cesarean section. Jlumhs 9:151-154.

7. Zahir J, Syed S, Jabeen N, Anjum Q, Shafiq UR, et al. (2011) Maternal and neonatal outcome after spinal versus general anaesthesia for caesarean delivery. Ann. Pak. Inst. Med. Sci. 7: 115-118.

8. Kosam D, Kosam A, Murthy M (2014) Effect of various techniques of anesthesia in elective caesarian section on short term neonatal outcome. international journal of medical research and review 2: 480-486.

9. Martin TC, Bell P, Ogunbiyi O (2007) Comparison of general anaesthesia and spinal anaesthesia for caesarean section.west indian medical journal 56: 330-333.

10. Odd DE, Rasmussen F, Gunnell D, Lewis G, WhitelawA (2008) A cohort study of low Apgar scores and cognitive outcomes. Arch Dis Child Fetal Neonatal Ed 93: F115-F120.

11. Rasooli S, Moslemi F (2014) Apgar scores and cord blood gas values on neonates from cesarean with general anesthesia and spinal anesthesia. J Anal Res Clin Med 2: 11-16.

12. Solangi SA, Siddiqui SM, Khaskheli MS, Siddiqui MA (2012) Comparison of the effects of general vs spinal anesthesia on neonatal outcome. Anaesth Pain & Intensive Care 16: 18-23.

13. Sungur Mo, Karaden M, Kili M, Seyhan Z (2013) Spinal anesthesia for elective cesarean section is associated with shorter hospital stay compared to general anesthesia 25: 55-63.

14. Tabassum R, Sabbar S, Khan FA, Shaikh JM (2010) Comparison of the eff ects of general and spinal anaesthesia on apgar score of the neonates in patients undergoing elective caesarean section: Pakistan j surg 26: 46-49.

15. Visalyaputra S, Rodanant O, Somboonviboon W, Tantivitayatan K, Thienthong S, et al. (2005) Spinal versus epidural anesthesia for cesarean delivery in severe preeclampsia: A prospective randomized, multicenter study. Anesth Analg 101: 862-868.

16. Kolatat T, Somboonnanonda A, Lertakyamanee J, Chinachot T, Tritrakarn T, et al. (1999) Effects of general and regional anesthesia on the neonate. j med assoc Thai 82: 40-45.

17. Tonni G, Ferrari B, Felice C de, Ventura A (2007) Fetal acid-base and neonatal status after general and neuraxial anesthesia for elective cesarean section. international journal of obstetrics and gynecology 97: 143-146.

18. Amiel-Tison C, Barrier G, Shnider SM, Levinson G, Hughes SC, et al. (1982) Anew Neurologic and Adaptive Capacity Scoring System for

Evaluation obstatric medication in full term New born Anesthesiology 56: 340-350.

19. Abboud Tk, Nagappala S, Murakawa K, David S, Haroutunian S, et al. (1985) Comparison of the effects of general and regional anesthesia for cesarean section on neonatal neurologic and adaptive capacity scores. journal of anesthesia analgesia 64: 996-1000.

20. Abdissa Z, Awoke T, Belayneh T, Tefera Y (2013) Birth Outcome after Caesarean Section among Mothers who Delivered by Caesarean Section under General and Spinal Anesthesia at Gondar. J Anesthe Clinic Res 4: 335.

21. Martin TC, Bell P, Ogunbiyi O (2007) Comparison of general anaesthesia and spinal anaesthesia for caesarean section. West Indian med. j. 56: 330-333.

22. Yeğin A, Ertuğ Z, Yilmaz M, Erman M (2003) The effects of epidural anesthesia and general anesthesia on newborns at cesarean section. Turk J Med Sci 33: 311-314.

23. Ahsan-ul-haq M (2004) Analysis of outcome of general versus spinal anaesthesia for caesarean delivery in severe pre-eclampsia with foetal compromise 20.

24. Fabris LK, Mareti A (2009) Effects of general anaesthesia versus spinal Anaesthesia for caesarean section on postoperative analgesic consumption and postoperative pain. Periodicum Biologorum 111: 251-255.

25. Saatsaz S, Moulookzadeh S, Rezaei R, Khani N (2014) Comparison of neonatal apgar score in general. Ind. J. Fund. Appl Life Sci. 4: 351-357.

26. Schewe JC, Komusin A, Zinserling J, Nadstawek J, Hoeft A, et al. (2009) Effects of spinal anaesthesia versus epidural anaesthesia for caesarean section on postoperative analgesic consumption and postoperative pain. Eur J Anaesthesiol 26: 52-59.

27. Siddiqi R, Jafri A (2009) Maternal satisfaction after spinal anaesthesia for caesarean deliveries. J Coll Physicians Surg Pakistan 19: 77-80.

28. Akyol A, Akgun A, Gedikbasi A, Agrali G, Ceylan Y (2006) Effects of general and spinal anesthesia on APGAR scores and Umbilical cord blood gases in elective cesarean operations. Cochrane register of controlled trials. Jinekoloji Ve Obstetrik Dergisi 20: 32-37.

Efficacy and Safety of Dexamethasone as an Adjuvant to Local Anesthetics in Lumbar Plexus Block in Patients Undergoing Arthroscopic Knee Surgeries

Bassant M Abdelhamid[1]*, Inas Elshzly[2], Sahar Badawy[2] and Ayman Yossef[3]

[1]*Lecturer of anesthesia, Cairo University, Egypt*

[2]*Professor of anesthesia Cairo University, Egypt*

[3]*Assistant Lecturer of Anesthesia, Cairo University, Egypt*

***Corresponding author:** Bassant Mohamed Abdelhamid, Department of anesthesia, Lecturer of anesthesia, Faculty of medicine, Cairo University, Egypt, E-mail: bassantmohamed197@yahoo.com

Abstract

Background: The benefit of adding dexamethasone in regional anesthesia has recently been the focus of investigation as clinical reports suggest improved block characteristics. The aim of this study is to evaluate whether perineural administration of dexamethasone is more effective in prolonging the duration of lumbar plexus block than giving it systemically.

Methods: 60 (out of 72) patients were recruited to undergo arthroscopic knee surgery using lumbar plexus block. These patients were divided randomly into 3 groups, 20 patients in each; group L (combined lumbar plexus and sciatic nerve block with bupivacaine 0.5%), group D (combined lumbar plexus and sciatic nerve block with bupivacaine 0.5%+8mg dexamethasone in LPB) and group S (combined lumbar plexus and sciatic nerve block with bupivacaine0.5% +8mg intravenous dexamethasone).

Results: patients showed statistically significant enhanced onset of sensory loss in group D when compared to group L (p value=0.04) but no statistically significant difference found between groups S and L (p value=0.13) or between groups D and S (p value=0.86). Regarding onset of motor loss it was found that group D enhanced onset of motor block significantly (p value<0.01) when compared to group L, while group S showed statistically insignificant enhancement of onset of motor block when compared to group L (p value=0.15) or group D (p value=0.71). Regarding sensory block duration (Postoperative analgesia), both groups D and S showed significant prolonged duration of analgesia (p value<0.01and0.04 respectively) when compared to group L, but no statistically significance detected when compared to each other (p value=0.24) which means they both similarly prolong duration of analgesia clinically. Motor block duration was significantly prolonged in group D when compared to groups L and group S (p value≤0.01).While group S didn't show statistically significant prolongation of motor block when compared to group L (p value=0.4).

Conclusion: Both perineural and IV administration of dexamethasone improve the efficacy of lumbar plexus block by prolonging the duration of analgesia, enhancing onset action of local anesthetics, and reducing postoperative analgesic requirements without increasing the incidence of complications.

Keywords: Dexamethasone; Lumbar plexus block; Arthroscopic knee surgeries

Key messages

To produce safe and efficient anesthesia with decreased perioperative pain score, early ambulation and hospital discharge.

Background

Over the last decades, the numbers of total knee arthroplasty procedures performed have increased dramatically. This very successful intervention, however, associated with significant postoperative pain and adequate postoperative analgesia, is mandatory in order to allow for successful rehabilitation and recovery [1].

Compared with neuroaxial (spinal/epidural) anesthesia, peripheral nerve blocks minimizes hypotension, urinary retention and eliminates the risk of spinal hematoma and infection that might occur with central neuraxial blocks [2].

Looking at the clinical efficacy, there is substantial evidence that a posterior approach of the lumbar plexus block has significant advantages compared to the anterior approach (femoral nerve block or "3-in-1 block") of the lumbar plexus. As the posterior approach is more effective in blocking the obturator nerve (the articular branches innervate the anteromedial capsule of the hip joint [3].

Dexamethasone appears to be the best method to prolong analgesia as an adjuvant over clonidine, epinephrine, or midazolam. The value of several additional hours of analgesia is a risk/benefit discussion that anesthesiologists must have with their patients, given the off-label use of perineural dexamethasone. [4].

The aim of this study is to evaluate whether perineural administration of dexamethasone is more effective in reducing the onset, prolonging the duration of lumbar plexus block and decrease the requirement of post operative systemic analgesia than giving it systemically.

Patients and Methods:

Approval of the ethical and research committees of our hospital was obtained. Prospective randomized controlled trial was conducted in orthopedic operating theater in the period from May 2014 to December 2014. Patients were radomized using concealed envelope method. The informed consent of the participants was taken after describing the steps of the procedure.

Preoperative assessment was done as follows; full explanation of type of anesthesia planned, history taking, laboratory investigations including; full blood count, liver and kidney functions, coagulation profile and blood sugar.

Patients with ASA (American Society of Anesthesiologists) physical class I or II undergoing endoscopic knee procedures. Patients of both genders and aged 18-50 years old were included in the study.

Patients with cardiopulmonary diseases, hypovolemia, coagulopathy, any contraindication to regional anesthesia or fever were excluded.

60 patients were assigned randomly using concealed envelop method to one of three groups. Each group consisted of 20 patients: Group L (combined lumbar plexus and sciatic nerve block without adjuvant), Group D (combined lumbar plexus and sciatic nerve block +perineural 8mg dexamethasone in LPB) and Group S (combined lumbar plexus and sciatic nerve block+intravenous 8mg dexamethasone).

IV cannula 18 G was inserted and midazolam 0.02mg/kg was given IV for sedation.

Lumbar plexus block was done using Capdevila's approach. The Patient was placed in the lateral decubitus position with a slight forward tilt. The foot on the side to be blocked was positioned over the dependent leg so that twitches of the quadriceps muscle and patella could be easily noted. Palpation of the anterior thigh was useful to make sure the motor response was indeed that of the quadriceps muscles. Identification of the iliac crest was by palpating hand over the ridge of the pelvic bone and pressing firmly against it. The spinous process of L4 was identified. A line was drawn from the center of the L4 spinous process laterally, to intersect with a line that passes through the posterior superior iliac spine parallel to the vertebral column on the side to be blocked. The puncture point was at the junction of the lateral one third and medial two thirds of the line joining L4 to the line passing through the PSIS.

After sterilization of the skin and under full aseptic precautions; the needle was advanced at right angles to the skin until the transverse process of L4 was encountered. The needle was then directed caudally, no more than 20mm; the accepted end point for the lumbar plexus was stimulation of the femoral nerve, observed by contraction of the quadriceps muscle. Quadriceps contraction which produced patella twitching was sought with an initial current of 1.5mA, and once elicited; the current was reduced until contraction was at 0.5mA. Motor response should not be present at a current less than 0.5 mA. 20ml of 0.5% Bupivacaine was injected slowly in increments of 5 mL after negative aspiration.

Sciatic nerve block was performed using parasacral approach just to cover the tourniquet pain by the use of nerve stimulator and injection

of 10 ml 0.5% bupivacaine after obtaining appropriate muscle response (planter flexion and inversion of the due to stimulation of the tibial nerve and dorsiflexion and eversion due to stimulation of common peroneal).

To determine loss of motor function Bromage scale from 1 to 3 (1=lack of hip flexion, 2=loss of knee extension, 3-loss of ankle dorsiflexion) was used. Sensory block was assessed by pinprick (using a 25 gauge hollow needle) every five minutes in the L1-S1 dermatomes. Failure to achieve motor or sensory loss after 30 min was considered block failure.

The measured parameters were; heart rate and mean blood pressure in preoperative, at skin incision, after 15, 30, 60min, 2, 4, 6, 12 and 24 hrs after block application, Pain assessment by the aid of Visual analogue scale recorded postoperative after 30 min., 2, 4, 6, 8, 12 and 24 hours after block application, onset of both sensory and motor block and duration of sensory and motor block, the total doses of paracetamol used as additional analgesia during the 1st 24 hours, incidence of Complications and patients' satisfaction using 5 point Likert scale [5].

Statistical analysis

SPSS statistics v.17.0 for windows was used. Data was summarized and analyzed; and the results were reported as mean ± SD. Comparison of the means of the 3 study groups was done using the ANOVA test. Non parametric variables were compared using Kruskal Wallis test. For all statistical tests, the level of significance was fixed at the 5% level. A p-value <0.05 indicated significant difference. The smaller the p-value obtained, the more significant was the difference.

Sample size

Given that the duration of thelumbar plexus sensory block is reported to be 18 ± 2 hours, a total sample size of 57 patients randomly allocated into three equal groups (19 patients per group) will have 80% power to detect a clinically significant difference of 10%or more in the mean duration of sensory block (effect size f=0.424, α error=0.05, β error=0.2). Statistical power calculations was performed using computer program G*Power 3 for Windows. (Franz Faul, Universität Kiel, Germany).

Results:

60 (out of 72) patients were recruited to undergo arthroscopic knee surgery using lumbar plexus block.12 patients were excluded from this study (5 patients showed failure of sensory block for 30 min after block application and 7 patients didn't complete the study due to early hospital discharge).

The demographic data of the patients, their baseline hemodynamic parameters, temperature and type of operation showed no statistical significant difference among the three study groups (Table1).

	Group L (n=20)	Group D (n=20)	Group S (n= 20)
Age (years)	33 ± 14	32 ± 13.6	34 ± 15
Gender	8 (40%)	11 (55%)	12(60%)
Male no. (%)	12(60%)	9 (45%)	8(40%)
Female no. (%)			

Weight (Kg)	70 ± 0.6	69 ± 0.8	71 ± 0.3
Duration of surgery(hrs)	2 ± 0.6	1.9 ± 0.8	2.1 ± 0.2
Data was presented as mean ± SD or no. (%)			

Table 1: Demographic data of the three studied groups.

The mean heart rate and the mean arterial blood pressure (MAP) preoperatively and intraoperative showed no significant variations between the 3 groups and within each group (Tables 2 and 3).

	Group L (n=20)	Group D (n=20)	Group S (n=20)	P value
T0	81.7 ± 11.4	83.7 ± 10.7	74 ± 11.12	®0.748 ©0.111 §0.07
T1	80.7 ± 5.6	83.7 ± 4.7	86.25 ± 5.3	®0.189 ©0.08 §0.28
T2	81.7 ± 6.1	81.3 ± 5.7	84 ± 6.1	®1 ©0.406 §0.39
T3	78.9 ± 6.9	79.7 ± 7.2	81.7 ± 5.7	®0.92 ©0.36 §0.59
T4	79.5 ± 6.9	79.3 ± 6.2	81.3 ± 7.3	®0.9 ©0.71 §0.63
T5	74.5 ± 5.8	75.3 ± 6.4	76.4 ± 6.1	®0.91 ©0.59 §0.84
T6	77.1 ± 4.1	76.9 ± 5.8	78.2 ± 4.2	®0.99 ©0.76 §0.70
T7	68.6 ± 6.8	78.3 ± 7.1	79.9 ± 6.8	®0.98 ©0.79 §0.70
T8	77.6 ± 7.5	81.6 ± 8.1	81.3 ± 7.6	®0.33 ©0.29 §0.99
T9	76.1 ± 7.1	79.2 ± 7.4	81.1 ± 7.6	®0.37 ©0.08 §0.68

T0=preoperative; T1=skin incision, T2=15 minutes thereafter; T3=30 minutes thereafter; T4=60 minutes thereafter; T5=4 hours thereafter; T6=6 hours thereafter; T7=8 hours thereafter; T8=12 hours thereafter; T9=24 hours thereafter, Data was presented as mean ± SD; ®=p value between Group L and D; ©= p value between Group L andS,§= p value between Group D and S; *=Significant

Table 2: Mean heart rate intraoperative and postoperative for the three groups.

	Group L (n=20)	Group D (n=20)	Group S (n=20)	p value
T0	92.3 ± 5.7	93.7 ± 4.5	95.4 ± 4.1	®0.60 ©0.1 §0.50
T1	93.3 ± 5.6	92.8 ± 4.4	91.1 ± 4.8	®0.95 ©0.33 §0.49
T2	96.1 ± 3.8	94.8 ± 4.4	96.5 ± 3.1	®0.50 ©0.95 §0.34
T3	95.3 ± 3.6	94.5 ± 4.1	94.6 ± 4.1	®0.82 ©0.86 §0.99
T4	94.4 ± 5.3	94.1 ± 3.9	96.1 ± 3	®0.96 ©0.41 §0.28
T5	94.1 ± 4.5	94.6 ± 4.1	95.6 ± 3	®0.91 ©0.45 §0.7
T6	94.4 ± 3.8	93.5 ± 4.6	94.2 ± 4.6	®0.79 ©0.99 §0.85
T7	93.3 ± 4.5	93.2 ± 5.4	94.6 ± 4.8	®0.99 ©0.65 §0.63
T8	93.6 ± 5.8	93.7 ± 4.7	93.3 ± 5.3	®0.99 ©0.97 §0.96
T9	93.8 ± 5.3	93.5 ± 4.1	92.2 ± 5.4	®0.97 ©0.57 §0.71

T0=preoperative; T1=skin incision, T2=15 minutes thereafter; T3=30 minutes thereafter; T4=60 minutes thereafter; T5=4 hours thereafter; T6=6 hours thereafter; T7=8 hours thereafter; T8=12 hours thereafter; T9=24 hours thereafter. Data was presented as mean ± SD; ®=p value between Group L and D; ©= p value between Group L and S; §= p value between Group D and S; *=Significant

Table 3: Mean ABP intraoperative and postoperative (mmHg) for the three studied groups.

By comparing the visual analogue score (VAS) of the 3 groups; 30 min, 2, 4, 6, 8, 12 and 24 (hours) postoperatively, results revealed non-significant variation between the 3 groups at T0,T1,T2,T3,T4 and T5.

But there was a statistically significant difference between the 3 groupS at T6 and T7 with less VAS observed in both groups D and S (p value<0.02) when compared to group L and non-significant difference between groups D and S (Table 4).

Time	Group L (n=20) Median/range	Group D (n=20) Median/range	Group S (n=20) Median/range	p value
T1	0/(0-0)	0/(0-0)	0/(0-0)	®1 ©1 §1
T2	0/(0-0)	0/(0-0)	0/(0-0)	®1 ©1 §1
T3	0/(0-10)	0/(0-0)	0/(0-0)	®0.32 ©0.32 §1
T4	0/(0-10)	0/(0-0)	0/(0-0)	®0.08 ©0.08 §1
T5	0/(0-30)	0/(0-0)	0/(0-0)	®0.08 ©0.08 §1
T6	0/(0-80)	0/(0-0)	0/(0-0)	®0.01* ©0.01* §1
T7	40/(0-90)	5/(0-50)	0/(0-50)	®0.02* ©0.01* §0.7

T1=30 min after block application, T2=2 hrs after block application, T3=4 hrs after block application, T4= 6 hrs after block application, T5= 8 hrs after block application, T6= 12 hrs after block application, T7= 24 hrs after block application. VAS was measured in mm. Data was presented as median /range; ®=p value between Group L and D; ©= p value between Group L and S; §= p value between Group D and S; *=Significant

Table 4: Visual analogue score 30 min, 2, 4, 6, 8, 12, 24 (hrs) after block application.

Regarding onset of sensory loss, results showed statistically significant enhanced onset of sensory loss in group D when compared to group L (p value=0.04) but no statistically significant difference found between groups S and L (p value=0.13) or between groups D and S (p value =0.86) (Table 5).

Regarding onset of motor loss it was found that group D enhanced onset of motor block significantly (p value<0.01) when compared to group L, while group S showed statistically insignificant enhancement of onset of motor block when compared to group L(p value=0.15) or group D (p value=0.71) (Table 5).

Regarding sensory block duration (Postoperative analgesia), both groups D and S showed significant prolonged duration of analgesia (p value<0.01and0.04 respectively) when compared to group L, but no statistically significance detected when compared to each other (p value=0.24) which means they both similarly prolong duration of analgesia clinically (Table 5).

Motor block duration was significantly prolonged in group D when compared to groups L and group S (p value≤0.01).While group S didn't show statistically significant prolongation of motor block when compared to group L (p value=0.4) (Table 5).

	Group L (n=20)	Group D (n=20)	Group S (n=20)	p value
Sensory loss onset(min)	15.4 ± 5.3	12.7 ± 1.3	14.1 ± 5.2	®0.04* ©0.13 §0.86
Motor loss onset(min)	25.1 ± 6.4	15.3 ± 1.8	16.5 ± 5.1	®0.00* ©0.15 §0.71
Sensory block duration (hrs)	18.9 ± 3.5	24 ± 1.2	21.7 ± 2.5	®0.00* ©0.04* §0.24
Motor block duration (hrs)	21.4 ± 3.2	26.4 ± 1.3	22.4 ± 2.1	®0.00* ©0.40 §0.00*

min=minutes, hrs=hours, Data was presented as mean ± SD; ®=p value between Group L and D; ©= p value between Group L and S; §= p value between Group D and S; *=Significant

Table 5: Sensory and motor loss onset (min) and regression (hrs).

Concerning postoperative analgesic requirements, it was noted that patients in groups D and S significantly required less analgesic doses in the first 24 hours postoperatively(p value=0.05), when compared with those in group L.

However there were no statistical significant differences between group D and group S (p value=1). One patient in group D and eight patients in group S required extra doses of analgesics (in the form of 1 gm paracetamol), compared to ten patients in group L (9 patients required 2 gm paracetamol and 1 patient required 3 gm paracetamol) (Table 6).

	Group L (n=20)	Group D (n=20)	Group S (n=20)	p value
Paracetamol (gm/24 hrs)	2.05 ± 0.3	0.05 ± 0.01	0.4 ± 0.09	®0.05* ©0.05* §1
hrs=hours; Data was presented as mean ± SD; *=Significant				

Table 6: Dose of paracetamol used in the first 24 (hours) postoperative.

There were two recorded complications in (groups S and D) in the form of hemodynamic instability after epidural spread that lead to anaesthesia for both limbs, and was managed by giving 500 ml crystalloids and 5 mg ephedrine increments till stabilizing blood pressure.

12 patients were excluded from this study as they showed failure of the block that was considered when failure of sensory block for 30 min after block application (Table 7).

Complications	Group L (n=20)	Group D (n=20)	Group S (n=20)
Yes	1(5%)	1(5%)	1(5%)
No	19(95%)	19(95%)	19(95%)
Data was presented as n (%)			

Table 7: Incidence of complications.

(Table 8) demonstrates patient satisfaction with lumbar plexus block in the three studied groups using Likert scale of satisfaction and it was mostly ranging between satisfied and completely satisfied.

Patients satisfaction	Group L (n=20)	Group D (n=20)	Group S (n=20)
Completely satisfied	2 (10%)	5 (25%)	2 (10%)
Satisfied	18 (90%)	14 (70%)	18 (90%)
Not Satisfied nor Dissatisfied	0 (0%)	1 (5%)	0 (0%)
Data was presented as n (%) using 5 point Likert scale.			

Table 8: Patient's satisfaction.

Discussion

Evidently the dexamethasone was proven superior in prolonging the duration of analgesia when compared to other adjuvants such as clonidine, neostigmine and tramadol [6].

Regarding hemodynamic changes (heart rate and mean blood pressure intra and postoperative), results of the present study showed hemodynamic stability in the three groups.

In addition, Siamak Y et al. [7] who enrolled 78 patients received axillary block for forearm fracture operation in 3 groups; [(group L) received 40 ml lidocaine and 2 ml distilled water, (group LD) received 40 ml lidocaine and 2 ml dexamethasone and (group LF) received 40 ml lidocaine and 2 ml fentanyl]. They found no difference between the groups in regards to hemodynamics.

Regarding onset of sensory loss, results of this study showed that both perineural and IV dexamethasone enhanced the onset of sensory block. But only perineural dexamethasone enhanced the onset of motor block not the IV administration.

These results were consistent with Yadav RK. et al. [8] study that included 90 patients received supraclavicular brachial plexus block and randomized into 3 groups; [(group A) received 24 ml lignocaine (1.5%) with adrenaline, (group B) received 24 ml lignocaine (1.5%) with adrenaline +500 µg Neostigmine, and (group C) received 24 ml lignocaine (1.5%) with adrenaline +4 mg Dexamethasone perineural]. Results showed enhanced onset of both sensory and motor block and prolonged duration dexamethasone group compared to the other two groups.

In addition the results of the present study were consistent with Prashant A. et al. [9] who evaluated the effect of dexamethasone added to lidocaine regarding onset of action and duration. They enrolled 60 patients received supraclavicular brachial plexus block for elective hand, forearm and elbow surgeries. They concluded that addition of dexamethasone to 1.5% lidocaine with adrenaline speeds the onset and prolongs the duration of sensory and motor blockade.

However this study results disagreed with the study done by Knezevic NN. et al. [10] who performed a meta-analysis (included 1022 patients) in order to assess the effects of different doses of dexamethasone added to LA for brachial plexus blocks either alone or with epinephrine. The latter study concluded that perineural dexamethasone injection significantly delayed the onset of sensory and motor block regardless of the dose.

Effect of different doses of dexamethasone (either perineuraly or IV) was not included in this study, but Yadav et al. [8] used lignocaine with smaller doses of dexamethasone (4 mg) than that used in the present study (8 mg); and found that low dose of dexamethasone also enhanced onset of motor and sensory blocks. Moreover, Knezevic NN. et al. proved that smaller doses of dexamethasone (4-5 mg) were as effective as higher ones (8-10 mg).

The results of the present study showed that both perineural and IV dexamethasone prolong the duration of analgesia similarly. That was consistent with Desmet M. et al. [11] who enrolled 150 patients presenting for arthroscopic shoulder surgery with inter scalene block and divided them into 3 groups; [(group R) received 30 ml ropivacaine 0.5%, (group RD) received 30 ml ropivacaine 0.5% and perineural dexamethasone 10 mg and (group RDiv) received 30 ml ropivacaine 0.5% with i.v. dexamethasone 10 mg]. The latter study proved that both IV and perineural dexamethasone has similar effects in prolonging analgesia after inter scalene block.

As for duration of analgesia, results of the present study were consistent with Abdallah F. et al. [12] who enrolled 75 patients divided into 3 groups 25 patients each, randomized to receive supraclavicular block using either [30-mL bupivacaine 0.5% alone (control group) or with concomitant intravenous dexamethasone 8 mg (DexIV group), or with perineural dexamethasone 8 mg (DexP group)]. Duration of analgesia was designated .Their results showed duration of analgesia was prolonged in the IV group (25 hours) compared with Control (13.2 hours), but similar to the perineural group (25 hours). Both IV and Perineural groups had reduced pain scores, reduced postoperative opioid consumption, and improved satisfaction compared with control group.

With regards to duration of the motor block, our results showed that both perineural and IV dexamethasone prolong the duration of motor block. It was found that perineural group showed prolongation of motor block duration when compared to IV administarion. These results were however against Abdallah F. et al. [12] who found that the IV group experienced longer motor block (30.1 hours) compared with perineural group (25.5 hours) and control groups (19.7 hours),although they used the same dose of dexamethasone and the same volume and concentration of bupivacaine used in the present study. Regarding analgesic requirements, results of this study showed that both IV and perineural dexamethasone when given with LPB reduced the analgesic requirements. That was consistent with Desmet M. et al. [11] and Abdallah F. et al. [12] who proposed that IV dexamethasone should be considered for routine use in patients having regional analgesia for the postoperative pain management.

Results of this study showed similar and significant reduction in VAS measurements at 12 and 24 hrs postoperative for both perineural and IV dexamethasone administration. These results were consistent with Desmet M. et al. [11] who found that both perineural and IV dexamethasone had reduced pain scores, reduced postoperative opioid consumption, and improved satisfaction.

In the present study no adverse effects were detected by adding dexamethasone as an adjuvant to local anesthetics in lumbar plexus block application.

That was consistent with Choi S. et al. [4] who enrolled 393 patients receiving dexamethasone (4–10 mg) as an adjuvant to LA used in brachial plexus block (BPB) and found that perineural administration of dexamethasone had no observed adverse events.

The results of the current study were consistent with Noss et al. [6] who made 11 randomized clinical trials (for 456 patients) evaluating adverse effects of variable doses of dexamethasone (ranging between 4

to 10 mg) as adjuvant to different types of LA (lidocaine, mepivacaine, bupivacaine and ropivacaine) in brachial plexus nerve blocks. They reported no major complications at one year when dexamethasone was added perineuraly.

Furthermore the results of the present study were consistent with Parrington et al. [13] who enrolled 45 adult patients undergoing elective hand or forearm surgeries under supraclavicular brachial plexus blockade, and were randomized to receive either [30 mL mepivacaine 1.5% plus dexamethasone 8 mg (4 mg/mL), or 30 mL mepivacaine 1.5% plus 2 mL normal saline]. They reported that the most frequent adverse effect in their study was numbness or tingling in the hand, which was transitory and was not significantly different between dexamethasone and control groups.

Knezevic NN. et al. [10] considered the excessively prolonged nerve block that was observed predominantly in the dexamethasone-adjuvant group as a complication.

Regarding patients' satisfaction, this study's results showed that all patients (100%) in groups S and L were satisfied, meanwhile (95%) of patients in group D were satisfied with (5%) neutral (not satisfied nor dissatisfied).

These results were in accordance with Desmet et al. [11] who found that both perineural and IV dexamethasone had reduced pain scores and improved patient satisfaction postoperative.

The results were also consistent with Ironfield et al. [14] questionnaire for 9969 patients (had operations done using peripheral nerve blocks). He stated that if they were willing to repeat the PNB they had or not, (90%) of respondents were satisfied or completely satisfied with the information provided about the nerve block, as well as the anesthesiologist-patient interaction.

Conclusion

Perineural dexamethasone when given as adjunct to LPB was found to enhance the action of LA by enhancing onset of action and prolonging duration for both sensory and motor blocks with significant less need for postoperative rescue analgesia, as well lower pain scores up to 24 hours postoperative, better patient satisfaction with no evidence to increase incidence of complications.

Moreover, it was found in this study that IV dexamethasone causes prolonged duration of analgesia but didn't found to enhance onset of action.

References

1. Thomas D, Mathias O, Stavros GM (2014) Perioperative pain control after total knee arthroplasty: An evidence based review of the role of peripheral nerve blocks. World J Orthop 5: 225-227.

2. Young TJ (2012) Peripheral nerve block for anesthesia in patients having knee arthroplasty. Korean J Anesthesiology 62: 403-411.

3. Ganidağli S, Cengiz M, Baysal Z, Baktiroglu L, Sarban S. (2005) The comparison of two lower extremity block techniques combined with sciatic block: 3-in-1 femoral block vs. psoas compartment block. Int J Clin Pract 59: 771-775.

4. Choi S, Rodseth R, McCartney CJL (2014) Effects of dexamethasone as a local anesthetic adjuvant for brachial plexus block: a systematic review and meta-analysis of randomized trials. Br J Anaesth 112: 427-439.

5. Likert R (1932) "A Technique for the Measurement of Attitudes". Archives of Psychology 140: 1-55.

6. Noss C, Lindsay M, Mark K (2014) Dexamethasone a Promising Adjuvant in Brachial Plexus Anesthesia? Journal of Anesthesia and Clinical Research 5: 7.

7. Siamak Y, Mahyar S, Zohreh Y (2013) Comparison of Postoperative Analgesic Effect of Dexamethasone and Fentanyl Added to Lidocaine through Axillary Block in Forearm Fracture.

8. Yadav RK, Sah BP, Kumar P, Singh SN (2013) Effectiveness of addition of neostigmine or dexamethasone to local anaesthetic in providing perioperative analgesia for brachial plexus block: A prospective, randomized, double blinded, controlled study. Kathmandu Univ Med J 6: 302-309.

9. Prashant AB, Padmanabha K, Kannappady G (2013) Effect of dexamethasone added to lidocaine in supraclavicular brachial plexus block. Indian journal of anesthesia 57.

10. Knezevic NN, Utchariya A, Kenneth DC (2015) Perineural Dexamethasone Added to Local Anesthesia for Brachial Plexus Block Improves Pain but Delays Block Onset and Motor Blockade Recovery Pain Physician 18: 1-14.

11. Desmet M, Braems H, Reynvoet M, Plasschaert S, Van Cauwelaert J (2013) I.V. and perineural dexamethasone are equivalent in increasing the analgesic duration of a single-shot interscalene block with ropivacaine for shoulder surgery: a prospective, randomized, placebo-controlled study. Br J Anaesth111: 445-452.

12. Abdallah FW, Johnson J, Chan V, Murgatroyd H, Ghafari M (2015) Intravenous Dexamethasone and Perineural Dexamethasone Similarly Prolong the Duration of Analgesia After Supraclavicular Brachial Plexus Block: A Randomized, Triple-Arm, Double-Blind, Placebo-Controlled Trial. Reg Anesth Pain Med 40: 125-132.

13. Parrington SJ, O'Donnell D, Chan VW, Brown-Shreves D, Subramanyam R (2010) Dexamethasone added to mepivacaine prolongs the duration of analgesia after supraclavicular brachial plexus blockade. Reg Anesth Pain Med 35: 422-426.

14. Ironfield CM, Barrington MJ, Kluger R, Sites B (2014) Are Patients Satisfied After Peripheral Nerve Blockade? Results from International Registry of Regional Anesthesia. Reg Anesth Pain Med 39: 48-55.

23

Enhanced Recovery after Surgery Pathway: How its Implementation Influenced Digestive Surgery Outcomes?

Carolina Tintim and Humberto S Machado*

Largo Professor Abel Salazar, Centro Hospitlar do Porto, Serviço de Anestesiologia, Portugal

***Corresponding author:** Humberto S Machado, Largo Professor Abel Salazar, Centro Hospitlar do Porto, Serviço de Anestesiologia, Portugal, E-mail: hjs.machado@gmail.com

Abstract

Introduction: In recent years, enhanced recovery after surgery protocols have increasingly been integrated into perioperative care of patients undergoing digestive surgery.

Aims: To conduct a non-systematic literature review related to the integration of enhanced recovery after surgery protocols in elective gastrectomy, colonic and rectal surgery, and the impact this had on outcomes.

Methods: The PubMed database was searched to identify studies that focused on the integration of enhanced recovery after surgery protocols in clinical practice, as well as their outcomes. 37 studies fulfilled the inclusion criteria and were reviewed accordingly between the years of 2007 and 2017.

Results: The enhanced recovery after surgery pathway has shown to reduce time to return of bowel function and to minimize length of hospital stay by at least one day, when compared to conventional care, in colorectal surgery and gastrectomy for gastric cancer. Optimal results are achieved with maximum compliance rates.

Conclusions: The enhanced recovery after surgery protocols may be safely implemented in colorectal surgery and gastrectomy for gastric cancer, producing improved patient outcomes. An adequate integration of the enhanced recovery after surgery protocols in these areas, with a high compliance rate, is a step towards a faster return of patients to their baseline activity.

Keywords: Enhanced recovery after surgery; Digestive; Gastrectomy; Colorectal; Colonic; Rectal; Gastrointestinal

Abbreviations: ERAS: Enhanced Recovery After Surgery; CHO: Complex Carbohydrates; ASA: American Society of Anesthesiologists; MBP: Mechanical Bowel Preparation; DVT: Deep Venous Thrombosis; LMWH: Low Molecular Weight Heparin; VTE: Venous Thromboembolism; LOSH: Length of Stay in Hospital; PONV: Postoperative Nausea and Vomiting; EDA: Epidural Analgesia; RCT: Randomized Controlled Trial; PCA: Patient Controlled Analgesia; BIS: Bispectral Index; TAP: Transversus Abdominis Plane; ED: Esophageal Doppler; NG: Nasogastric; BD: Bladder Drainage; UTI: Urinary Tract Infection; NSAIDs: Non-steroidal Anti-inflammatory Drugs; ICU: Intensive Care Unit; POD: Postoperative Day; IL: Interleukin; QR: Quality of Recovery.

Introduction

Despite steady advances in surgical and anesthetic techniques over the years, postoperative complications remain one of the major concerns regarding surgical procedures, not only because of the impact on the patient, but also on the health care system in general.

The ERAS programs, originally based on the "fast track" surgery concept introduced by Henrik Kehlet [1], were developed as multimodal perioperative pathways that include multiple interventions that individually produce small insignificant effects, but collectively have a strong synergistic impact on the patients' homeostasis [2]. These protocols strike to attenuate the metabolic stress through perioperative measures, and simultaneously to support the patient's rapid return to baseline function, producing therefore a decrease in complication rates and lessening the recovery time after surgery.

The present literature review aims to gather current scientific knowledge regarding outcomes of ERAS programs in digestive surgery. It was considered important to first briefly review the ERAS items, as it allows for a better comprehension of results. This review focuses on elective digestive surgery, more specifically on gastrectomy and colorectal surgery, for which the ERAS Society published guidelines for perioperative care.

Materials and Methods

This literature review is based on a PubMed search with the following instructions: Title/abstract: ("enhanced recovery after surgery" OR "eras") AND ("gastrectomy" OR "gastric" OR "colon" OR "colonic" OR " colorectal" OR "rectal"). The following filters were applied to the search: species: human; date: 2007-2017.

From the 131 articles found, 37 were selected for review. The excluded papers regarded non-elective surgery (e.g. emergency context), surgery of fields other than colorectal and gastric (bariatric surgery not included), studies that focused on the elderly or on the pediatric population, studies that used modified ERAS protocols, publications related to cost-effectiveness of ERAS protocol implementations, or because they did not adjust to the topics reviewed in this article. No procedure specific ERAS items have been revised.

Additional articles were referenced as they were found relevant for the debate of the state of the art of the subject.

Results

Surgical stress

The stress response to surgery is activated through the nervous system, which mainly results in hematological, immunological and endocrinological responses. The extent of this response correlates with the degree of tissue injury, which may be posteriorly amplified by postoperative complications [2,3].

Stress response is proportional to the extension of the surgical wound, the degree of internal organ manipulation and tissue dissection and reflects increased demands on organ function [2].

The hormonal changes produced result, as an overall, in a hypermetabolic status where most biochemical reactions are accelerated. In evolutionary terms, it seems likely that this stress response was developed as a protective mechanism that aims to provide maximum chances of survival, through the increase of cardiovascular functions, volume preservation and mobilization of substrates [3-5]. In current surgical and anesthetic practice, it is questionable if this stress response is necessary as it turns out that a prolonged hypermetabolic state may result in the body's exhaustion, causing loss of weight, decreased resistance, delayed ambulation and increased morbidity and mortality [3,5]. This considered, in modern surgical practice, efforts are made to minimize the stress response [6].

Minimizing surgical injury through the eras pathway

The ERAS pathway strike to attenuate the physiological stress response to surgery and maintain preoperative organ function. The ERAS protocols include measures integrated before, during and after the surgical procedure.

Preoperative Items:- 1. Information, education and counseling: Preoperative anxiety, emotional distress and depression have been associated with higher complication rates, greater postoperative pain, cognitive disturbances and delayed convalescence [2].

Giving the patient, as well as of the caregivers, information about the surgical and anesthetic procedures is essential to reduce anxiety and to facilitate active participation in the recovery process [2,7-9]. Indicating specific daily targets for the postoperative period may facilitate eating, mobilization, pain control and respiratory function, therefore reducing complication risk [8].

In the case of patients undergoing rectal surgery, it is important to add specific information regarding the marking and management of stomas [9].

2. Preoperative medical optimization: The impact of preoperative physical conditioning on surgical outcomes is controversial, and increasing exercise preoperatively may benefit the patient's recovery [7-9].

Preoperative optimization also involves alcohol and smoking cessation and abstinence for at least 4 weeks before the surgery, to reduce the incidence of complications related to these habits [7-10]. Alcohol abusers have a two-to-threefold increase in postoperative

morbidity, the most frequent complications being bleeding, wound and cardiopulmonary complications. Smokers have an increased risk for postoperative pulmonary and wound complications [7].

3. Fasting and carbohydrate loading: Standard care follows fasting guidelines supported by multiple anesthesia societies, that recommend that clear fluids and solid food should not be ingested 2 h and 6 h, respectively, before the induction of anesthesia. Although this is the recommendation, it is not uncommon for patients scheduled for elective surgery to fast since midnight [7,10]. There is no scientific evidence that fasting from midnight reduces the risk of pulmonary aspiration in elective surgery [7], and this practice has been shown to increase insulin resistance, produce patient discomfort [8] and potentially decrease intravascular volume [7,10].

Preoperative treatment with complex carbohydrate (CHO) drinks attenuates the catabolic state induced by overnight fasting and surgery, allowing patients to undergo surgery in a metabolically fed state [9]. The increase of preoperative insulin levels, reduces postoperative insulin resistance [9], maintains glycogen reserves, decreases protein breakdown and reduces the loss of muscle strength [2,7,9,10]. In addition to this, treatment with CHOs also has been shown to reduce preoperative thirst, hunger and anxiety [7,9]. Faster surgical recovery, as a consequence of this practice, still remains controversial [10].

Preoperative treatment with CHO drinks, following the "preoperative fasting status" ASA recommendations, is advised for all non-diabetic patients [9], and may be safely administered except in emergency surgeries [10,11], and in patients with documented delayed gastric emptying or gastrointestinal motility disorders [10,11]. Obese patients have been shown to have the same gastric-emptying characteristics as slim individuals. Diabetic patients with neuropathic affectation may have delayed gastric emptying for solids, which may increase the risk of regurgitation and aspiration. There isn't any conclusive data relating to delayed fluid emptying. In diabetic patients without neuropathy, gastric emptying has been reported as normal, and CHO drinks may be given along with diabetic medication [7].

4. Bowel preparations: Lately, the use of mechanical bowel preparation (MBP) has been strongly questioned. This practice, not only is distressing to the patient, but also causes dehydration and is associated with prolonged ileus after colonic surgery. In addition to this, the use of MBPs, on colorectal surgery, has been shown to increase the incidence of spillage of bowel contents, increasing the risk of postoperative complications [7]. However, when a diverting ileostomy is planned, MBP may be necessary [9]. If, for any reason, intraoperative colonoscopy might be carried out, MBP is also advised.

Most of the randomized control trials conducted on this matter, are focused on open colorectal surgery, therefore, extrapolating these results to laparoscopic surgery may be questionable [7].

According to ERAS Society recommendations, in gastrectomy, MBP should not be used [8].

5. Antibiotic prophylaxis and skin preparation: The use of prophylactic antibiotics with aerobic and anaerobic coverage, in colorectal surgery, has shown to reduce postoperative infectious complications. In gastrectomy and colorectal surgery, intravenous antibiotics should ideally be administered 30-60 min before the first surgical incision [7,8]. A multidose regimen may be preferred in prolonged surgeries (>3 h), whenever it is appropriate considering the antibiotic's pharmacokinetics [7-9]. The optimal combination of antibiotics is still not defined, however the combination of

metronidazole and an aerobic antibiotic is often recommended. New generation drugs should be reserved for infectious complications [9].

A study comparing the use of povidone-iodine and chlorhexidine-alcohol in skin cleansing concluded that the latter is superior in preventing infectious complications [8,9], being associated with a 40% lower prevention of surgical site infections. The use of chlorhexidine-alcohol, however, may be a risk factor for burn injuries whenever diathermy is used [7].

6. Thromboprophylaxis: All patients undergoing abdominal or pelvic surgery should receive mechanical thromboprophylaxis with well-fitted stockings, as they have been shown to significantly reduce the incidence of deep venous thrombosis (DVT) in hospitalized patients. Intermittent pneumatic compression should be considered, above all, in patients with risk factors for thromboembolic events [7-9]. Risk factors include previous pelvic surgery, preoperative treatment with corticosteroids, malignant disease [7,9], major surgery, long periods of recumbence, chemotherapy [8] and other hypercoagulable states.

The benefits of pharmacological prophylaxis with low-molecular-weight heparin (LMWH) or unfractionated heparin in the prevention of venous thromboembolism are well established [7,8], they reduce the prevalence of symptomatic venous thromboembolism (VTE) without increasing side effects such as bleeding [9]. However, the benefit of extended (28 days) prophylaxis after discharge, is less consensual. Extended prophylaxis has been shown to significantly reduce the prevalence of symptomatic DVT, but, due to a very low prevalence of this complication in patients who did not receive prophylactic treatment, it is questionable whether a large number of patients should receive thromboprophylaxis to prevent a few symptomatic events [7]. Current ERAS Society guidelines advocate that this treatment should be reserved for patients who had major cancer surgery in the abdomen or pelvis or who have other important risk factors for VTE [7].

It is unknown if the implementation of ERAS protocols and/or the use of laparoscopic surgery, through the promotion of an early recovery, reduce the risk of VTE and, therefore, the need for pharmacological prophylaxis [9].

Incidence of asymptomatic DVT in colorectal surgical patients without thromboprophylaxis is approximately 30%, with fatal pulmonary embolus occurring in 1% of individuals [7].

8. Preanesthesia medication: Data from studies on abdominal surgery, show no evidence of clinical benefit from preoperative use of long-acting sedatives [8]. Their administration is associated with impaired postoperative mobilization and direct participation, resulting in prolonged length of stay in hospital (LOSH) [7,10]. Short-acting anesthetic drugs (e.g. fentanyl combined with small incremental doses of midazolam or propofol) may be safely administered, under monitorization, to facilitate anesthetic procedures (e.g. epidural or spinal anesthesia) previously to the induction of anesthesia, with minimal residual effect at the end of surgery [7].

Preoperative education and counseling may help reduce the need for anxiolytic medication, as well as other ERAS elements, such as the avoidance of MBP and prolonged fasting, and preoperative treatment with CHOs [7].

Intraoperative Items: 1. Laparoscopy: Laparoscopy is a minimally invasive surgical technique that has been shown to decrease inflammatory response to surgery when compared to open approaches. The ERAS Society guidelines recommend that proctectomy and proctocolectomy for benign disease, colonic resection and early gastric cancer gastrectomy be done laparoscopically, if an experienced surgeon is available. In this setting, laparoscopic surgery has shown to be safe and may lower hospital stay and decrease complication rates. However, ERAS Society guidelines do not recommend laparoscopic resection of rectal cancer outside a trial setting, due to lack of equivalent data on oncological outcomes, nor laparoscopically assisted total gastrectomy for advanced cancer, as there is inconclusive data as to the safety of this procedure [7-9].

2. Anesthetic management: Although there are no trials comparing general anesthetic techniques for gastrointestinal surgery [7,8,10], ERAS protocols aim for a minimal impact of anesthetic agents and techniques on organ function, and for a rapid awakening, allowing an early return to baseline activity [10]. To do so, it is sensible to assume that short-acting agents should be preferred.

Short-acting induction agents, such as propofol, combined with short-acting opioids, such as fentanyl or remifentanil, are widely used, as well as short-acting muscle relaxants [7,8,10]. Recently, a review on the use of continuous intravenous lidocaine infusion in the perioperative of abdominal surgery concluded that it provides significant pain relief, reduces postoperative opioid consumption, decreases opioid-induced nausea and vomiting, and promotes a faster return of bowel function, allowing for reduced LOSH. There is a continuous effort to reduce opioid administration because they are associated with several complications, such as respiratory depression, sedation, postoperative nausea and vomiting (PONV), ileus and urinary retention [11,12]. A recent RCT in patients undergoing colorectal surgery with the ERAS program, showed no difference between continuous lidocaine infusion and thoracic epidural analgesia (EDA), in return of bowel movements and LOSH, whilst another RCT focused on patients undergoing laparoscopic gastrectomy showed a reduction in postoperative fentanyl consumption and pain with lidocaine infusion by patient-controlled analgesia (PCA) [8].

Muscle relaxants can be titrated using neuromuscular monitoring, allowing for administration of the minimal dose necessary to produce the intended effect. The maintenance of a deep neuro-muscular blockage is essential to allow adequate vision and surgical access [7], particularly in laparoscopic surgery [8]. Despite this, reversal of profound muscle relaxation, can occasionally be incomplete. In these cases, the use of sugammadex to counter act the action of large doses of muscle relaxants, has proven to facilitate recovery [9].

The maintenance of anesthesia can be made using inhalation anesthetics or intravenous anesthesia, in which case, target controlled pumps may be used. These are especially useful in patients with susceptibility to PONV [7]. Short-acting agents should also be used in maintaining anesthesia, always adjusted the estimated duration of surgery.

Depth of induction and maintenance anesthesia can be monitored using the bispectral index (BIS) monitor, which enables titration of the minimum amount of anesthetic necessary to avoid complications [7-10]. Anesthetic depth guided by BIS is a key aspect in preventing awareness and in allowing for a faster immediate recovery, although time to discharge home seems unaffected [10]. To this effect, BIS index should be between 40 and 60. Studies have highlighted that too deep anesthesia should be avoided, as this reflects increased suppression of brain activity and can lead to postoperative confusion, mainly in the elderly [10].

Regional anesthetic blockage, used in addition to general anesthesia, can minimize the need for postoperative intravenous opiates and reduce the stress response. This includes a reduction in insulin resistance, an important causing mechanism of postoperative hyperglycemia [7].

Another important component of the anesthetic management is the regulation of ventilation and airway. Attention to intubation techniques is important to reduce risk of micro-aspiration and subsequent postoperative lung infection. To this end, adequate sized endotracheal tubes with cuff-pressure control should be used [7]. Lung ventilation with low tidal volumes, limiting peak air pressure, is suggested to reduce the risk of barotraumas [9].

Surgical stress demands for an increased fraction of inspired oxygen, to overcome hypoxia under anesthesia. It has been suggested that, in patients undergoing general anesthesia, high inspired oxygen concentrations (>80% [9]) reduces the prevalence of surgical site infections. Other than this, it is also said to reduce the incidence of late (>24 h postoperatively) nausea and vomiting, in patients receiving volatile anesthesia without antiemetic prophylaxis [10]. It has been suggested that excessive use of high concentrations of inspired oxygen on cancer patients undergoing abdominal surgery can have deleterious long-term effects and that using 100% inspired oxygen may be associated with an increased risk of atelectasis. Therefore, inspired oxygen concentration should be titrated to produce normal oxygen saturations, avoiding both hypoxia and hyperoxia [10].

3. Regional anesthetic techniques: Insertion of a thoracic epidural catheter is useful in open and laparoscopic procedures to provide improved pain management. Local anesthetics can be administered throughout the procedure, either in bolus or in a continuous infusion [9]. An optimal postoperative analgesia provides an adequate pain relief, early mobilization, early return of gut function and feeding, without associated side effects [7]. Interestingly, a RCT [13] in context of colectomy, showed that, although EDA produces superior pain control, LOSH is not reduced [7].

For open midline laparotomy, EDA has been established as the ideal. EDA using local analgesics (e.g. lidocaine) and low-dose opioids has shown to be superior to intravenous opioid-based alternatives, regarding outcomes such as postoperative pain [7,8] (superior analgesia in the first 72 h following surgery), PONV and pulmonary complications [7]. In this context, EDA was also associated with improved postoperative pulmonary function, decreased risk of pneumonia, improved arterial oxygenation, reduced insulin resistance and a lower rate of postoperative ileus [8].

In laparoscopic surgery, studies regarding colorectal surgery have shown that different epidural blockage levels produce different effects on gastrointestinal function: low-thoracic epidural wasn't associated with benefits, on the contrary, mid-thoracic epidural showed significantly earlier return of flatus, defecation and tolerance of oral diet, when compared to intravenous opioid analgesia [7]. Another study [14], comparing spinal analgesia, PCA with intravenous morphine, and low thoracic epidural anesthesia concluded that patients with the latter had a longer LOSH [7].

EDA causes an extended sympathetic block, which may compromise tissue perfusion. The adequate use of vasopressors to prevent this side effect, provided that the patient is not hypovolemic [7], allows for EDA to be safely used and to its full potential [8]. This adverse effect appears to be attenuated using a combination of low-dose local analgesics and opioids [7]. Other concerns regarding EDA

lie with the fact that up to one-third of epidurals are dysfunctional, possibly due to catheter misplacement, inadequate dosing or pump failure. To ensure that the catheter is well placed, sensory blockage should be tested previously to anesthesia induction [8].

Perioperative transversus abdominis plane (TAP) blocks have been used in laparoscopic colonic surgery, alongside intravenous paracetamol, to cover lower abdominal incisions. TAP blocks have the disadvantage of being short-acting and that no significant RCT has yet compared the use of TAP with epi- or subdural analgesia [7]. There is limited information regarding the use of this technique in rectal surgery and gastrectomy [8,9].

Subarachnoid long-acting local anesthetics and opioids have been successfully used for colonic and colorectal resection [9]. A recent study [15], in the context of laparoscopic colorectal surgery, concluded that this anesthetic technique allows for earlier mobilization and hospital discharge, when compared to EDA [7].

4. Fluid management: Normovolemia is essential for an adequate organ perfusion. Overload of salt/water and hypovolemia both increase postoperative complication rates [8]. Use of goal-directed fluid therapy using minimally invasive cardiac output monitoring, such as the esophageal Doppler (ED), can help optimize fluid management [7,9]. Use of ED in major surgery has demonstrated reduced LOSH and complication rate [8,9], faster return of bowel function, less PONV, and lower incidence of acute kidney injury [7]. Balanced crystalloids have proved to be superior to 0.9% saline solution for the maintenance of the electrolyte balance, and should therefore be preferred [7-9].

Attention to arterial pressure values is especially important when epidural anesthesia is administered, due to its effect on vascular tone [7]. Once normovolemia has been established, vasopressors such as neosynephrine or low doses of norepinephrine [9], should be used to avoid intraoperative hypotension and secure adequate organ perfusion.

Fluid shifts should be minimized by avoiding bowel preparation, maintaining preoperative hydration, as well as minimizing bowel handling and exteriorization outside the abdominal cavity [7,9]. Overload of fluids increases the risk of pulmonary interstitial edema, postoperative hypoxia and cardiopulmonary complications, and exacerbates gastrointestinal edema, which may delay recovery of gut function [16].

In colorectal surgery, assuring an adequate gut perfusion is highly important for the integrity of the anastomosis. It depends on mean arterial pressure and cardiac output, since the splanchnic circulation isn't capable of autoregulation [7,9].

Postoperative intravenous fluids should be minimized to avoid fluid excess. The enteral route should be preferably used [7].

5. Nasogastric intubation: Strong evidence supports that routine nasogastric (NG) decompression, following gastrectomy and colorectal surgery, should be avoided. NG tubes placed during surgery (to evacuate air), should be removed before reversal of anesthesia [7-10]. Gastroesophageal reflux is increased during laparotomy if NG tubes are used [9], as well as complications such as fever, atelectasis and pneumonia [7,9]. The avoidance of NG tubes was associated with a faster return of bowel movements [7-9]. LOSH and gastric discomfort also showed data supporting no NG decompression [7].

6. Maintenance of normothermia: Numerous meta-analysis and RCTs have related hypothermia (definition <36ºC), during major

abdominal surgery, with higher rates of would infections, cardiac complications, bleeding, pain sensibility [7,9] and transfusion requirements [8]. Warming in the preoperative period is especially beneficial for patients who will be exposed due to prolonged anesthetic procedures [7,8]. Temperature maintenance during procedure can be achieved by using forced-air warming blankets, heating mattresses, circulating water garment systems [7]; evidence supports that the latter offers superior temperature control than forced-air warming systems [8]. Also, intravenous fluids should be warmed prior to administration [7]. Patient core temperature should be monitored and maintained in an adequate range [7,9]. Heating or humidifying the carbon dioxide used for insufflation in laparoscopic surgery has not improved temperature maintenance or pain scores postoperatively [7].

7. Urinary drainage: Bladder drainage (BD) is used during and after major abdominal surgery to monitor urine output and prevent urinary retention [7]. Increased BD duration is associated with increased rates of urinary tract infection (UTI) [7]. Early removal is recommended, ideally ≤ 24 h postoperatively [8,9]. If EDA is used, there is an increased risk of urinary retention [17], but, after 24 h of catheterization, this risk is low [9].

Several RCTs have reported that suprapubic catheterization, compared to transurethral, causes less discomfort and is associated with lower rates of UTI, however, the duration of catheterization in these studies was ≥ 4 days [7-9]. This method is recommended for patients with increased risk of prolonged postoperative urinary retention [9].

Postoperative items: 1. Perianastomotic Drainage: ERAS Society Guidelines for perioperative care in elective gastrectomy, colonic and rectal surgery agree that abdominal drains should be avoided to reduce drain-related complications and reduce LOSH [7-9]. Studies presented in the gastrectomy guidelines state that, after gastrectomy, there is no significant difference in postoperative course, namely in time to first bowel movement, oral intake of light diet or LOSH between patients in whom drains were and were not used. In fact, it is even defended that drainage increases LOSH, postoperative morbidity, time to oral intake and causes more frequent reoperations [8].

In colorectal surgery, it was costume to drain the abdominopelvic cavity to prevent accumulation of fluids and anastomotic leakage. However, studies have found that the use of drains after colorectal surgery doesn't affect the rate of anastomotic dehiscence or overall outcomes [7,9]. ERAS Society Guidelines for perioperative care in elective colonic surgery state that drainage systems are a setback to independent mobilization [7].

2. Analgesia: Adequate postoperative pain management may reduce the extent of surgery-induced immunosuppression and inflammation. Patients who experience adequate analgesia, demonstrate decreased levels of pro-inflammatory cytokines and increased lymphocyte activity [6]. Postoperative analgesia is based on a multimodal regimen that aims to avoid the use of opioids [7], due to their multiple adverse effects, which may prolong the LOSH [12].

When EDA is used in abdominal surgery, it should be maintained for at least 48h and, after a successful stop test, replaced by oral analgesia. If necessary, EDA may be prolonged [8]. In the context of colorectal surgery, the aim is to remove the catheter ≈ 48-72 h postoperatively, by the time the patient has had bowel movements [7,9]. In rectal surgery, there is extensive tissue dissection and many patients will even have preoperative pain which may be neuropathic, partially due to neoadjuvant treatments, which will difficult pain management and require a multi-pharmacological approach that includes, for example, the combination of EDA with systemic opioids [9].

A RCT [18], for patients submitted to gastrectomy in gastric cancer context, concluded that patient-controlled EDA is more effective in pain control, and in reducing stress response, than patient-controlled intravenous analgesia, enabling a faster return of normal bowel activity [8].

In the context of laparoscopic surgery, the duration of postoperative pain that requires major analgesics is much shorter than for open surgery, which allows for discharge as soon as 23 h following surgery [7]. The faster recovery associated with this technique, allows for toleration of early feeding, which implies that analgesic requirements can be met through oral multimodal analgesia, avoiding the need for regional blocks or strong analgesics [7].

Multimodal analgesia with paracetamol and non-steroidal anti-inflammatory drugs (NSAIDs) has shown to spare opioid use by 30% [9]. Paracetamol may be administered up to 4 times a day, in an intravenous preparation of 1 g. Clinical trials, in colorectal surgery, have related the use of NSAIDs (diclofenac and celecoxib) with an increased risk of anastomotic dehiscence [7,9]. Nowadays, there isn't enough evidence supporting that NSAIDs should be abandoned, more studies regarding this question are needed [7]. No medication has yet been recommended for routine use [7,9], however, there are several ongoing studies on opioid alternatives for the relief of postoperative pain [7].

3. Control of glucose: In surgical stress context, there is a generalized catabolic, hyperglycemic response that leads to insulin resistance [4,5]. Insulin resistance is associated with increased morbidity and mortality after major gastrointestinal surgery [7,8]. Hyperglycemia is a major predictor of adverse post-surgical outcomes, exerting inflammatory action and possibly increasing predisposition to infection. Hypoglycemia is equally dangerous as this state adversely affects the circulatory and both the autonomic and central nervous systems [19].

Several ERAS items attenuate insulin resistance, the most obvious ones being: no preoperative fasting and MBP; oral CHO treatment and stimulation of bowel movements through optimal fluid balance; avoidance of systemic opioids; early mobilization; and lessening of the overall stress response by using EDA whenever possible [7,8]. These treatments have the added advantage of not carrying risk of hypoglycaemia [7].

Treatment of hyperglycemia in postsurgical patients in the intensive care unit (ICU) may require the need for insulin, however, this carries the risk of hypoglycemia and, therefore, should only be used when strictly necessary [7]. The optimal target glucose levels remain uncertain [7-9].

4. Prevention of nausea and vomiting: PONV following a standard anesthetic procedure using inhalational anesthetics and opioids, and without any PONV prophylaxis, affects up to 30% of all surgical patients. PONV is an important cause of delay in postoperative feeding and recovery [9]. There are several PONV scoring systems (e.g. Apfel score) stratifying patients from low-to-high risk groups. These scoring systems serve to help guide antiemetic prophylaxis, and in several RCTs have proven to reduce PONV, however, they still haven't been widely implemented in routine practice [7]. Multimodal regimens should be adopted in patients with ≥ 2 risk factors undergoing major

colorectal surgery or gastrectomy [8,9]. A multimodal approach to PONV includes antiemetic medication and non-pharmacological techniques, as the avoidance of inhalational anesthetics and of increased propofol doses in induction/maintenance, minimal preoperative fasting, carbohydrate loading and adequate hydration [7].

5. Perioperative nutritional care: An early resumption of normal oral feeding following major abdominal surgery is associated with a decreased rate of infectious complications and faster recovery, however early feeding seems to be associated with an increased risk of vomiting [9].

An RCT, in colorectal surgery context, that combined preoperative treatment with oral CHO, EDA and early oral feeding showed an improved nitrogen equilibrium whilst maintaining normal glucose concentrations, without the need for insulin administration [7].

ERAS Society guidelines for patients submitted to rectal surgery, recommend that this group of patients begin oral ad libitum diet 4h after surgery [9], whilst ERAS Society guidelines for patients who underwent colonic surgery state that, in the postoperative phase, patients can drink and eat normal hospital food, immediately after recovery from anesthesia [7]. Early oral diet has been shown to be safe in patients with a non-diverted colorectal anastomosis [9], not affecting the risk of anastomotic dehiscence [7]. There is doubt if normal food intake is enough to prevent postoperative weight loss and, therefore, it is recommended that patients be offered oral nutritional supplements to maintain adequate protein and energy intake [7].

Patients subjected to total gastrectomy are probably at a greater risk of malnutrition and cachexia at the time of surgery [8]. All patients with risk of malnutrition/nutrient deficit should receive special nutritional considerations. In severely malnourished patients, supplements have a greater effect if initiated 7-10 days preoperatively [7]. A prospective observational study [19,20] of an ERAS program for colorectal surgery concluded that malnourished patients were at risk for delayed recovery of gastrointestinal function, prolonged LOSH and increased postoperative morbidity.

No trial has reported adverse effects from the attempt of introducing early introduction of oral feeding in patients who underwent gastrectomy [8]. ERAS Society [8] recommendations for gastrectomy state that patients should be offered drinks and food at will from postoperative day (POD) 1, with the advice to begin cautiously and increase intake according to tolerance. Malnourished patients or patients unable to meet 60% of daily requirements by POD6, should be given nutritional support.

In several studies in the context of traditional care, immunonutrition diets (special preparations to enhance immune function in surgical patients) have shown to reduce the rate of complications and shorten LOSH, but results are heterogeneous. Evidence suggests that it is more effective in malnourished patients. There are no RCTs conducted in the ERAS setting [7].

6. Stimulation of gut movement and prevention of postoperative ileus: Postoperative ileus is one of the most common occurrences after abdominal surgery, causing delayed recovery, increased LOSH and medical costs [21]. The elimination of ileus, allows for earlier initiation of enteral nutrition, which is essential to reduce risk of infection [5]. Strategies to reduce the risk of postoperative ileus, included in the ERAS pathway, are balancing fluids, avoiding nasogastric tubes [7,9], opioid analgesia, and PONV [2,9].

EDA, compared with intravenous opioid analgesia is highly effective in reducing ileus occurrence [7]. Laparoscopic colonic resection is also associated with a faster return of gut movement, when compared to laparotomy [7,9].

Use of oral laxatives such as oral magnesium oxide or bisacodyl has demonstrated, in different RCTs, a 1-day reduction in time to first defecation. Other outcomes (toleration of oral food, LOSH, morbidity and mortality) weren't altered. In colonic resection, administration of oral laxatives has been associated with faster normalization of gastrointestinal transit [7,9]. No RCTs to this matter have been conducted specifically in rectal surgery, so further studies are needed [9]. Oral alvimopan, approved for clinical use in postoperative ileus, has shown to accelerate gastrointestinal recovery, whilst reducing the LOSH in patients who underwent open colonic resection, having postoperative opioid analgesia [7]. Current recommendations state that oral laxatives should only be used when opioid analgesia is administered [7]. It is not yet known if stimulant laxatives are associated with an increased risk of anastomotic dehiscence, further studies are necessary [9].

Chewing gum is a safe strategy that seems to have a positive effect on postoperative duration of ileus after gastrointestinal surgery [7], reducing time to first bowel movement by 1-day [9]. This strategy has shown no impact on LOSH [9]. Efficacy on colorectal surgery has been demonstrated, but RCTs specifically concerning gastrectomy are lacking [8].

8. Early mobilization: Prolonged bed rest is a risk factor for several complications, such as thromboembolism, prolonged ileus, increased insulin resistance, loss of muscle and strength, pulmonary depression and reduced tissue oxygenation [7,9]. Early mobilization should be encouraged since the first postoperative day, but for a limited number of hours [7-9].

Available RCTs show no direct clinical advantage of early mobilization, however disadvantages of prolonged immobilization are well supported [7].

Postdischarge Items: 1. Audit of compliance and outcomes: Auditing of compliance and outcomes is the last phase of the ERAS protocol. Regular auditing and standard measuring is essential to determine clinical outcome and confirm the adequate implementation of the protocol. It is crucial though to distinguish an unsuccessful implementation from lack of aimed results [8].

Auditing ERAS protocols has three main dimensions: measurement of clinical outcomes such as LOSH, complication and readmission rates; evaluation of patient experience and functional recovery; assessment of degree of compliance [7].

The ERAS Society has created an online interactive software, the ERAS* Interactive Audit System, to facilitate protocol implementation. This tool not only collects data on the patient, treatment and outcomes, but also provides relevant feedback on clinical outcomes that are important for the patient and the healthcare team [7].

Systematic audit has shown to improve compliance and clinical outcomes [8], and helps to understand where there is space for modifications and improvements.

Outcomes

Colonic surgery

A comprehensive medical record review, developed by Haverkamp et al. [22] for laparoscopic colectomy, stated a significant difference in LOSH in patients who received the ERAS perioperative care (median: 4 days *vs.* 6 days, p<0.007). Time to return of bowel function was 1 day less in the ERAS group (p<0.001). No significant differences were noted in postoperative procedure-related complications, 30-day morbidity and mortality, readmission and reoperation rates. Haverkamp et al. [22] suggest that these results are the effect of the combination of the ERAS protocol with laparoscopic colectomy. The design of this study is limited by the fact that it lacks both blinding and randomization, but results are in agreement with data from other studies.

Bakker et al. [23] studied, over the course of 8 years, the impact that adherence levels to ERAS protocols had on LOSH, following colon cancer resection, concluding that they relate inversely. Years with high adherence to protocol had a shorter LOSH than years with low adherence (5.7 days *vs.* 7.3 days, p<0.001). It was noted, however, that there was a variation in the percentage of laparoscopic resections over the 8 years, which may have influenced results on LOSH. Cakir et al. [24] also reported that strict adherence to the ERAS protocol resulted in lower LOSH and improved outcomes in colon surgery for malignancy. In colorectal laparoscopic surgery, Pisarska et al. [25] reported consistent findings by showing that improvement of protocol compliance leads to better treatment results and convalescence parameters, even when groups with high and very-high compliance rate are compared. Pisarska et al. [25] only analyzed short-term results, whereas Gustafsson et al. [26] demonstrated that the risk of 5-year cancer-specific death in colorectal cancer is lower by 42% in groups with ≥ 70% compliance in comparison to <70%. Although this last study demonstrates a striking relationship between adherence to protocol and cancer survival, this may not imply a cause and effect association between them – the study doesn't present evidence of mechanisms behind this effect. Several other studies have demonstrated that an improved adherence to the ERAS protocol, is associated with lower LOSH and improved clinical outcomes following colorectal surgery [27-30].

Rectal surgery

Recently, two cohort studies comparing ERAS and conventional perioperative care reported similar results: Teeuwen et al. [31] studied results in open rectal surgery, and Huibers et al. [32] in laparoscopic total mesorectal excision for rectal cancer. Both studies showed significantly shorter LOSH in the ERAS group [(median: 8 days *vs.* 12 days, p<0.005) and (median: 7 days *vs.* 10 days, p<0.001, respectively)], with no significant difference in mortality, morbidity, and readmission rates between groups. Functional recovery was also faster in the ERAS groups, with reduced time to first bowel movement (p<0,001, for both studies). Teeuwen et al. [31] noted a trend towards more readmissions in the ERAS group, however this difference was not significant (17.1% *vs.* 7.3%; p<0.203). While these studies demonstrated a benefit in terms of LOSH in the ERAS group, caution must be exercised in interpreting these results due to their lack of randomization, which gives room for potential bias and confounding.

Colorectal surgery

In a RCT, Mari et al. [33] demonstrated that the ERAS protocol, applied to colorectal laparoscopic procedures, reduces the surgical stress response by diminishing levels of important proinflammatory elements, more specifically IL-6 and C-reactive protein. This attenuates the liver's protein synthesis switch from physiological to acute phase inflammatory proteins, allowing for an earlier liver function resumption.

Ren et al. [34] concluded, in a 597-patient RCT, that the ERAS protocol attenuates the surgical stress response, by reducing the postoperative insulin resistance index, and cortisol and cytokine levels in the ERAS group, comparing with the control group (p<0.001). The ERAS group had decreased LOSH (5.7 ± 1.6 days *vs.* 6.6 ± 2.4 days) in comparison with the controls. This study, however, modified one item of the ERAS protocol: traditional Chinese herbal medicine with acupuncture was used to promote gut motility, instead of common drugs such as magnesium oxide. It is not known to what extent this may have influenced results.

Zhuang et al. [35], in a meta-analysis of 13 RCTs (total 1910 patients) found that, in comparison to conventional care, ERAS programs in colorectal surgery are associated with significantly lower LOSH (weighted mean difference, -2.44 days; 95% CI, -3.06 to -1.83 days; p<0.00001). No significant differences were found for readmission rates, surgical complications and mortality. This review found several other studies with consistent conclusions in colorectal surgery, reporting that ERAS programs reduce LOSH [36-42]. Shida et al. [43] found these same results in patients operated for obstructed colorectal cancer. Keane et al. [37] added that time to tolerate light diet and first bowel movements were also significantly reduced in the ERAS group.

In a retrospective review, Smart et al. [44], found that deviation from certain ERAS items at the end of POD1 predicted a delayed discharge after colorectal surgery and consequent ERAS failure: sustained intravenous fluid infusion, dysfunctional epidural, failure to mobilize, vomiting demanding nasogastric tube insertion and re-insertion of urinary catheter, were strongly associated with delayed discharge.

In an interesting study, Shida et al. [45], studied if the lower LOSH associated with the implementation of ERAS programs in colorectal cancer patients is compatible with a better outcome from the patients' point of view. To do so, a 40-item quality of recovery score (QoR-40) was used. QoR-40 measures five dimensions: physical comfort, physical independence, emotional state, psychological support and pain, on the preoperatory and on POD 1, 3, 6 and one month later. On POD6 the global QoR-40 was not significantly different from the baseline level (p=0.06), and one month after surgery the score was almost the same as the baseline score (p=1.00).

A meta-analysis developed by Keane et al. [37] for patients undergoing colorectal surgery, concluded that median primary LOSH (duration of postoperative hospital stay until discharge) and total LOSH (primary LOSH plus any additional days during hospital readmission) were significantly shorter in the ERAS group by one (p<0.004) and three days (p<0.003), respectively, than in the conventional care group. In a subgroup analysis for patients undergoing colonic and rectal surgery, it was noticed that in the latter subgroup, differences in length of stay were less pronounced, probably due to special requirements of this group of patients, namely regarding stoma management and urinary catheter removal.

Pędziwiatr [46] investigated if there were differences in short-term outcomes between laparoscopic surgery for colonic and rectal carcinoma, in the context of an ERAS program and concluded that LOSH was significantly lower for patients treated for colonic cancer than for those treated for rectal cancer (median LOSH: 4 *vs.* 5; p<0.0464). No statistical difference was found in postoperative complications between groups, nor in the 30-day readmission rates. The study points out as explanations for this difference the fact that there was a higher percentage of patients with stomas in the rectal group, which may prolong LOSH once these patients require training on how to handle the stoma; and the significantly increased use of MBP and postoperative drainage in the rectal cancer group.

Gastrectomy

Unlike with colorectal surgery, ERAS protocols have been less implemented in gastric surgery, and, consequently, there are less studies in this field.

The works published on this area, show that the ERAS protocol can be safely implemented for gastric cancer surgery [47,48]. Makuuchi et al. [49], in a 300-patient case-control study, concluded that the use of the ERAS protocol for gastrectomy in patients with gastric cancer shortened LOSH by 1 day (p<0.001) without increasing complications. The main reason for the shortened stay being the introduction of oral feeding one day earlier. This approach was safely adopted without increased incidence of anastomotic leakage.

Abdikarim et al. [16], in an RCT conducted in patients submitted to laparoscopic assisted radical gastrectomy, showed that time to first ambulation, oral food intake, and time do defecation were significantly sorter in the ERAS group, compared to the conventional one (p=0.04, 0.003, 0.01 respectively). LOSH was also significantly lower in the ERAS group (6.8 ± 1.1 days *vs.* 7.7 ± 1.1 days, p=0.002). Incidence of complications between groups wasn't significantly different (p=1).

Jeong et al. [50] found that female sex and age (≥ 65 years) were significantly associated with a delay in recovery of oral intake, and that total gastrectomy was significantly associated with delayed achievement of adequate pain control.

Discussion

It was noted that, for studies evaluating the same operated organ (stomach, rectum or colon), works related to laparoscopic surgery, when compared to laparotomy, showed lower LOSH [37]. Although this tendency was noticed, no definite conclusions can be drawn, nor is this the aim of the present review. It is also important to consider that in studies comparing ERAS to conventional care in terms of outcomes, if laparoscopic surgery is significantly more common in the ERAS group, this may confound results [37,49].

In most patients, achieving total protocol compliance isn't possible. Even in centers that use ERAS protocols on a routine basis, compliance rate round 60-80% [25]. Many studies do not specify the compliance rate of the ERAS protocols and, between the ones who do, there is lack of uniformity in compliance definitions, which are frequently defined by different cutoff points for common analyzed parameters. A good example of this lies in the definition of early mobilization, which is subjectively determined by authors [25]. A lack of standardization may result in bias when trying to evaluate overall compliance rates.

Most studies concerning ERAS protocols in colorectal surgery include heterogeneous groups of patients operated for colonic/rectal disease, creating a potential bias. There is lack of research focusing specifically on the outcomes of rectal and colonic surgery, under ERAS programs. Each group has special postoperative requirements [37]. Namely regarding urinary catheterization. Rectal dissection involves a greater risk of pelvic autonomic neuropraxia, making this group of patients more likely to suffer urinary retention after and anticipated catheter removal. In addition to this, this type of surgery is more likely to require stoma formation. Stoma-related complications are a common cause for delay in discharge. It seems that rectal surgery patients have longer LOSH than colonic surgery patients, but that they equally benefit from the implementation of the ERAS protocols.

All studies that came up in the PUBMED search for this literature review relate to cancer related gastrectomies [16,47-50]. Therefore, further studies are needed to conclude if the ERAS protocols are safe and effective in gastrectomies due to a different etiology.

Teeuwan et al. [31], in a study focused on rectal surgery patients, noticed a trend towards an increased readmission rate in the ERAS group, although the difference was not significant. This raises the question if early discharge is likely to raise readmission rates. An adequate use of proper discharge criteria should prevent increased readmission rates in fast-track surgery. Other than this, several RCTs [16,31,49] studying the impact of the ERAS protocols did not include the discharge criteria in the publication. It is important for the discharge decision to be made according to standardized criteria and by clinicians who are not involved in the study, to secure that this decision is solemnly based on the patients' condition, and not influenced by the fact that the patient was randomized to the ERAS program.

Given that factors such as sex and age influence recovery time after gastrectomy [50], studies with uneven samples for these two aspects, may have achieved lower/higher results that are influenced by these factors, and not solemnly dependent on the implementation of the ERAS protocol.

It would be interesting to know which key elements of ERAS protocols are mainly responsible for the overall reduction in LOSH, although work developed by Watt et al. [51] states that there is limited evidence of the effect of individual ERAS protocol items in reducing the stress response following colorectal surgery.

Using LOSH as a measure of recovery may be problematic, as this value is influenced by several non-clinical factors, including patient expectations, traditions, availability of communitarian or familial support, insurance status and discharge destination [45]. Furthermore, LOSH is largely dependent on discharge criteria, which still lack standardized uniformization.

Conclusions

The ERAS pathway has shown to be safe and to improve outcomes in gastrectomy (due to gastric cancer) and colorectal surgery, by minimizing length of stay in hospital by at least one day as well as time to return of bowel function.

This was achieved without an increase in complications, readmissions, morbidity and mortality rates, whilst maintaining quality of care.

This multimodal approach reaches optimal perioperative management and results when the compliance level is high.

The implementation of the ERAS pathway in colorectal surgery has shown to successfully reduce the stress response to surgery and to help maintain homeostasis perioperatively, information is lacking regarding impact from this point of view in gastrectomy within an ERAS protocol.

Conclusions on which ERAS pathway elements contribute the most to a reduction in postsurgical hospital stay can't be made from this review. It seems that the collective implementation of the ERAS items is what contributes to a significant impact in length of hospital stay, as opposed to the implementation of the ERAS items individually.

References

1. White PF, Kehlet H, Neal JM, Schricker T, Carr DB, et al. (2007) The role of the anesthesiologist in fast-track surgery: from multimodal analgesia to perioperative medical care. Anesth Analg 104: 1380-1396.

2. Scott MJ, Baldini G, Fearon KC, Feldheiser A, Feldman LS, et al. (2015) Enhanced Recovery After Surgery (ERAS) for gastrointestinal surgery, part 1: pathophysiological considerations. Acta Anaesthesiol Scand 59: 1212-1231.

3. Singh M (2003) Stress Response and Anaesthesia: Altering the Peri and Post-Operative Management. Indian J Anaesth 47: 427-434.

4. Burton D, Nicholson G, Hall G (2004) Endocrine and metabolic response to surgery. Contin Educ Anaesth Crit Care Pain 4: 144-147.

5. Desborough JP (2000) The stress response to trauma and surgery. Br J Anaesth 85: 109-117.

6. Scholl R, Bekker A, Babu R (2012) Neuroendocrine and Immune Responses to Surgery. Int J Anaesthesiol 30.

7. Gustafsson UO, Scott MJ, Schwenk W, Demartines N, Roulin D, et al. (2013) Guidelines for Perioperative Care in Elective Colonic Surgery: Enhanced Recovery After Surgery (ERAS*) Society Recommendations. World J Surg 37: 259-284.

8. Mortensen K, Nilsson M, Slim K, Schafer M, Mariette C, et al. (2014) Consensus guidelines for enhanced recovery after gastrectomy: Enhanced Recovery After Surgery (ERAS(R)) Society recommendations. Br J Surg 101: 1209-1229.

9. Nygren J, Thacker J, Carli F, Fearon KC, Norderval S, et al. (2012) Guidelines for perioperative care in elective rectal/pelvic surgery: Enhanced Recovery After Surgery (ERAS(R)) Society recommendations. Clin Nutr 31: 801-816.

10. Feldheiser A, Aziz O, Baldini G, Cox BPBW, Fearon KCH, et al. (2016) Enhanced Recovery After Surgery (ERAS) for gastrointestinal surgery, part 2: consensus statement for anaesthesia practice. Acta Anaesthesiol Scand 60: 289-334.

11. Apfelbaum JL, Caplan RA, Connis RT, Epstein BS, Nickinovich DG, et al. (2010) Practice Guidelines for Preoperative Fasting and the Use of Pharmacologic Agents to Reduce the Risk of Pulmonary Aspiration: Application to Healthy Patients Undergoing Elective Procedures. Anesthesiology 114: 495-511.

12. McCarthy GC, Megalla SA, Habib AS (2010) Impact of intravenous lidocaine infusion on postoperative analgesia and recovery from surgery: a systematic review of randomized controlled trials. Drugs 70: 1149-1163.

13. Senagore AJ, Delaney CP, Mekhail N, Dugan A, Fazio VW (2003) Randomized clinical trial comparing epidural anaesthesia and patient-controlled analgesia after laparoscopic segmental colectomy. The British journal of surgery 90: 1195-1199.

14. Levy BF, Scott MJ, Fawcett W, Fry C, Rockall TA (2011) Randomized clinical trial of epidural, spinal or patient-controlled analgesia for patients undergoing laparoscopic colorectal surgery. Br J Surg 98: 1068-1078.

15. Virlos I, Clements D, Beynon J, Ratnalikar V, Khot U (2010) Short-term outcomes with intrathecal versus epidural analgesia in laparoscopic colorectal surgery. Br J Surg 97: 1401-1406.

16. Abdikarim I, Cao XY, Li SZ, Zhao YQ, Taupyk Y, et al. (2015) Enhanced recovery after surgery with laparoscopic radical gastrectomy for stomach carcinomas. World J Gastroenterol 21: 13339-13344.

17. Stubbs BM, Badcock KJ, Hyams C, Rizal FE, Warren S, et al. (2013) A prospective study of early removal of the urethral catheter after colorectal surgery in patients having epidural analgesia as part of the Enhanced Recovery After Surgery programme. Colorectal Dis 15: 733-736.

18. Zhu Z, Wang C, Xu C, Cai Q (2013) Influence of patient-controlled epidural analgesia versus patient-controlled intravenous analgesia on postoperative pain control and recovery after gastrectomy for gastric cancer: a prospective randomized trial. Gastric Cancer 16: 193-200.

19. Finnerty CC, Mabvuure NT, Ali A, Kozar RA, Herndon DN (2013) The Surgically Induced Stress Response. JPEN J Parenter Enteral Nutr 37: 21S-29S.

20. Lohsiriwat V (2014) The influence of preoperative nutritional status on the outcomes of an enhanced recovery after surgery (ERAS) programme for colorectal cancer surgery. Tech Coloproctol 18: 1075-1080.

21. Lubawski J, Saclarides T (2008) Postoperative ileus: strategies for reduction. Ther Clin Risk Manag 4: 913-917.

22. Haverkamp MP, de Roos MA, Ong KH (2012) The ERAS protocol reduces the length of stay after laparoscopic colectomies. Surg Endosc 26: 361-367.

23. Bakker N, Cakir H, Doodeman HJ, Houdijk AP (2015) Eight years of experience with Enhanced Recovery After Surgery in patients with colon cancer: Impact of measures to improve adherence. Surgery 157: 1130-1136.

24. Cakir H, van Stijn MF, Lopes Cardozo AM, Langenhorst BL, Schreurs WH, et al. (2013) Adherence to Enhanced Recovery After Surgery and length of stay after colonic resection. Colorectal Dis 15: 1019-1025.

25. Pisarska M, Pędziwiatr M, Małczak P, Major P, Ochenduszko S, et al. (2016) Do we really need the full compliance with ERAS protocol in laparoscopic colorectal surgery? A prospective cohort study. Int J Surg 36: 377-382.

26. Gustafsson UO, Oppelstrup H, Thorell A, Nygren J, Ljungqvist O (2016) Adherence to the ERAS protocol is Associated with 5-Year Survival After Colorectal Cancer Surgery: A Retrospective Cohort Study. World J Surg 40: 1741-1747.

27. Gustafsson UO, Hausel J, Thorell A, Ljungqvist O, Soop M, et al. (2011) Adherence to the enhanced recovery after surgery protocol and outcomes after colorectal cancer surgery. Arch Surg 146: 571-577.

28. Pędziwiatr M, Kisialeuski M, Wierdak M, Stanek M, Natkaniec M, et al. (2015) Early implementation of Enhanced Recovery After Surgery (ERAS(R)) protocol - Compliance improves outcomes: A prospective cohort study. Int J Surg 21: 75-81.

29. Ahmed J, Khan S, Lim M, Chandrasekaran TV, MacFie J (2012) Enhanced recovery after surgery protocols - compliance and variations in practice during routine colorectal surgery. Colorectal Dis 14: 1045-1051.

30. Pędziwiatr M, Pisarska M, Kisielewski M, Matlok M, Major P, et al. (2016) Is ERAS in laparoscopic surgery for colorectal cancer changing risk factors for delayed recovery? Med Oncol 33: 25.

31. Teeuwen PH, Bleichrodt RP, de Jong PJ, van Goor H, Bremers AJ (2011) Enhanced recovery after surgery versus conventional perioperative care in rectal surgery. Dis Colon Rectum 54: 833-839.

32. Huibers CJ, de Roos MA, Ong KH (2012) The effect of the introduction of the ERAS protocol in laparoscopic total mesorectal excision for rectal cancer. Int J Colorectal Dis 27: 751-757.

33. Mari G, Crippa J, Costanzi A, Mazzola M, Rossi M, et al. (2016) ERAS Protocol Reduces IL-6 Secretion in Colorectal Laparoscopic Surgery: Results From a Randomized Clinical Trial. Surg Laparosc Endosc Percutan Tech 26: 444-448.

34. Ren L, Zhu D, Wei Y, Pan X, Liang L, et al. (2012) Enhanced Recovery After Surgery (ERAS) program attenuates stress and accelerates recovery in patients after radical resection for colorectal cancer: a prospective randomized controlled trial. World J Surg 36: 407-414.

35. Zhuang CL, Ye XZ, Zhang XD, Chen BC, Yu Z (2013) Enhanced recovery after surgery programs versus traditional care for colorectal surgery: a meta-analysis of randomized controlled trials. Dis Colon Rectum 56: 667-678.

36. Teeuwen PH, Bleichrodt RP, Strik C, Groenewoud JJ, Brinkert W, et al. (2010) Enhanced recovery after surgery (ERAS) versus conventional postoperative care in colorectal surgery. J Gastrointest Surg 14: 88-95.

37. Keane C, Savage S, McFarlane K, Seigne R, Robertson G, et al. (2012) Enhanced recovery after surgery versus conventional care in colonic and rectal surgery. ANZ J Surg 82: 697-703.

38. Bona S, Molteni M, Rosati R, Elmore U, Bagnoli P, et al. (2014) Introducing an enhanced recovery after surgery program in colorectal surgery: a single center experience. World J Gastroenterol 20: 17578-17587.

39. Geltzeiler CB, Rotramel A, Wilson C, Deng L, Whiteford MH, et al. (2014) Prospective study of colorectal enhanced recovery after surgery in a community hospital. JAMA Surg 149: 955-961.

40. Lv L, Shao YF, Zhou YB (2012) The enhanced recovery after surgery (ERAS) pathway for patients undergoing colorectal surgery: an update of meta-analysis of randomized controlled trials. Int J Colorectal Dis 27: 1549-1554.

41. Varadhan KK, Neal KR, Dejong CH, Fearon KC, Ljungqvist O, et al. (2010) The enhanced recovery after surgery (ERAS) pathway for patients undergoing major elective open colorectal surgery: a meta-analysis of randomized controlled trials. Clin Nutr 29: 434-440.

42. Paton F, Chambers D, Wilson P, Eastwood A, Craig D, et al. (2014) Effectiveness and implementation of enhanced recovery after surgery programmes: a rapid evidence synthesis. BMJ Open 4: e005015.

43. Shida D, Tagawa K, Inada K, Nasu K, Seyama Y, et al. (2017) Modified enhanced recovery after surgery (ERAS) protocols for patients with obstructive colorectal cancer. BMC Surg 17: 18.

44. Smart NJ, White P, Allison AS, Ockrim JB, Kennedy RH, et al. (2012) Deviation and failure of enhanced recovery after surgery following laparoscopic colorectal surgery: early prediction model. Colorectal Dis 14: e727-e734.

45. Shida D, Wakamatsu K, Tanaka Y, Yoshimura A, Kawaguchi M, et al. (2015) The postoperative patient-reported quality of recovery in colorectal cancer patients under enhanced recovery after surgery using QoR-40. BMC Cancer 15: 799.

46. Pędziwiatr M, Pisarska M, Kisielewski M, Major P, Mydlowska A, et al. (2016) ERAS protocol in laparoscopic surgery for colonic versus rectal carcinoma: are there differences in short-term outcomes? Medical Oncol 33: 56.

47. Sugisawa N, Tokunaga M, Makuuchi R, Miki Y, Tanizawa Y, et al. (2016) A phase II study of an enhanced recovery after surgery protocol in gastric cancer surgery. Gastric Cancer 19: 961-967.

48. Yamada T, Hayashi T, Aoyama T, Shirai J, Fujikawa H, et al. (2014) Feasibility of enhanced recovery after surgery in gastric surgery: a retrospective study. BMC Surg 14: 41.

49. Makuuchi R, Sugisawa N, Kaji S, Hikage M, Tokunaga M, et al. (2017) Enhanced recovery after surgery for gastric cancer and an assessment of preoperative carbohydrate loading. Eur J Surg Onco 43: 210-217.

50. Jeong O, Ryu SY, Park YK (2016) Postoperative Functional Recovery After Gastrectomy in Patients Undergoing Enhanced Recovery After Surgery: A Prospective Assessment Using Standard Discharge Criteria. Medicine (Baltimore) 95: e3140.

51. Watt DG, McSorley ST, Horgan PG, McMillan DC (2015) Enhanced Recovery After Surgery: Which Components, If Any, Impact on The Systemic Inflammatory Response Following Colorectal Surgery?: A Systematic Review. Medicine (Baltimore) 94: e1286.

24

Evaluation of TEE Training for Chinese Anesthesiology Residents using Two Various Simulation Systems

Fei Liu[1], Fu S Lin[2], Yong G Peng[3], Li Liu[4], Massimiliano Meineri[5], Hai B Song[1*] and Jin Liu[1]

[1]Department of Anesthesiology, West China Hospital, Sichuan University, Chengdu, Sichuan 610041, People's Republic of China

[2]College of Medicine, Sichuan University, Chengdu, Sichuan 610041, People's Republic of China

[3]Department of Anesthesiology, College of Medicine, University of Florida, Gainesville, Florida, USA

[4]School of Computing, National University of Singapore, 117417, Singapore

[5]Department of Anesthesia and Pain Management , Toronto General Hospital, University Health Network, 200 Elizabeth Street EN 3-442, Toronto, ON, M5G 2C4, Canada

*Corresponds author: Hai B Song, Attending Physician, Department of Anesthesiology, West China Hospital, Sichuan University, Chengdu, Sichuan 610041, People's Republic of China, E-mail: pdasonghaibo@163.com

Abstract

Objective: This study was designed to compare the efficacy of simulator-based VRSim TEE training system and web-based virtual TEE program in training anesthetic residents.

Methods: 28 second-year anesthetic trainees with no record of TEE experience were randomly assigned to two groups: simulator group and e-learning group. The simulator group undertaken training via simulator-based VRSim TEE training system. In contrast, e-learning group received training via web-based virtual TEE training program. At the end of the training, all participants were examined aiming to find if there is a difference between these two training systems and which is better for use in training future anesthetic Resident.

Results: Average scores in the final exam were compared for the two groups using two independent samples t-test accepting a $p < 0.05$. Anesthetic resident in simulation group received scores an average of 63.75 ± 3.96, which was significant high comparing to the e-learning group (46.61 ± 2.67).

Conclusion: This study suggests that simulator-based VRSim TEE training is more effective in training anesthetic residents in understanding TEE imaging and manipulation of the TEE probe compared to the web-based TEE modules alone.

Keywords: Transesophageal echocardiography; Simulator-based education; Web-based education

Introduction

Transesophageal echocardiography (TEE) has become a standard practice in cardiac operation room attributed to its major advantages of noninvasiveness, real-time assessment of cardiac function and accurate evaluation of cardiac anatomy [1-3]. In recent years, TEE has also been widely used as an intraoperative monitoring tool in high-risk, non-cardiac surgeries [4] as well as in intensive care units [5]. As TEE becomes more utilized and accepted, it is of great interest for anesthesiologists to acquire the basics techniques of TEE. For this reason, basic TEE training is being integrated into anesthesia residency training programs in many countries [6-11].

In performing basic TEE and meet the criteria of basic intraoperative TEE competency, a minimum of 150 to 180 cases of TEE examination should be performed [12] under supervision, while present TEE training is designed to be one patient-one procedure paradigm. However, there are many limitations and disadvantages involved in this model. Limited opportunities of onsite practice for anesthesia residents due to medical ethics restriction. Time constraints in surgical theatre also restrict the training efficiency. Training may also distract medical staff's attention from important patient care. Prolonging and repeating of the TEE examination cause unnecessary risk and complications to the patients [13].

As trainee has minimal opportunities to perform a TEE exam in the operation room, simulator-based TEE training is developed and introduced as a new training method [14]. Several TEE simulators have been tested in the past few years, such as a web-based training system or a mannequin- and computer-assembled simulation training module [15]. In comparing with traditional TEE training, both web simulator based TEE training and mannequin based TEE training module greatly simplify the understanding of TEE anatomy, image orientation and significantly reduce the learning time and curve [6, 16]. There are few disadvantages of these simulators, for example, using web based TEE simulator, trainees is not allowed to have onsite practice in actual probe manipulations and image acquisition, while mannequin based TEE training module is very expensive and such high cost prohibit its widespread use. Moreover, these two TEE simulators only provide normal anatomy, but sometimes, "abnormal" anatomy and function is more important in training.

Many previous reports have confirmed that simulator (web-based or mannequin) is better than the traditional method in training program. However, to our knowledge, no studies yet compared the effectiveness of a web-based training system with the mannequin-assembled computer, simulation-based training module. Virtual TEE, a web-based TEE training program developed by the Department of Anesthesia and Pain Management of Toronto General Hospital, has been translated into several languages and is the most popular program in world [17]. The VRSim TEE training system, developed by the Department of Anesthesiology in the West China Hospital of Sichuan University and the Chengdu Branch of Chinese Academy of Sciences in 2010, is the first Chinese TEE simulator [6]. In the present study, we compared these two TEE training systems and analysed the effectiveness of the two simulator training system for TEE beginners in basic TEE skills.

Materials and Methods

This study was approved by the West China Hospital ethic committee 2013(15). Written informed consents were obtained from all 28 anesthesia residents who were recruited in May 2014. For this study, 14 anesthesia residents per group allowed us to detect a 20% difference between two training systems (α=0.05; β=0.8, power calculation n=5). All of the participants were second year residents who never received any training and inexperience in intraoperative TEE or cardiac operation room rotations. Participants were randomly assigned to two groups: Virtual TEE group and VRsim TEE group. The randomization sequence was generated using online randomization software (www.randomization.com). All participants were requested to study the "American Society of Echocardiography for Intraoperative Echocardiography and the Society of Cardiovascular Anesthesiologists (ASE/SCA) guidelines" for TEE exam 2 hours prior to simulation training.

In the e-learning group, an experienced perioperative trasesophagel echocardiographer was a demonstrator and showed the group of basic techniques of probe manipulation, image orientation, anatomy 20 standard views on the Virtual TEE program which was developed by Toronto General Hospital group (http://pie.med.utoronto.ca/TEE) (Figure 1). The training session was finished in 60 minutes. Participants in the simulator group were exposed to the VRSim TEE training system -a simulator-based TEE training module. The training was supervised as same as the demonstrator in e-learning group and also finished in 60 minutes (Figure 2). Immediately after the training session, a 30-minute anonymous multiple choice question (MCQ) test was administered to all study subjects. The test was designed according to ASA/SCA T EE exam guidelines and consists of two sections with a total score of 100 points. The first section involved the recognition of cardiac anatomy on 20 standard views, and the second section was related to orientation of TEE views and manipulation of the TEE probe to get a particular TEE view. The study flow is shown in Figure 3.

Statistics

The mean scores of the written test for the two groups were compared using two independent-sampled t tests with P<0.05 considered significant. All the statistical evaluations were estimated by using SPSS 19.0.

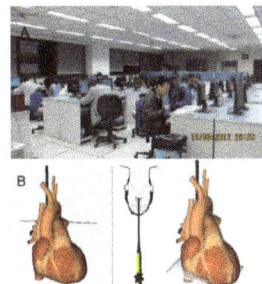

Figure 1: Teaching mode in the control group. A: Every resident has a computer and link to an internet-based TEE learning resource. B: Relationship of TEE probe and three-dimensional heart model shown in the Virtual TEE program.

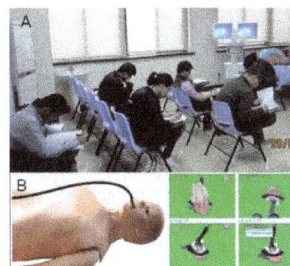

Figure 2: Teaching mode in the study group. A: Residents sit in a classroom and watch the tutor use the VRSim TEE training system to show them basic technique of TEE. B: TEE probe and three-dimensional heart model shown in the VRSim TEE training system with a dummy probe and mannequin.

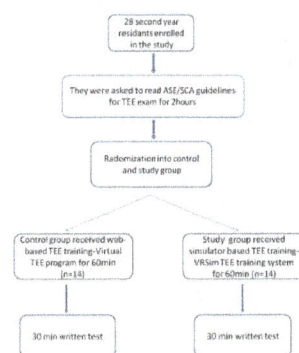

Figure 3: Study flow chart. ASE/SCA, American Society of Echocardiography/Society of Cardiovascular Anesthesiologists.

Results

The mean score of the e-learning group was recorded at 46.61 ± 2.67, comparing to the simulator group score at 63.75 ± 3.96 (P<0.05), with the 95% confidence interval of the difference being -27.03, -7.25. Results for both first and the second MCQ sections indicated a statistically significant difference between the e-learning group (25.18

in Section 1 and 21.43 in Section 2) and the simulator group (34.11 in Section 1 and 29.64 in Section 2). The simulator group achieved significantly higher scores in average comparing to the e-learning group (Figure 4).

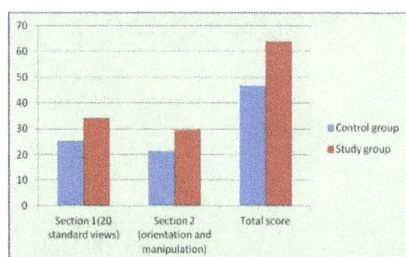

Figure 4: Comparison of the effectiveness of the Virtual TEE and VRSim TEE training systems.

Discussion

It has been reported that simulator training compared with traditional methods could enhance resident performance in transesophageal echocardiography [13,16-18]. However, there have been no previous reports to compare the efficiency among different simulator training modes. Our presented study compared two simulator training modes for the efficiency of the training, which showed that mannequin-based TEE simulator substantially improved the ability of residents for the recognition of cardiac anatomy, orientation of TEE views and manipulation of the TEE probe.

Virtual TEE use, which consists of 20 standard cross-sections as well as 19 non-standard was recommended by ASE/SCA but only used two-dimensional TEE views [9]. In this virtual scenario, trainees can learn the spatial relationship between the probes, the anatomic structures of the (three-dimensional) heart, and the cross-section of cardiac anatomy relevant to echocardiographic views. This design can help for improving a trainee's spatial cognition and implementing their mental model transformation from two-dimensional echocardiographic planes to a three-dimensional heart remodeling. Training guide for the 20 standard cross-sections TEE view also facilitates a trainee's understanding of the relationship between these views with easy memorization. Jerath and his colleagues reported a significant improvement in TEE learning for 10 trainees using this system [9]. Jerath's study suggested that Virtual TEE was a useful adjunctive tool for learning TEE [17] without hand-on experience Moreover, this team also found that 1 hour training using the virtual TTE simulation is essential for improving the knowledge of navigation among the 20 standard views for the trainees [18]. However, limited number of participants in both studies and no control group may not precisely validate if virtual TEE system can replace traditional TEE methods for training purpose

Another prospective randomized study was reported to evaluate the effects of Virtual TEE and simulation-based training on TEE learning for anesthetic trainees [19]. The results showed that trainees who received TEE training via Virtual TEE acquired better image recognition skills compared to those who used traditional methods. In the second part of this study, all participants undertake simulation-based echocardiography training before a test, suggesting that simulation training on subjects with previous experience of e-learning could further improve a trainee's echocardiography knowledge. Bose at

al found that simulation-based TEE training can significantly benefits junior anesthesiology trainee compared with conventional methods [20]. The TEE simulator that was used in both Sharma and Bose' studies and the Heart work TEE simulator was developed by Heart works (Inventive Medical, Ltd, London, UK).

The VRSim TEE Simulator used in our study consists of a mannequin, a probe, and a machine with two split screens. When the trainee manipulates the probe on the mannequin, echocardiographic views appear on the left side of the screen, and a corresponding three-dimensional heart model, together with the visible probe, showing on the right side of screen. This set of VRSim TEE simulator provides a friendly environment without pressure and time limitations for hands-on TEE training in the operation room.

The real grayscale images of VRSim TEE obtained from volunteers' TEE exam data have made our simulator unique. The VRSim system images are easy for the instructor and trainees to discuss on echo image manipulation and acquisition.

To the best of our knowledge, our study is the first to compare the training effectiveness of a web-based TEE training system with simulator-based TEE training module. The reason for choosing the Virtual TEE system is because, Virtual TEE uses real grayscale images from volunteers' TEE exam data, unlike the CT2TEE web-based training program [21]. We assume that the use of Virtual TEE will avoid the color image differences and visual effect bias between the two groups, which can potentially enhance the training outcomes. In addition, the Virtual TEE system, which has already been translated into Chinese, also prevents any misunderstanding via a language barrier.

The results of our study shows that residents who received one hour simulator-based VRSim TEE training system performed better in the written test compared to the residents who were only undertaken to web-based Virtual TEE at same time. The written test included factual information, cognitive imaging recognition, descriptive probe manipulation to acquire appropriate images (acquisition and interpretation).

The main difference between these two training methods is that the simulator-based method is able to provide an opportunity for hands-on practice with probe manipulation and image acquisition. Moreover, there are a great amount of echocardiographic views on every aspect of the heart in the VRSim system, which allows the trainees to be able to repeat a simulated comprehensive TEE examination. Hand-eye coordination can also enhance memory and helps to develop spatial orientation. This method is user-friendly for trainees to achieve a visual picture in mind and understanding between probe position, heart anatomy, and two-dimensional images [6]. In addition, VRSim system is the first mannequin- and computer-assembled TEE simulator including a Chinese interface while CAE VImedix and Heartworks has English interface only that are not suitable for most Chinese aneshthesiologists.

Despite these results, the web-based TEE training also has its characteristic advantages. For instance, web-based training does not require any expensive or sophisticated devices. It is available to all students who wish to learn TEE online, with no require on space, facility or supervision. Few limitations in our study need to be concerned. Firstly, we only conducted a short-term experiment and focused on certain learning objectives and teaching points. The impact of long-term learning process on these two methods needs to be investigated in future. In addition, no test was conduct for participants before the training program, therefore, if any of them has knowledge or experience of TEE was unknown. The different knowledge backgrounds of the participants may also lead to the heterogeneity of the residents that were enrolled in the study. Furthermore, the sample size of the study was small, which limits the extrapolation of the results to a larger population. Only MCQ examination was used to investigate if the simulator is good for improving trainees' knowledge, but in reality about the master of TEE is not sure.

TEE has become a routine check in cardiac and non-cardiac surgeries. However, education on how to use TEE for anesthesiologist residents become a challenge. Simulation-based medical education has been widely accepted as an effective training approach and has been adapted by many subspecialties such as laparoscopic procedures, robotic surgery, basic and advanced life support, and cardiovascular medicine. Simulation-based medical education has achieved remarkable results in last decade [22]. Nowadays, development of a TEE simulator is still in its early stage with only few options of TEE simulators commercially available. In addition to the Virtual TEE and VRSim TEE systems mentioned in our study, similar TEE training devices and programs have been reported previously [20-21,23,24]. A TEE simulator training system provides a friendly, comprehensive learning environment that can reduce the TEE "learning curve" [16]. The application of a TEE simulator is an innovative advancement of simulation-based medical training. Further studies are needed to further validate simulation and e-learning training program on trainees curricula.

Acknowledgement

This study was funded by the National Natural Science Foundation (Grant no. NSF30700781), the Sichuan Science and Technology Support Project (grant no. 2012SZ01333) and by the Technology Innovation Fund of West China Hospital (Grant no. 124060113). No other financial interest was included in this article.

All authors of this article work contribute equally.

Financial supports

National Natural Science Foundation, China (NSF30700781); Sichuan Science and Technology Support Project (2008SZ0100); Technology Innovation Fund of West China Hospital (134060113).

References

1. Practice guidelines for perioperative transesophageal echocardiography. An updated report by the American Society of Anesthesiologists and the Society of Cardiovascular Anesthesiologists Task Force on Transesophageal Echocardiography. Anesthesiology 11: 1084-1096.

2. Hahn RT, Abraham T, Adams MS, Bruce CJ, Glas KE, et al. (2013) Guidelines for performing a comprehensive transesophageal echocardiographic examination: recommendations from the American Society of Echocardiography and the Society of Cardiovascular Anesthesiologists. J Am Soc Echocardiogr 26: 921-964.

3. Reeves ST (2013) Basic and comprehensive perioperative transesophageal echocardiography consensus statement documents. J Am Soc Echocardiogr 26: 25A.

4. Rebel A, Klimkina O, Hassan ZU (2012) Transesophageal echocardiography for the noncardiac surgical patient. Int Surg 97: 43-55.

5. Côrte-Real H, França C (2011) The transoesophageal echocardiography in the general intensive care: its utility in the ventilated critically ill patient. Acta Med Port 24 Suppl 4: 747-754.

6. Song H, Peng PG, Liu J (2012) Innovative transesophageal echocardiography training and competency assessment for Chinese anesthesiologists: role of transesophageal echocardiography simulation training. Curr Opin Anaesthesiol 25: 686-691.

7. Peng YG, Janelle GM (2012) Emergent limited perioperative transesophageal echocardiography: should new guidelines exist for limited echocardiography training for anesthesiologists? Front Med 6: 332-337.

8. Cardiovascular Section of the Canadian Anesthesiologists' Society; Canadian Society of Echocardiography, Béïque F, Ali M, Hynes M, Mackenzie S, et al. (2006) Canadian guidelines for training in adult perioperative transesophageal echocardiography. Recommendations of the Cardiovascular Section of the Canadian Anesthesiologists' Society and the Canadian Society of Echocardiography. Can J Cardiol 22: 1015-1027.

9. Aronson S, Thys DM (2001) Training and certification in perioperative transesophageal echocardiography: a historical perspective. Anesth Analg 93: 1422-1427, table of contents.

10. Denault AY, Rochon AG (2011) Transesophageal echocardiography training: looking forward to the next step. Can J Anaesth 58: 1-7.

11. [No authors listed] (2000) Intraoperative transesophageal echocardiography: basic aspects and recommendations for the training of the anesthesiologist. Joint Working Group of the Section on Echocardiography and Other Imaging Techniques of the Spanish Cardiology Society and the Cardiac Anesthesia Section of the Spanish Society for Anesthesiology, Resuscitation and Pain Management]. Rev Esp Anestesiol Reanim 47: 363-366.

12. Finley A, Reeves ST (2011) Basic perioperative transesophageal echocardiography certification. J Am Soc Echocardiogr 24: A38.

13. Fox KF (2012) Simulation-based learning in cardiovascular medicine: benefits for the trainee, the trained and the patient. Heart 98: 527-528.

14. Shook DC (2010) Basic perioperative transesophageal echocardiography: an education opportunity and a dilemma. J Am Soc Echocardiogr 23: 34A, 34A.

15. Maus TM (2011) Simulation: the importance of "hands-on" learning. J Cardiothorac Vasc Anesth 25: 209-211.

16. Bose R, Matyal R, Panzica P, Karthik S, Subramaniam B, et al. (2009) Transesophageal echocardiography simulator: a new learning tool. J Cardiothorac Vasc Anesth 23: 544-548.

17. Jerath A, Vegas A, Meineri M, Silversides C, Feindel C, et al. (2011) An interactive online 3D model of the heart assists in learning standard transesophageal echocardiography views. Can J Anaesth 58: 14-21.

18. Vegas A, Meineri M, Jerath A, Corrin M, Silversides C, et al. (2013) Impact of online transesophageal echocardiographic simulation on learning to navigate the 20 standard views. J Cardiothorac Vasc Anesth 27: 531-535.

19. Sharma V, Chamos C, Valencia O, Meineri M, Fletcher SN (2013) The impact of internet and simulation-based training on transoesophageal echocardiography learning in anaesthetic trainees: a prospective randomised study. Anaesthesia 68: 621-627.

20. Bose RR, Matyal R, Warraich HJ, Summers J, Subramaniam B, et al. (2011) Utility of a transesophageal echocardiographic simulator as a teaching tool. J Cardiothorac Vasc Anesth 25: 212-215.

21. Kempny A, Piórkowski A (2010) CT2TEE--a novel, internet-based simulator of transoesophageal echocardiography in congenital heart disease. Kardiol Pol 68: 374-379.

22. Okuda Y, Bryson EO, DeMaria S Jr, Jacobson L, Quinones J, et al. (2009) The utility of simulation in medical education: what is the evidence? Mt Sinai J Med 76: 330-343.

23. Matyal R, Bose R, Warraich H, Shahul S, Ratcliff S, et al. (2011) Transthoracic echocardiographic simulator: normal and the abnormal. J Cardiothorac Vasc Anesth 25: 177-181.

24. Ferrero NA, Bortsov AV, Arora H, Martinelli SM, Kolarczyk LM, et al. (2014) Simulator Training Enhances Resident Performance in Transesophageal Echocardiography. Anesthesiology 120:149-159.

Evaluation of USG Guided Transversus Abdominis Plane Block for Post-Operative Analgesia in Total Abdominal Hysterectomy Surgeries

Natesh Prabu, Alok Kumar Bharti*, Ghanshyam Yadav, Vaibhav Pandey, Yashpal Singh, Anil Paswan, Bikram Kumar Gupta and Dinesh Kumar Singh

Institute of Medical Sciences, Banaras Hindu University, Varanasi, India

Corresponding author: Alok Kumar Bharti, Department of Anesthesiology, Institute of Medical Sciences, Banaras Hindu University, Varanasi, India, E-mail: alok.bharti48@gmail.com

Abstract

Introduction and aims: Transversus abdominis plane (TAP) block is a fascial plane block providing postoperative analgesia in patients undergoing surgery with infraumbilical incision. This single blind prospective randomized control study aimed to evaluate the effectiveness of the TAP block for postoperative pain, as part of a multimodal analgesic regimen in patients undergoing TAH.

Material and methods: Sixty adult female patients undergoing Total Abdominal Hysterectomy (TAH) under general anaesthesia were randomizedto undergo TAP block with Ropivacaine along with intravenous paracetamol and diclofenac in group I (n=30) verses group II (n=30) with intravenous paracetamol and diclofenac alone. All patients were given inj.paracetomol 1gm infusion and inj.diclofenac 75 mg intravenously along with induction of anaesthesia. Group I patients additionally received ultrasound guided TAP Block bilaterally with Ropivacaine (0.25%) (25 ml on either side). Each patient was accessed separately by blinded observer at regular intervals upto 24 h for visual analogue scale (VAS), analgesic requirement, PONV and level of sedation using Ramsay sedation scale. If patients complained of pain or VAS>3, inj.Morphine 0.1 mg/kg was given. The observation in two groups was compared statistically using chi-square test and Paired t-test and analysed by SPSS version 18 software.

Result: Result showed that the mean visual analogue score (VAS) of group1 was statistically less than group 2 (P<0.001). Mean analgesic requirement in mg for first 24 h postoperatively was significantly less in group 1 (5.40 ± 3.701) than group 2 (9.40 ± 3.856).

Conclusion: TAP Block is easy to perform under ultrasound guidance without complication and it provides effective analgesia. TAP Block is effective holds good as a part of multimodal analgesia regimen for patients undergoing Total Abdominal Hysterectomy.

Keyword:

Total abdominal hysterectomy; Transversus abdominis plain block; Ropivacaine; Multimodal analgesia

Introduction

Total abdominal hysterectomy (TAH) is a commonly performed major surgical procedure that results in substantial postoperative pain and discomfort [1]. These patients require a multimodal postoperative pain treatment regimen that provides high quality analgesia with minimal side effects. A substantial component of the pain experienced by patients after abdominal surgery is derived from the abdominal wall incision [2]. A promising approach to the provision of postoperative analgesia after abdominal incision is to block the sensory nerve supply to the anterior abdominal wall [3]. However, the clinical utility of current approaches to the blockade of these nerve afferents, such as abdominal field blocks is limited, and the degree of block achieved can be unpredictable. So Rafi in 2001 first introduced the TAP block [4] and described it as block delivering local anaesthetics in the TAP using the iliac crest as anatomical landmarks by identifying the lumbar triangle of Petit. Hebbard et al. introduced the First USG guided approach for TAP block in 2007 [5].

Recent published clinical trials involving patients undergoing both major abdominal [6] as well as gynecological surgery have demonstrated promising results with this technique as part of a multimodal post-operative pain treatment. TAP block has been used for various abdominal procedures other than total abdominal hysterectomy such as large bowel resection, open/laparoscopic appendectomy, laparoscopic cholecystectomy, and open prostatectomy, abdominoplasty with or without flank liposuction, inguinal hernia and iliac crest bone graft [7-13].

This study was designed to evaluate the effectiveness of the TAP block for postoperative pain, as part of a multimodal analgesic regimen in patients undergoing TAH.

Material and Method

After obtaining approval from Institutional ethics committee and written informed consent, sixty ASA I and II adult patients undergoing elective total abdominal hysterectomy were included in prospective randomized single blinded control study which was completed over a period of 12 month.

Patients who had H/O allergy to Ropivacaine, diclofenac, pregnancy, BMI>35 chronic opioid use and who refused after inclusion were excluded.

Patients between age group between 30-65 years were randomly allocated into two group having 30 patients in each group. Patients were randomized by sealed envelopes, to undergo TAP block or to receive standard care. Group I (n=30) received intravenous paracetomol 1 gm 6th hourly and intravenous diclofenac 75 mg 12th hourly and Transverses Abdominis Plane block.

Group II (n=30) received paracetomol 1 gm 6th hourly and diclofenac 12th hourly only. After routine preoperative evaluation and machine check, surgery was performed under general anaesthesia with controlled ventilation. All Patients were premedicated with ondensetron 0.1 mg/kg. Anaesthesia was induced with Fentanyl 2 μg/kg, propofol 1-2.5 mg/kg and Endotracheal tube placement was facilitated with vecuronium 0.1 mg/kg. The Anaesthesia was maintained using Oxygen, Nitrous Oxide (30%:70%), Isoflurane 1%, and intermittent Fentanyl 1 μg/kg, Vecuronium 0.01 mg/kg as and when required.

Standard ASA monitors were used. All patients were given inj.paracetomol 1 gm infusion and inj.diclofenac 75 mg intravenously along with induction of anaesthesia. Group I patients additionally received Transversus Abdominis Plane Block with Ropivacaine 0.25%, 25 ml on both sides under USG guidance.

The patients randomized to undergo the TAP block underwent USG guided TAP block after induction of anaesthesia using linear array Transducer probe (Sono Site M-Torbo, SonoSite, Inc., Bothwell, MO, USA) of frequency 10-15 MHz by posterior approach on both side of Transversus Abdominis Plane.

Patient's vital parameters like Heart Rate, Blood pressure, oxygen saturation were noted on induction of anaesthesia and during surgery. Recordings were made by a blinded observer. After completion of the surgical procedure and emergence from anaesthesia, patients were transferred to the postoperative recovery room.

In postoperative recovery room all patients were monitored for Heart Rate, Blood Pressure, Saturation, Pain (VAS) PONV, Sedation and other complaints on immediate post-operative, 1, 2, 4, 6, 12, 24 h. If patients complained of pain or VAS>3 inj.Morphine 0.1 mg/kg was given. All recordings were done by a blinded observer. Pain and sedation were assessed by Visual analogue scale and Ramsay sedation scale respectively.

The statistical analysis was done using SPSS for Windows version 18.0 software. For non-continuous data Chi-square test was used. The mean and standard deviation of the parameters studied during observation period were calculated for two treatment groups and compared using Paired 't' test. The critical value of 'p' indicating the probability of significant difference was taken as<0.05 for comparisons.

Results

Sixty patients were registered in the study. Thirty Patients were randomized to undergo TAP blockade with 0.25% ropivacaine along with parenteral diclofenac 75 mg and paracetomol 1 gm, and remaining 30 were randomized as a control group receiving parenteral diclofenac 75 mg and paracetomol 1 gm only.

Groups were comparable in terms of age, weight, height, and BMI, surgery and anaesthesia time [Table 1]. In all patients randomized to

undergo TAP block, transversus abdominis Plane was located under the guidance of ultrasound and 0.25% ropivacaine was deposited on both sides without any complication.

Patients in TAP group had less heart rate and mean arterial pressure throughout 24 h. The Patients in TAP group had reduced VAS Score than control group all the time [Table 2]. The mean VAS Score was 2. Patients in TAP group had reduced mean morphine requirement (5.40 mg *vs.* 9.40 mg) in 24 h period [Table 3] and found to be statistically significant (P<0.001) consumption of morphine was significantly lower during immediate postoperative period (0-6 h).

There was no significant difference in sedation scores between both groups at any point of time except at 6hrs, where control group had more sedation score [Table 4]. The patients in TAP group had reduced incidence of postoperative nausea and vomiting at 2, 4, and 12 h and at rest of time there was no significant difference in the incidence [Table 5]. The patients in control group had high PONV scores (1 or more).

Parameters	Tap group (N=30)	Control group (N=30)	P-value
Age (yrs)	41.47 ± 5.501	43.20 ± 2.124	0.113
Weight (kg)	53.87 ± 7.829	55.10 ± 5.081	0.472
Height (cms)	153.30 ± 3.583	153.90 ± 2.881	0.478
BMI (kg/m^2)	23.80 ± 4.55	22.86 ± 1.70	0.29
Surgery time (min)	45.17 ± 9.436	45.47 ± 8.713	0.899
Anaesthesia time (min)	63.13 ± 10.504	62.13 ± 7.583	0.674

Tables 1: Demography and patients characteristic were comparable.

Vas Score	Group 1 (TAP)	Group 2 (Control)	P value
Immed Postop	2.53 ± 3.082	3.10 ± 1.768	0.386
1 h	2.80 ± 2.511	3.60 ± 1.773	0.159
2 h	1.93 ± 0.980	3.13 ± 1.279	<0.001
4 h	2.23 ± 0.679	3.40 ± 1.610	0.001
6 h	2.53 ± 1.408	3.67 ± 1.647	0.006
12 h	2.90 ± 1.729	3.97 ± 1.771	0.022
24 h	2.27 ± 0.640	3.17 ± 1.440	0.003

Tables 2: Comparison of Vas score between Group 1 and Group 2.

	Total analgesic req	P value
Group 1	5.40 ± 3.701	<0.001
Group 2	9.40 ± 3.856	

The cumulative morphine requirement is significantly lower in TAP Group. There is 57% reduction in mean morphine requirement in TAP group.

Table 3: Mean morphine requirement in milligram in first 24 h after TAH.

Sedation scores (>3)	Tap group (no of patients)	Control group (no of patients)	p-value
Immed Postop	4	2	0.389
1 h	0	1	0.315
2 h	3	3	1.000
4 h	0	0	-
6 h	0	0	-
12 h	0	0	-
24 h	0	0	-

Ramsay sedation scale was used. Only few patients were found to have Scores>3. There was no significant difference in sedation scores between two groups.

Tables 4: Ramsay sedation scale.

PONV (>1)	Tap group		Control group		P-value
	No.	%	No.	%	
Immed postop	0	0	0	0	---
1 h	3	10	1	3.3	0.302
2 h	0	0	5	16.7	0.019
4 h	1	3.3	9	30	0.005
6 h	0	0	1	3.3	0.315
12 h	0	0	6	20	0.009
24 h	0	0	3	10	0.075

The incidence of PONV was found to be more in control Group (p < 0.05) particularly during 2, 4 and 12th h.

Table 5: PONV score.

Discussion

This Randomised single blinded controlled clinical trial demonstrates that the TAP BLOCK when used as a part of multimodal analgesia provides effective analgesia for patients undergoing Total Abdominal Hysterectomy. It reduced the intensity of breakthrough pain and requirement of morphine. All blocks were done under ultrasound guidance which ensured the exact location. There was no block related complication. The standard regimen of injection paracetomol and diclofenac intravenously at our institution didn't provide good postoperative pain relief in all patients following TAH.

So a multimodal analgesia regimen is needed for providing effective postoperative pain relief. Substantial component of pain experienced by the patient is from abdominal wall incision in abdominal surgeries. So, any interventions that block pain from abdominal wall will provide good post-operative pain relief. TAP Block is a type of abdominal field block that anaesthetizes the nerve supplying the abdominal wall and being used for providing post-operative pain relief after abdominal surgeries both in adults and children.

In a systematic review, Moiniche et al. [14] found little evidence to support the use of instillation of local anesthetics into the wound incision. In contrast, the combination of intraperitoneal and incisional bupivacaine did provide some analgesia in this patient. However, more effective strategies are required for patients undergoing TAH.

TAP Block group had reduced VAS Scores throughout the 24 h postoperative period. The patients in TAP Group had significantly decreased VAS scores (p<0.05) for 24 h period except at 0, 1 h postoperative period with a mean VAS Score of 2. Similar decreased VAS Scores were also observed by John carney [15], Mc Donnell et al. [16], G. Niraj et al. [17]. In our study, the patients who received the TAP block had significantly reduced post-operative morphine consumption (p<0.03) at 2,4 and 6 h. TAP Block reduced the mean morphine consumption (mg) 5.40 mg *vs.* 9.40 mg in control group (p<0.001). TAP block had reduced the morphine requirement by 57% in our study and it is par with many clinical studies in patients who underwent laparotomy, caesarean surgeries. This shows the effectiveness of TAP block as a part of multimodal analgesia regimen and its ability of reducing opioid requirement and opioid related adverse effects.

In our study we found that addition of TAP Block to paracetomol and diclofenac showed reduced VAS Scores and morphine requirement for 24 h period. The addition of TAP block reduced the pain scores due to its ability to block transmission of nociceptive impulse from abdominal wall. This shows that single shot application of TAP Block can provide good pain relief for a period of 24 h. Many studies had showed beneficial effect of TAP Block in providing postoperative pain relief.

The TAP block has been demonstrated to provide excellent analgesia to the skin and musculature of the anterior abdominal wall in patients undergoing colonic resection surgery involving a midline abdominal wall incision, patients undergoing cesarean delivery (McDonnell JG et al.) [18] and patients undergoing radical prostatectomy (O'Donnell BD et al.) [19].

TAP Block also reduced the incidence of PONV. This may be due to the amount of morphine consumed in the TAP block group was sufficiently less compared to control group. In calculating the incidence of PONV, any score of above zero at any time point was taken as indicating that the patient had PONV. The control group had higher PONV scores (>1) particularly in early postoperative period (1-6 hrs) reflecting the use of morphine at similar period. Many clinical studies also observed similar reduced PONV incidence (McDonnell JG, Curley GCJ et al.) [19].

TAP block didn't made impact on sedation score. Both groups had accepted sedation scores (3 or less) and there was no significant difference in sedation scores between two groups. Even though control group patients had higher morphine consumption; there was no increase in sedation scores. This may be due to higher pain scores and PONV scores in these patients.

Limitations of Our Study

First we restricted our study period up to 24 h postoperative analgesia, however many studies have shown that TAP Block provides analgesia for around 48 h. Second, blinding was not perfect as sensations were lost over the abdomen and is a single blinded.

Future Recommendations

Further studies should be undertaken to evaluate the effectiveness of adding various drugs (opioid, dexmedetomidine) with local anaesthetics in Transversus Abdominis Plane block.

Conclusion

TAP Block is easy to perform under ultrasound guidance and it provides effective analgesia. TAP Block is effective holds good as a part of multimodal analgesia regimen for patients undergoing Total Abdominal Hysterectomy.

References

1. Ng A, Swami A, Smith G, Davidson AC, Emembolu J (2002) The analgesic effects of intraperitoneal and incisional bupivacaine with epinephrine after total abdominal hysterectomy. Anesth Analg 95: 158-162.

2. Wall PD, Melzack R (1999) Pain measurements in persons in pain. Textbook of pain (4thedn). Edinburgh, UK: Churchill Livingstone 409-426.

3. Kuppuvelumani P, Jaradi H, Delilkan A (1993) Abdominal nerve blockade for postoperative analgesia after caesarean section. Asia Oceania J Obstet Gynaecol 19: 165-169.

4. Rafi AN (2001) Abdominal field block: a new approach via the lumbar triangle. Anaesthesia 56: 1024-1026.

5. Hebbard P, Fujiwara Y, Shibata Y, Royse C (2007) Ultrasound-guided transversus abdominis plane (TAP) block. Anaesth Intensive Care 35: 616-617.

6. Abrahams MS, Aziz MF, Fu RF, Horn JL (2009) Ultrasound guidance compared with electrical neurostimulation for peripheral nerve block: a systematic review and meta-analysis of randomized controlled trials. Br J Anaesth 102: 408-417.

7. Bharti N, Kumar P, Bala I, Gupta V (2011) The efficacy of a novel approach to transversus abdominis plane block for postoperative analgesia after colorectal surgery. Anesth Analg 112:1504-1508.

8. Niraj G, Searle A, Mathews M, Misra V, Baban M, et al. (2009) Analgesic efficacy of ultrasoundguided transversus abdominis plane block in patients undergoing open appendicectomy. Br J Anaesth 103: 601-615.

9. El Dawlatly AA, Turkistani A, Kettner SC, Machata AM, Delvi MB, et al. (2009) Ultrasoundguided transversus abdominis plane block: Description of a new technique and comparison with conventional systemic analgesia during laparoscopic cholecystectomy. Br J Anaesth 102: 763-767.

10. O'Donnell BD, McDonnell JG, McShane AJ (2006) The transversus abdominis plane (TAP) block in open retropubic prostatectomy. Reg Anesth Pain Med 31: 91.

11. Araco A, Pooney J, Memmo L, Gravante G (2010) The transversus abdominis plane block for body contouring abdominoplasty with flank liposuction. Plast Reconstr Surg 125: 181e-182e.

12. Heil JW, Ilfeld BM, Loland VJ, Sandhu NS, Mariano ER (2010) Ultrasoundguided transversus abdominis plane catheters and ambulatory perineural infusions for outpatient inguinal hernia repair. Reg Anesth Pain Med 35: 556-558.

13. Chiono J, Bernard N, Bringuier S, Biboulet P, Choquet O, et al. (2010) The ultrasoundguided Transverse abdominis plane block for anterior iliac crest bone graft postoperative pain relief: A prospective descriptive study. Reg Anesth Pain Med 35: 520-524.

14. Moiniche S, Mikkelsen S, Wetterslev J, Dahl JB (1998) A qualitative systematic review of incisional local anaesthesia for postopera-tive pain relief after abdominal operations. Br J Anaesth 81: 377-383.

15. Carney J, McDonnell JG, Ochana A, Bhinder R, Laffey JG (2008) The transversus abdominis plane block provides effective postoperative analgesia in patients undergoing total abdominal hysterectomy. Anesth Analg 107: 2056-2060.

16. McDonnell JG, O'Donnell B, Curley G, Heffernan A, Power C, et al. (2007) The analgesic efficacy of transversus abdominis plane block after abdominal surgery: a prospective randomized controlled trial. Anesth Analg 104: 193-197.

17. Niraj G, Searle A, Mathews M, Misra V, Baban M, et al. (2009) Analgesic efficacy of ultrasound-guided transversus abdominis plane block in patients undergoing open appendicectomy. Br J Anaesth 103: 601-605.

18. McDonnell JG, Curley G, Carney J, Benton A, Costello J, et al. (2008) The analgesic efficacy of transversus abdominis plane block after cesarean delivery: a randomized controlled trial. Anesth Analg 106: 186-191.

19. O'Donnell BD, McDonnell JG, McShane AJ (2006) The transversus abdominis plane (TAP) block in open retropubic prostatectomy. Reg Anesth Pain Med 31: 91.

26

Fluid Optimization in Liver Surgery

Levantesi Laura[1], Oggiano Marco[1], Fiorini Federico[1], Sessa Flaminio[1], De Waure Chiara[2*], Congedo Elisabetta[1] and De Cosmo Germano[1]

[1]*Institute of Anaesthesiology and Intensive Care, Catholic University of Sacred Heart, Rome, Italy*

[2]*Department of Public Health, Catholic University of Sacred Heart, Rome, Italy*

[*]**Corresponding author:** Levantesi Laura, Institute of Anaesthesiology and Intensive Care, Catholic University of Sacred Heart, Rome, Italy, E-mail: laule82@hotmail.com

Abstract

Study's purposes: To reduce bleeding, hepatectomies are usually performed maintaining low central pressure (CVP) combined with extrahepatic control flow and this management can lead hemodynamic instability and reduction in oxygen delivery. This study analyzes hemodynamic changes and so the derived fluid management, in patients undergoing liver resection, through the Vigileo/FloTrac system.

Basic procedures: Seventeen patients were included. Low CVP, below 4 mmHg, was reached by loop diuretics. Hemodynamic parameters were recorded and blood gas analysis was also performed. At the end of resection, fluid replacement was carried out with 500 ml of crystalloid solution in 20 minutes evaluating changes in CVP, Cardiac Index (CI) and Stroke Volume Variation (SVV).

Main findings: During Pringle maneuver, Cardiac Index resulted stable through a modification in heart rate and vascular resistances (p<0.01). Only SVV significantly changed during Pringle maneuver (p=0.03) and not CVP (p=0.8). In all patients the oxygen delivery was maintained upper 600 ml/min/m^2. Fluid optimization was performed with 1917 ml ± 1161 ml of crystalloid solution with a significant reduction in SVV (p<0.01) about 7% despite a CVP of 5 mmHg.

Conclusions: We suppose that SVV can replace CVP in major hepatectomy management. Regarded results we can conclude that a good peripheral perfusion can be reached also with a fluid restrictive regimen avoiding overload and postoperative edema.

Keywords: Cardiovascular system-responses; Fluid therapy; Heart-cardiac output

Introduction

Blood loss is the major complication during liver resection and morbidity and mortality are directly related with bleeding and transfusions [1,2]. To avoid this, hepatic surgery is performed with the maintenance of a low central pressure combined with extrahepatic control flow. The intermittent Pringle maneuver (IPM), which consists in clamping the hepatoduodenal ligament and blocks the hepatic inflow [3], is frequently applied. However the combination between low CVP and vascular exclusion can determine hemodynamic instability and systemic hypoperfusion that can persist at the end of resection and increase mortality according to the new concept of goal directed therapy.

Goal directed therapy (GDT) is a perioperative management that improve tissue perfusion and outcome, through cardiac output or oxygen delivery optimization [4]. Actually, dynamic hemodynamic parameters such as SVV (stroke volume variation), have been shown to be superior to CVP in predicting fluid responsiveness. According to this idea, in this surgery, a monitoring more advanced then CVP, avoiding pulmonary artery catheterization, results essential. In fact, Swan-Ganz remains a gold standard but with limitations in the use for invasiveness and complications such as arrhythmias, valvular lesions and rupture of the pulmonary artery [5].

Consequently the technique of arterial waveform analysis, considered minimally invasive, was developed. FloTrac/Vigileo is one of available devices for the assessment of hemodynamic parameters through the minimal invasive methods of analysis of arterial pressure waveform. FloTrac/Vigileo provides continuous cardiac output (CO), stroke volume (SV) and stroke volume variation (SVV) through an existing arterial line. Potential advantages of this system are the absence of manual calibration, the need of a peripheral artery and also an automatic recalibration every 60 sec to assess changes in arterial compliance.

The purpose of this study is the analysis of hemodynamic status in patients undergoing major hepatic surgery, optimizing fluid replacement at the end of resection using Vigileo/FloTrac system hemodynamic monitoring.

Methods

Permission was obtained from the local Ethical Committee (ID 656/11). After written informed consent was obtained from all subjects, patients, aged 30-70 years, with American society of anesthesiologist physical status I-III, scheduled for elective major hepatic surgery, from September 2011 to February 2012 were enrolled in this study.

Exclusion criteria were refusal of enrolment, cirrhosis, systolic ventricular contractility or diastolic relaxation alterations, ischemic or valvular diseases, absence of sinusal rhythm and impaired renal function.

General anesthesia was induced with propofol 2 mg/kg IV, and sufentanil 0.5 mcg /kg IV, and tracheal intubation was facilitated with cisatracurium 0.15 mg/kg IV, then maintained with a continuous infusion of 0.3 mcg/Kg/h IV.

Anaesthesia maintenance was performed with sevoflurane (in an oxygen/air mixture) and sufentanil in continuous infusion (3-5 mcg/Kg/min). The minimum alveolar concentration of sevoflurane was set to achieve a Bispectral Index (BIS) value between 40 and 60 [6].

Mechanical ventilation was set with a tidal volume of 8 ml/kg, PEEP 0 cmH$_2$O and with an inspiration/expiration rate of 1:2. These parameters remained stable during the procedure. The respiration rate was adjusted to obtain an etCO$_2$ between 38-45 mmHg. The monitoring was performed with ECG, pulse oximetry and non-invasive blood pressure before induction and after a 20 G catheter was placed in left radial artery and connected to Vigileo/FloTrac system, and after zeroing CO was displayed with SVV.

A double-lumen venous catheter was placed in right internal jugular vein to monitor CVP, venous oxygen saturation (Svo2) and for rapid infusion. Initially, to achieve a low CVP (between 2 and 4 mmHg), loop diuretics were administrated; norephinephrine was infused if mean arterial pressure was less than 60 mmHg or oxygen deliveries below 600 ml/m^2.

The intermittent Pringle maneuver (IPM), which consists in clamping the hepatoduodenal ligament and blocks the hepatic inflow [3] is applied during surgery [7].

Hemodynamic parameters and BIS were recorded every 15 min during 3 periods: before (Time 1), during (Time 2) and after pedicle clamping (Time 3). Arterial and venous blood gas analysis was performed during surgical intervention. At the end of resection, a fluid replacement was carried out with 500 ml of crystalloid solution in 20 minutes evaluating changes in CVP, CI and SVV.

The algorithm used in this study, was based on a cutoff for SVV of 13% to distinguish between fluid responders and not [8]. Specifically, if SVV is greater than 13%, patients should respond to fluid replacement with an increase in Stroke Volume.

Statistical analysis

A general linear model for repeated measurements was applied in order to evaluate the relationship between time and the following parameters: MAP, heart rate (HR), systemic vascular resistance index (SVRI), CI, SV, SVV, CVP. A post-hoc analysis with Bonferroni correction was carried out too.

Mean and Standard Deviations (SD) were used to report data. The statistical significance level was set at $p=0.05$ and SPSS software 12.0 was used to perform the analysis.

Results

17 patients (9 men and 8 women) undergoing liver surgery (13 for liver metastases and 4 for primitive liver cancer), were enrolled. They were 58 ± 10 years old; the median body surface area was 1.89 ± 0.3 m^2 with body weight 75 ± 14 kg and height 167 ± 7 cm.

The maintenance of anaesthesia with sevoflurane with a median MAC of 1.6% resulted adequate with a median BIS value of 41. During anaesthesia a mean diuresis of 2 ml/kg/h was maintained. No patients need norephinephrine infusion. In Table 1 data of parameters under study are shown with respect to Time.

	PAM	FC	RSVI	CI	SV	SVV	PCV
Time 1	83.65 (8.99)	71.20 (8.08)	1290.18 (224.37)	2.60 (0.34)	64.03 (7.05)	12.15 (3.80)	2.08 (1.29)
Time 2	87.06 (12.96)	79.20 (10.48)	1480.00 (323.17)	2.51 (0.36)	62.49 (7.36)	14.65 (4.24)	1.85 (1.31)
Time 3	80.24 (9.93)	70.60 (12.87)	1125.06 (223.10)	2.89 (0.44)	72.53 (9.19)	7.47 (1.51)	5.23 (1.80)

Table 1: Mean (SD) of parameters at the three points in time.

As far as changes in time are concerned, no significant associations with time were found with respect to MAP. So despite low CVP, MAP resulted stable within normal range of values also during clamping without relevant changes with a median of 87 ± 12.96 mmHg. Moreover CI resulted stable during extrahepatic control flow (p=0.71). The results of the post hoc analysis are shown in Table 2. During Pringle maneuver we noted a significant increase in HR and in systemic resistances (respectively p<0.01 and 0.02).

	FCT	RSVI	CI	SV	SVV	PCV
Time 1 vs. Time 2	<0.01	<0.02	0.71	0.35	0.03	0.80
Time 1 vs. Time 3	1	<0.01	<0.01	<0.01	<0.01	<0.01
Time 2 vs. Time 3	0.03	<0.01	<0.01	<0.01	<0.01	<0.01

Table 2: Post hoc analysis (p-values).

Furthermore between Time 1 and 2 we did not observe a statistical signification in CVP variation but in SVV (p=0.8 and 0.03).

At the end of liver resection, fluid replacement was carried out with 500 ml of crystalloid solution in 20 minutes with a median of 1917 ml ± 1161 ml of crystalloid solution and during this stage, SVV significantly changed (p<0.01) and resulted in a reduction about 7% in all patients demonstrating an adequate fluid replacement despite a median CVP of 5 mmHg. Median estimated blood loss is 335 ml ± 319 ml so no patient needed blood transfusion.

Discussion

Blood loss is the major complication during liver resection and morbidity and mortality are directly related with bleeding and transfusions [2,9]. Hepatectomies can be complicated also by an important hemodynamic instability resulting from low CVP and Pringle maneuver.

In fact a CVP of 5 mmHg or less is considered optimal and has been showed to be associated with less bleeding during parenchymal transection and reduced need of transfusion [10,11] but it should increase the risk of air embolism and systemic tissue hypoperfusion.

Ya Guo et al. evaluated the influence of different values of low CVP on hemodynamic parameters, oxygen transport and the rate of blood loss during partial hepatectomy in pig models [12]. They founded that blood loss in the CVP $\geq$ 5 cmH_2O group was more significant and also that there was a significant reduction in MAP, CO and CI with CVP<2 cmH_2O.

DO_2 decreased when CVP<2 cmH_2O, VO_2 when CVP <1 cmH_2O, and ERO_2 when CVP<1 cmH_2O. So they concluded that a CVP at 2 to 3 cmH_2O seems to be optimal for hepatic resection to avoid bleeding, hemodynamic instability and also failure in oxygen delivery.

So this management minimize mortality, facilitates operative control of hemorrhage, but also preserves renal function [13].

In this study we describe hemodynamic changes that occur during major liver resections, performed in non-cirrhotic patients, associating to traditional monitoring the Vigileo/FloTrac system. Actually dynamic parameters such as SVV (stroke volume variation), have been shown to be superior to CVP and static data in predicting fluid responsiveness so Swan-Ganz is rarely used for limitations in invasiveness and complications such as arrhythmias, valvular lesions and rupture of the pulmonary artery [14]. Consequently the technique of arterial waveform analysis, considered minimally invasive, was developed. FloTrac/Vigileo provides continuous cardiac output (CO), stroke volume (SV) and stroke volume variation (SVV) through an existing arterial line. Potential advantages of this system are the absence of manual calibration, the need of a peripheral artery and also an automatic recalibration every 60 sec to assess changes in arterial compliance. This system is validated by various studies, for example Hofer et al. compared FloTrac/Vigileo system and PiCCO for prediction of fluid responsiveness using SVV and founded the same accuracy [15]. A meta-analysis published in 2009 on Journal of Cardiothoracic and Vascular Anesthesia conclude that, with the introduction of software version 1.07, there was an improvement of FloTrac/Vigileo that results comparable to thermodilution measurements [16]. Vigileo/FloTrac system seems adequate also in patients with circulatory failure after liver transplantation [17].

So SVV is a dynamic parameter helpful in determining fluid responsiveness with a cutoff of 13%. Previously, during liver resection with hepatic vascular exclusion, important hemodynamic changes were demonstrate with cardiac output reduction and increase in systemic vascular resistance with a compensatory role for arginine vasopressin and sympathetic systems [18] that explains the hemodynamic tolerance, despite the marked decrease in venous return, after caval clamping. We performed only portal triad clamping but also we observed a sympathetic compensatory phenomenon characterized by stability in Cardiac Index and in MAP balanced by a statistically significant modification in HR and SVRI despite a reduction in venous return.

Thanks to the use of the Vigileo/FloTrac we observed changes between CVP and SVV. Stroke volume variation seemed not to be in relationship, in any moment of liver resection, with central venous pressure. It is moreover important that this one, unlike SVV, did not result in statistical changes before and after Pringle maneuver.

A previous systematic review demonstrated a very poor relationship between CVP and blood volume and so CVP should not be used to make clinical decisions regarding fluid management [19]. In addition, in other studies SVV results usefulness in predict hypovolemia in septic shock, in reduced cardiac function and in cardiac surgical patients [20-22].

The same should be considered regard liver resection with next application of arterial waveform-derived dynamic variables for anesthesiology management [23], mentioning that SVV seems a predictor of blood loss as previously evaluated in donors undergoing right hepatectomy [24]. The use of SVV in major abdominal surgery improves outcome [25] and stability [26] related to the concept of goal directed therapy (GDT), in surgical patients. Goal directed therapy (GDT) is a perioperative management that improve tissue perfusion and outcome, through cardiac output or oxygen delivery optimization [26].

Shoemaker et al. introduced in 1980 the GDT into the perioperative care of high risk surgical patients [27] with a reduction in mortality from 38 to 21%.

We can identify high risk surgical patients such as patients with individual mortality risk greater than 5% (ASA IV mortality 18.3% and V mortality 93.3%) [28] or with a surgical risk greater than 5% [28,29]. In intra and postoperative period, the increase in oxygen consumption causes organ dysfunction and also morbidity and mortality especially in this kind of patients unable in provide for rising oxygen delivery. However, Hamilton et al. demonstrated an advantage with the application of GDT also in patients with moderate risk [30].

GDT is based on supranormal values of Cardiac Index and of Oxygen Delivery and consumption that we simply reached thought the use of Vigileo.

In this study, stability during Pringle maneuver allows maintaining a DO_2 greater than 600 ml/min/m^2 with a median VO_2 of 108 ml/min/m^2 and then an ERO_2 of 11%.

Blood gas analysis performed during Pringle maneuver demonstrated SvO_2 greater than 75% and pH within normal range showing a good peripheral perfusion. Blood lactate concentration achieved a maximum of 7 mmoli/L that, we suppose, resulted from a reduction in hepatic metabolism rather than from reduced perfusion.

So despite low CVP, in all patients oxygen delivery was maintained upper 600 ml/min/m^2; so we can conclude that a good peripheral perfusion can be reached also with a fluid restrictive regimen avoiding overload and postoperative edema.

For hemodynamic optimization, seems reasonable that indirect perfusion indexes should be used in low risk patients and/or surgery, while for high risk should be used a more advanced monitoring. This is true especially in liver resection where we reach initially an extreme hypovolemia until a fluid replacement at the end of surgery.

Funding

Only departmental funds were used for this study. No external funds were obtained

Implication Statement

Blood loss is the major complication during liver resection so hepatic surgery is performed with a low central pressure combined with extrahepatic control flow.

The purpose of this study is the analysis of hemodynamic status in patients undergoing major hepatic surgery using Vigileo/FloTrac monitoring.

Contributions

- De Cosmo Germano: Study design and writing up of the first draft of the paper.
- Levantesi Laura: Study design, patient recruitment, data collection and writing up of the first draft of the paper.
- Chiara de Waure: Data analysis with a results section review.
- Oggiano Marco: Patient recruitment, data collection and writing up of the first draft of the paper.
- Elisabetta Congedo: Patient recruitment, data collection and writing up of the first draft of the paper.
- Federico Fiorini: Patient recruitment, data collection and writing up of the first draft of the paper.
- Flaminio Sessa: Patient recruitment, data collection and writing up of the first draft of the paper.

References

1. de Boer MT, Molenaar IQ, Porte RJ (2007) Impact of blood loss on outcome after liver resection. Dig Surg 24: 259-264.
2. Kooby DA, Stockman J, Ben-Porat L, Gonen M, Jarnagin WR, et al. (2003) Influence of transfusions on perioperative and long-term outcome in patients following hepatic resection for colorectal metastases. Ann Surg 237: 860-869.
3. Pringle JH (1908) V. Notes on the Arrest of Hepatic Hemorrhage Due to Trauma. Ann Surg 48: 541-549.
4. Jhanji S, Pearse RM (2009) The use of early intervention to prevent postoperative complications. Curr Opin Crit Care 15: 349-354.
5. Sandham JD, Hull RD, Brant RF, Knox L, Pineo GF, et al. (2003) A randomized, controlled trial of the use of pulmonary-artery catheters in high-risk surgical patients. N Engl J Med 348: 5-14.
6. Punjasawadwong Y, Boonjeungmonkol N, Phongchiewboon A (2007) Bispectral index for improving anaesthetic delivery and postoperative recovery. Cochrane Database Syst Rev: CD003843.
7. Chouillard EK, Gumbs AA, Cherqui D (2010) Vascular clamping in liver surgery: physiology, indications and techniques. Ann Surg Innov Res 4: 2.
8. Cannesson M, Le Manach Y, Hofer CK, Goarin JP, Lehot JJ, et al. (2011) Assessing the diagnostic accuracy of pulse pressure variations for the prediction of fluid responsiveness: a "gray zone" approach. Anesthesiology 115: 231-241.
9. de Boer MT, Molenaar IQ, Porte RJ (2007) Impact of blood loss on outcome after liver resection. Dig Surg 24: 259-264.
10. Bhattacharya S, Jackson DJ, Beard CI, Davidson BR (1999) Central venous pressure and its effects on blood loss during liver resection. Br J Surg 86: 282-283.
11. Eid EA, Sheta SA, Mansour E (2005) Low central venous pressure anesthesia in major hepatic resection. Middle East J Anaesthesiol 18: 367-377.
12. Guo Y, Lin CX, Lau WY (2011) Hemodynamic and oxygen transport dynamics during hepatic resection at different central venous pressures in pig models. Hepatobiliary Pancreat Dis Int 10: 516-520.

13. Melendez JA, Arslan V, Fischer ME, Wuest D, Jarnagin WR, et al. (1998) Perioperative outcome of major hepatic resection under low central venous pressure anaesthesia: blood loss, blood transfusion, and the risk of postoperative renal dysfunction. J Am Coll Surg 187: 620-625.
14. Sandham JD, Hull RD, Brant RF, Knox L, Pineo GF, et al. (2003) A randomized, controlled trial of the use of pulmonary-artery catheters in high-risk surgical patients. N Engl J Med 348: 5-14.
15. Hofer CK, Senn A, Weibel L, Zollinger A (2008) Assessment of stroke volume variation for prediction of fluid responsiveness using the modified FloTrac and PiCCOplus system. Crit Care 12: R82.
16. Mayer J, Boldt J, Poland R, Peterson A, Manecke GR Jr (2009) Continuous arterial pressure waveform-based cardiac output using the FloTrac/Vigileo: a review and meta-analysis. J Cardiothorac Vasc Anesth 23: 401-406.
17. Biais M, Nouette-Gaulain K, Cottenceau V, Revel P, Sztark F (2008) Uncalibrated pulse contour-derived stroke volume variation predicts fluid responsiveness in mechanically ventilated patients undergoing liver transplantation. Br J Anaesth 101: 761-768.
18. Eyraud D, Richard O, Borie DC, Schaup B, Carayon A, et al. (2002) Hemodynamic and Hormonal Responses to the Sudden Interruption of Caval Flow: Insights from a Prospective Study of Hepatic Vascular Exclusion During Major Liver Resections. Anesth Analg 95: 1173-1178
19. Marik PE, Baram M, Vahid B (2008) Does Central Venous Pressure Predict Fluid Responsiveness?*: A Systematic Review of the Literature and the Tale of Seven Mares. Chest 134: 172-178.
20. Marx G, Cope T, McCrossan L, Swaraj S, Cowan C, et al. (2004) Assessing fluid responsiveness by stroke volume variation in mechanically ventilated patients with severe sepsis. Eur J Anaesthesiol 21: 132-138.
21. Reuter DA, Kirchner A, Felbinger TW, Weis FC, Kilger E, et al. (2003) Usefulness of left ventricular stroke volume variation to assess fluid responsiveness in patients with reduced cardiac function. Crit Care Med 31: 1399-1404.
22. Wiesenack C, Fiegl C, Keyser A, Prasser C, Keyl C (2005) Assessment of fluid responsiveness in mechanically ventilated cardiac surgical patients. Eur J Anaesthesiol 22: 658-665.
23. Marik PE, Cavallazzi R, Vasu T, Hirani A (2009) Dynamic changes in arterial waveform derived variables and fluid responsiveness in mechanically ventilated patients: a systematic review of the literature. Crit. Care Med 37: 2642-2647.
24. Kim YK, Shin WJ, Song JG, Jun IG, Hwang GS (2011) Does stroke volume variation predicts intraoperative blood loss in living right donor hepatectomy? Transpl Proc 43:1407-1411.
25. Benes J, Chytra I, Altmann P, Hluchy M, Kasal E, et al. (2010) Intraoperative fluid optimization using stroke volume variation in high risk surgical patients: results of prospective randomized study. Crit Care 14: R118.
26. Jhanji S, Pearse RM (2009) The use of early intervention to prevent postoperative complications. Curr Opin Crit Care 15: 349-354.
27. Shoemaker WC, Appel PL, Kram HB, Waxman K, Lee TS (1988) Prospective trial of supranormal values of survivors as therapeutic goals in high-risk surgical patients. Chest 94: 1176-1186.
28. Wolters U, Wolf T, Stützer H, Schröder T (1996) ASA classification and perioperative variables as predictors of postoperative outcome. Br J Anaesth 77: 217-222.
29. Boyd O, Jackson N (2005) How is risk defined in high-risk surgical patient management? Crit Care 9: 390-396.
30. Hamlton MA, Cecconi M, Rhodes A (2011) A systematic rewiev and meta-analysis on the use of preemptive hemodynamic intervention to improve postoperative outcome in moderate and high-risk surgical patients. Anaesth Analg 112:1392-1402.

27

Heart Rate Variability in Children Submitted to Surgery

Marta Joao Silva[1,2,3*], **Raquel Pinheiro**[1], **Rute Almeida**[3,4,5], **Francisco Cunha**[6,7], **Augusto Ribeiro**[2], **Ana Paula Rocha**[3,4] and **Hercília Guimaraes**[1,8]

[1]Faculdade de Medicina da Universidade do Porto (FMUP), Portugal

[2]Unidade de Cuidados Intensivos Pediatricos, Centro Hospitalar São João, Porto, Portugal

[3]CMUP-Centro de Matemática da Universidade do Porto, Departamento de Matemática da FCUP, Universidade do Porto, Porto, Portugal

[4]Faculdade de Ciências da Universidade do Porto (FCUP), Portugal

[5]BSICoS Group, Aragon Institute for Engineering Research (I3A), IIS Aragón, Universidad de Zaragoza and CIBER-Bioingeniría, Biomateriales y Nanomedicina, Communications Technology Group (GTC), Zaragoza University, Spain

[6]Centro da Criança e do Adolescente, Hospital Cuf Porto, Porto, Portugal

[7]Center for Health Technology and Services Research (CINTESIS), Portugal

[8]Unidade de Cuidados Intensivos Neonatais, Centro Hospitalar São João, Porto, Portugal

*Corresponding author: Marta Joao Silva, Unidade de Cuidados Intensivos Pediátricos, Centro Hospitalar São João and Departamento de Pediatria, Faculdade de Medicina da Universidade do Porto, Portugal, E-mail: martajoaosilva@gmail.com

Abstract

Objective: Heart Rate Variability (HRV) is known to reflect the sympathetic/parasympathetic interaction on several physiological and pathological conditions such as the cardiac activity responsiveness to physiological and environmental stimuli. Therefore, it has been widely used to assess nervous autonomic fluctuations and their influence on sinus node. Studies on children have demonstrated the correlation between HRV and different parameters like age, gender, physical activity and autonomic diseases whereas little evidence exists of the effects of surgery and residual anesthesic drugs on HRV. The aim of this study was to define the possible role of minor surgery in HRV in healthy children.

Design: Observational prospective cohort study.

Setting: Pediatric Surgery Department of a tertiary, university-affiliated hospital.

Patients: 47 healthy children who were scheduled for elective minor surgery.

Measurements and main results: HRV measurements of 10 to 15 minutes were obtained before and after surgery, using a Holter recorder and the BioSigBrowser® software. Results showed significant differences in HRV time domain indices before and after surgery in younger patients and in frequency domain in the older ones. They also demonstrated decreased HRV indices until one hour after being submitted to surgery in both time domain and LF parameters, reflecting a parasympathetic withdrawal and sympathetic predominance. Differences were also found when analyzing other variables such as anesthetic drugs.

Conclusion: This study demonstrated that surgery has impact on Autonomic Nervous System function in healthy children but, independently of anesthetic drugs, type of surgery, age and existence of pain 60 minutes after surgery no difference in HRV measures was found and autonomic homeostasis was re-established. However, further investigation in this area is required in order to a better support of the role of HRV monitoring on early prognosis prediction and risk stratification in the surgical context.

Keywords: Heart rate variability; Autonomic nervous system; Children; Surgery; Anesthesia; Healthy

Introduction

Heart Rate Variability (HRV), defined as the variation of the interval between consecutive R peaks of the electrical heart beat signal obtained through the electrocardiogram (ECG) reflects the heart's capacity to respond to physiological and environmental stimuli [1,2]. Heart Rate Variability is widely accepted as a valuable tool to investigate the sympathetic and parasympathetic contribution to regulation of heart rate rhythm. Variations in heart rate may be evaluated by a number of methods (Task Force, 1996). Time and frequency domain measures, determined by either the heart rate or the intervals between successive normal complexes, are a widely used tool in the investigation of autonomic cardiovascular control.

Three main spectral components are distinguished and usually differentiated in the spectral profile (Task Force, 1996): (a) the high frequency (HF) band (0.15 to 0.40 Hz); (b) the low frequency (LF) band (0.04 to 0.15 Hz); and (c) the very low frequency (VLF) band (<0.04 Hz). Evidence suggested that HRV was a tool to understand the interplay between the sympathetic and parasympathetic nervous system on the regulation of cardiac activity and on assessing cardiac health [3,5], so it was used as a marker of nervous autonomic modulation of sinus node [4], providing an insight into several conditions and enhancing risk stratification [2,5].

Reyes del Paso et al. [6], made a critically review of the state of research challenging the suitability of the LF component of HRV as an index of cardiac sympathetic control and the LF/HF ratio as an index of sympathovagal balance. They concluded that all HRV components predominantly relate to vagal control. However, it does not imply that they provide the same information about autonomic regulation. Each HRV component provides information about different physiological control mechanisms. HF oscillations relate to respiratory influences what reflect effects of respiration on heart rate (HR), also referred to as respiratory sinus arrhythmia (RSA). LF oscillations provide information about blood pressure control mechanisms such as the modulation of vasomotor tone including the so-called 0.1 Hz fluctuation. VLF power is related to kidney functioning and thermoregulation, meaning that HRV also gives information about sympathetic mechanisms (e.g., vasomotor tone fluctuations, rennin-angiotensin system) which manifest resonant phenomena through cholinergic oscillations in the sinus node [6].

Healthy children have higher ranges of normal respiratory rate and heart rate when compared to adults, which can interfere with Autonomic Nervous System (ANS) analysis [7,8]. Some authors suggest different ranges for heart rate and respiratory rate cited in international paediatric guidelines [8]. Since children can breathe at higher rates than 24 cpm we also calculated HFn+ corresponding to frequencies higher than 0.15 Hz (defined later) and can include all high rates of breathing.

Factors known to influence HRV indices includes age, gender, and physical activity [1] or non-physiological conditions, such as smoking, alcohol and drugs [3,5].

The main objective of the ANS is the maintenance of cardiovascular, respiratory, metabolic and thermal homeostasis, representing the primary defense against any internal or external factor jeopardizing systemic homeostasis [5]. The measurement of HRV from the ECG is a bedside, non-invasive and easy to perform method, which, by reflecting the balance of the ANS regulation of heart rate, detects the presence of ANS dysfunction [5].

In children, several studies have shown reduced or delayed cardio-vagal development in different pathologies such as diabetes mellitus [6-8], respiratory distress syndrome of the new-born [9-11], brain death [12] and sudden infant death syndrome [13,14]. There is also evidence of low HRV in functional pain conditions, anxiety and emotional disorders, which may indicate HRV as a potent biomarker of general stress and health [15-18].

Concerning the post-operative period, it is known, in adults, the correlation between ANS dysfunction and life-threatening complications after surgery [19-21]. The effect of anesthetics per se also affects ANS function. The ANS dysfunction represents a serious source of anesthetic risk affecting the outcome of patients undergoing surgery [5].

The aim of this study was to define the possible role of surgery in HRV in healthy children by HRV assessment both before and after minor surgery (76.7% correction of phimosis and/or inguinal, umbilical or abdominal wall hernia), accounting for several of its dimensions, namely, drugs involved, pain, airway access and surgical stress [5].

Methods

Study design

This observational prospective cohort study included a convenience cohort population of children who were scheduled for elective minor surgery at the Pediatric Surgery Department of a tertiary hospital, Sao Joao Hospital Center in Oporto, between September and November of 2015.

The study was conducted according to the Declaration of Helsinki and the Ethics Committee approved the project protocol. Written informed consent was obtained from the parents.

Sample

Participants included 47 subjects: 35 aged between 4 to 6 years (10 females and 25 males) and 12 aged between 14 to 16 years. Only healthy children, defined as children without any known congenital or chronic disease were enrolled in the study. Subjects under daily medication were also excluded.

Study measurement

HRV was assessed by high resolution 12 lead ECG acquired with a Holter H12+ Mortara recorder, exported using SuperECG propriety software from Mortara Rangoni, Italy and the BioSigBrowser software (BSB) [22,23]. Measurements of 15 minutes (min) were tentatively obtained at two different moments: the first before surgery, with the child seated in 45 degrees chair in the preoperative holding area and the second in the post-anesthesia care unit, with the subject still lying on the bed at 30 degrees. Both environments were dark and quiet. The time elapsed from the end of the anesthesia until the second HRV measurement was also registered.

Other study variables

Other variables were assessed as possible determinants, including physical activity [measured in hours per week (hours/week)] and Body Mass Index (BMI), calculated using the formula weight (Kg)/[height (m)] [2]. The percentiles of BMI were defined according to the growth charts developed by the National Center for Health Statistics in collaboration with the National Center for Chronic Disease Prevention and Health Promotion 2000 [21].

Pain after surgery was quantified in younger children according to a pain numeric rating scale (NRS) and in the older ones a visual analog scales (VAS).

Respiratory Rate (RespR) before and after surgery was collected. Heart Rate (HR) in beats per minute (bpm) and Systolic Blood Pressure (SBP) in mmHg before and after surgery were also collected and the difference between the pre and post-surgical values were calculated.

Information regarding the type of anesthesia and drugs used during the procedure was obtained from the anesthetic report.

In order to compare the differences between age and gender, the sample was divided into three groups: group A (n=10) including girls from 4 to 6 years old (yo), group B (n=25) including boys from 4 to 6 yo and group C (n=12) corresponding to male adolescents aged between 14 and 16 yo.

Data analysis

The graphical interface BSB [25] was used to perform the automatic ECG annotation and beat-to-beat series extraction. Namely, a multiscale wavelet-based ECG annotator previously developed and validated [26] was applied to obtain single lead (SL) based annotations and multilead based peak annotations obtained as the median mark of the 8 SL annotators for R peak from leads I, III, V1-V6. The interval RR(n) related to the nth beat is defined as the time from (n-1)th to the nth beat measured between consecutive R multilead based annotated R peaks.

The graphical interface BSB [22] was also used to obtain both "time domain" and "frequency domains" HRV measures following the standards defined by Task Force of the European Society of Cardiology and the North American Society of Pacing and Electrophysiology [2].

Series were then divided in short segments of a fixed duration of 5 min.

Each segment of analysis was detrended using the approach proposed by Tarvainen [28]. Series were assumed to be equally sampled at the local mean heart rate, as this has been shown acceptable for spectral analysis for frequencies far from Nyquist frequency [29].

HRV "time domain" local measures [2] were obtained over each available 5-min segment and includes "% HRM": mean heart rate (beats/min); "% SDNN": standard deviation of normal-to-normal (NN) intervals (milliseconds-ms); "% RMSSD": square root of the mean squared differences of successive NN intervals (ms) and "pNN50": the NN50 count divided by the total number of all NN intervals (%).

"Frequency domain" techniques, using a fast Fourier transform method applied to 5-min recording allow to estimate a spectrum in which two major bands of frequency assess ANS activity: low frequency (LF) band, from 0.04 to 0.15 Hz, is the expression of baroreceptor-mediated regulation and is mainly due to the contribution of sympathetic discharge; high frequency (HF) band, from 0.15 to 1.4 Hz, reflects the modulation of vagus nerve discharge caused by respiration [2]. We calculate also HFn+ (>0.15 Hz) since small children breathe faster and the window spanning of HF-HRV from 0.15 to 0.4 Hz could not be appropriate. This was calculated by the formula HFn ± (TP-VLF-LF)/TP.

Welch method in 64 points windows, with 50% overlap and 512 points for fast Fourier transform estimation was used over each segment. Non parametric (np) measures were taken as the power in each standard band (LF_np, HF_np), measured as the area under the spectra. LFn_np and HFn_np are power measures respectively at LF and HF bands, normalized by power in the band above 0.04 Hz, which is TP_np-VLF_np. Autonomic balance (B_np) was obtained as LF_np/HF_np and reflects the sympathovagal balance [5]. These measures were taken in normalized units.

Statistical analysis

Descriptive statistics are reported as frequencies for categorical variables and median (iIQR) or (minimum-maximum) for continuous variables. Patient and clinical characteristics were compared using Chi-square test or Fisher's exact test, as appropriate, for the categorical variables and Wilcoxon rank sum test or Kruskall Wallis test for continuous variables. All data were analyzed using SPSS ver. 22 (SPSS, Chicago, IL, USA). A P-value less than 0.05 were considered statistically significant.

Results

Characterization of each group relative to the parameters evaluated, including age, weight, BMI, physical activity, surgery duration and pre and post-surgical HR, respiratory rate (RespR) and systolic blood pressure (SBP) is shown at Table 1.

Group (n)	Age (yo)	Weight (kg)	BMI (kg/m^2)	Physical Activity (hours/week)	SBP (mmHg) Before Surgery	SBP (mmHg) After Surgery	Surgery Duration (min) Before Surgery	Respiratory Rate (cpm) After Surgery	Respiratory Rate (cpm) Before Surgery	Heart Rate (bpm) After Surgery	Heart Rate (bpm)
A (10)	5 (4-6)	20 (18-28)	15 (13.6-16.8)	2 (0-3)	99 (86-112)	102.5 (90-111)	36.5 (23-56)	19.5 (17-28)	18 (15-25)	94 (76-109)	100.5 (83-127)
B (25)	5 (4-6)	20 (11-34)	15 (11-29.9)	1 (0-3)	98.5 (86-120)	104 (84-123)	29 (18-103)	20 (16-26)	19.5 (13-23)	88.5 (61-110)	91 (72-113)
C (12)	15 (14-16)	64.5 (44-104)	20.9 (16.3-32.1)	4.5 (2-10)	124 (100-142)	126 (105-137)	29 (12-130)	18.5 (14-23)	17 (13-24)	75 (61-108)	71.5 (51-101)
Total (47)	6 (4-16)	21 (11-104)	15.8 (11-32.1)	2 (0-10)	104 (86-142)	106 (84-137)	29 (12-130)	19 (14-28)	18 (13-25)	88 (61-110)	88.5 (51-127)
Values are expressed as median (minimum-maximum)											

Table 1: Description of the sample and assessed variables.

When analyzing the nature of the surgeries, 76.7% of patients had phimosis and/or hernia correction (inguinal, umbilical and abdominal wall), three patients (11.6%) had winged ear correction, three (7.0%) cutaneous lesion extraction and two (4.7%) excision of sacroccygeal cyst.

Participants BMI was categorized according to CDC Growth Charts into percentile<5 (n=5; 10.6%), percentile 5 to percentile 85 (n=34; 72.3%) and percentile>85 (n=8; 17%).

Physical activity was divided in three groups: less than 2 hours/week (n=32; 68.1%), 2 to 5 hours/week (n=10; 21.3%) and more than 5 hours/week (n=5; 10.6%).

When studying the influence of physical activity, three groups were formed: children who practiced less than 2 hours/week (n=32; 68.1%), children who practiced from 2 to 5 hours/week (n=10; 21.3%) and children who practiced more than 5 hours/week (n=5; 10.6%).

They were also divided according to surgery duration into three groups: those whose surgery lasted less than 30 min (n=26; 55.3%), those surgeries lasted from 30 to 60 min (n=17; 36.2%) and those whose surgery lasted more than 60 min (n=4; 8.5%). The median time of surgery duration in minutes was 29 ranging from 12 to 130 minutes and with IQR of 26 and 40 minutes.

Concerning the effect of time between surgery and the second measurement of HRV and in order to simplify the analysis, participants were divided in three groups: those whose measurement was performed in less than 30 min (n=15; 31.9%) after surgery, those in which it was performed from 30 to 60 min after surgery (n=23; 48.9%) and those whose measurement was taken more than 60 min after surgery (n=9; 19.1%). The median time between registration and surgery in minutes was 43 (22-57) minutes ranging from 7 to 115 minutes.

Pain after surgery was reported only in 17 (36.2%) cases with a similar distribution between groups A, B and C.

With regard to the anesthesia, all of the participants from A and B group were submitted to induction with sevoflurane, ten of them were also submitted to fentanyl (eight from A group and two from B group) and none of them were submitted to propofol. In C group, sevoflurane was used to induce anesthesia in nine cases, associated to fentanyl in eight of them and to propofol in six. Three cases were submitted to intravenous induction with propofol and, in one of them, in association to fentanyl. In summary, sevoflurane was used in 44 subjects, propofol in nine and fentanyl in seventeen.

The values of HRV parameters comparing the different groups (A, B or C) before and after surgery are expressed in Table 2. Group A (girls from 4 to 6 yo) and group B (boys from 4 to 6 yo) presented significant lower values of HRV in the time domain measures after the surgery while no difference was found in spectral components except for Group B that showed a significant decrease of HFn+. On the other hand, group C (boys from 14 to16 yo) showed a decrease in HF component, non-significant in HFn but significant in HFn+, and an increase in LFn values after surgery and, consequently, in balance (B). Furthermore, no significant differences were found in the time domain measures. Globally, significant differences were found for HRV decrease in the time domain measures and HFn+ component and an increase in LF component.

Group (n)	Measure	Before surgery	After surgery	Difference (before-after)	P (Wilcoxon test)
A (10)	SDNN	57.6 (48.6-70.8)	42.3 (24.3-54.5)	25.2 (-0.1-30.2)	0.037*
	RMSSD	40.0 (19.6-60.8)	20.1 (11.6-32.2)	22.5 (2.6-39.0)	0.013*
	pNN50	11.4 (2.5-19.4)	2.4 (0.2-10.2)	10.8 (-0.3-15.3)	0.028*
	LFn	1.7 (1.4-3.5)	1.9 (1.5-3.1)	0.2 (-0.3-1.4)	0.553
	HFn	38.6 (24.8-50.5)	37.9 (24.7-64.7)	-0.1 (-5.9-7.9)	0.959
	B(LF/HF)	0.07 (0-0.1)	0.1 (0.0-0.1)	0.0 (-0.07-0.06)	0.914
	HF+	0.98 (0.97-0.99)	0.98 (0.97-0.99)	-0.001 (-0.01-0.01)	0.646
B (25)	SDNN	66.6 (58.6-85.2)	52.9 (40.4-84.6)	14.9 (-2.3-27.4)	0.028*
	RMSSD	56.2 (41.3-71.3)	29.3 (16.9-71.8)	18.2 (7.6-42.8)	0.011*
	pNN50	22.2 (16.1-34.3)	5.6 (0.9-27.5)	13.1 (1.2-23.7)	0.004*
	LFn	1.7 (1.4-2.3)	1.9 (1.3-3.9)	-0.2 (-1.3-0.3)	0.072
	HFn	30.9 (24.4-40.9)	37.9 (28.5-48.1)	-1.8 (-18.7-5.3)	0.166
	B(LF/HF)	0.1 (0.04-0.10)	0.1 (0.0-0.1)	0.0 (0.0-0.0)	0.221
	HF+	0.98 (0.97-0.99)	0.97 (0.96-0.99)	0.005 (-0.002-0.15)	0.026*
C (12)	SDNN	76.4 (52.3-93.2)	65.7 (44.5-98.3)	-4.6 (-22.5-21.6)	0.638
	RMSSD	43.7 (18.5-69.7)	22.1 (16.4-78.9)	2.9 (-42.8-24.6)	0.875
	pNN50	17.6 (2.4-42.3)	3.3 (0.9-36.7)	3.1 (-7.6-13.8)	0.583
	LFn	6.2 (3.9-9.8)	8.9 (5.6-26.2)	-4.1 (-14.7-0.2)	0.023*
	HFn	61.8 (42.2-70.7)	59.8 (52.4-63.9)	1.9 (-14.2-14.2)	1

	B(LF/HF)	0.1 (0.1-0.19)	0.2 (0.1-0.4)	-0.07 (-0.3-0.0)	0.017*
	HF+	0.93 (0.89-0-96)	0.90 (0.78-0.96)	0.03 (0.004-0.15)	0.028*
All	SDNN	66.6 (55.4-80.8)	53.6 (39.6-78.1)	9.4(-5.5-28.5)	0.021*
	RMSSD	48.6 (35.7-70.7)	23.4 (15.9-50.6)	17.7 (-3.6-36.7)	0.003*
	pNN50	18.9 (10.1-32.8)	3.9 (0.9-25.3)	42.2 (-1.1-18.7)	0.00*
	LFn	2.1 (1.6-5.0)	2.8 (1.6-5.0)	6.3 (-2.4-0.3)	0.024*
	HFn	39.1 (26.2-50.5)	43.2 (31.2-62.2)	61.5 (-16.8-7.8)	0.288
	B(LF/HF)	0.1 (0.05-0.1)	0.10 (0.0-0.1)	0.1 (-0.05-0.0)	0.272
	HF+	0.98 (0.95-0.99)	0.97 (0.94-0.98)	0.06 (-0.002-0.02)	0.005*

Values are expressed as median (IQR-interquartile range); *Significant difference between measures before and after surgery (p<0.05)

Table 2: HRV parameters by age and gender.

No significant difference was found on HRV measures when comparing them by BMI percentile.

With respect to physical activity influence on HRV parameters before and after surgery, statistically significant decreases were found in the time domain measures in children who practiced less than 2 hours/week (SDNN: 63.3 (53.4-76.8) versus 51.2 (40.6-73.9), p=0.02; RMSSD: 48.6 (36.6-65.8) versus 23.4 (15.2-48.9), p=0.003; pNN50: 19.4 (10.2-32.5) versus 3.7 (0.8-21.4), p=0.002). No other significant findings related to physical activity were observed.

Comparing the groups by the surgery duration significant differences were observed between pre and post-surgical HRV values only in the group in which it lasted from 30 to 60 min and in time domain parameters, with decreased values in SDNN [62.9 (54.3-70.2) versus 36.1 (26.9-53.6), p=0.002], RMSSD [46.3 (27.3-62.0) versus 17.1 (12.5-20.1), p=0.001] and pNN50 [14.8 (6.3-20.6) versus 0.58 (0.3-2.4), p=0.001]. No differences were found in the frequency domain parameters in any of the groups.

When analyzing the effect of the time occurred since the end of the surgery until the measurement of HRV (Figure 1), a statistically significant reduction in RMSSD [43.3 (19.7-52.1) versus 19.2 (12.7-32.1), p=0.003] and pNN50 [12.6 (2.5-26.4) versus 7.2 (1.9-12.2), p=0,005] was observed in those patients whose HRV measurement was taken in less than 30 min after surgery. Those whose measurement was taken between 30 to 60 min after surgery presented a statistically

significant decrease in pNN50 [28.7 (14.7-38.8) versus 8.4 (1.3-28.8), p=0.036] and LF [29.9 (23.8-39.4) versus 3.2 (1.6-5.3), p=0.013]. Beyond these, no other significant differences were found in the other HRV measures related to time after surgery.

The patients who have reported pain after surgery (Figure 2) showed a significant decrease in all time domain indices [SDNN: 63.3 (51.1-83.1) versus 48.7 (38.3-60.1), p=0.031; RMSSD: 44.1 (29.6-74.4) versus 19.2 (15.2-33.6), p=0.011; pNN50: 20.7 (6.3-36.4) versus 2.1 (0.5-11.9), p=0.002] while in those with no reported pain only pNN50 was significantly reduced [18.5 (12.9-32.5) versus 6.6 (0.9-28.5), p=0.043].

Analysis of propofol and fentanyl influence on HRV is presented in Table 3. Most of the patients (93.6%) were submitted to sevoflurane (only 3 were not) so the results of HRV parameters on sevoflurano are very similar to the general population posted on Table 2. In the group in which propofol was used there was only significant differences in LFn component, in balance (B) and in HFn+. Nevertheless, time domain parameters revealed to be significantly different among those cases in which propofol were not used during anesthesia. All patients that were submitted to propofol were from C group, they presented lower values of HR before and after surgery than the others were not submitted to propofol and HR lowered after surgery. SBP was lower in the patients who did propofol also.

		Measure	Before surgery	After surgery	p (Wilcoxon test)
Propofol (n)		HR	76 (68-106)	71 (60-88)	0.032*
		SBP	127 (119-133)	129 (122-135)	0.889
		RespR	19 (15-21)	17 (16-20)	0.669
		SDNN	67.9 (49.7-102.9)	59.8 (38.7-109.1)	0.767
		RMSSD	44.1 (12.9-66.8)	18.1 (15.6-73.8)	0.953
		pNN50	17.3 (0.5-41.6)	1.5 (0.6-31.2)	0.953
	Yes (9)	LFn	7.4 (4.5-10.7)	12.2 (8.0-29.5)	0.038*

		HFn	66.4 (43.3-70.1)	60.6 (47.3-64.2)	0.953
		B (LF/HF)	0.1 (0.1-0.2)	0.2 (0.2-0.6)	0.027*
		HFn+	0.92 (0.89-0.95)	0.87 (0.74-0.92)	0.038*
	No (38)	HR	96 (91-102)	99 (89-109)	0.049*
		SBP	100 (93-108)	104 (97-107)	0.081
		RespR	20 (18-22)	19 (17-22)	0.050*
		SDNN	65.3 (56.1-79.9)	51.2 (39.4-78.8)	0,007*
		RMSSD	50.9 (36.9-71.0)	25.2 (16.3-52.1)	0.001*
		pNN50	19.4 (12.0-32.8)	4.4 (0.9-25.6)	0.001*
		LFn	1.8 (1.5-3.6)	2.01 (1.6-3.9)	0.177
		HFn	33.7 (24.8-47.8)	39.6 (28.4-59.4)	0.252
		B (LF/HF)	0.1 (0.04-0.1)	0.1 (0.0-0.1)	0.573
		HFn+	0.98 (0.91-0.99)	0.97 (0.96-0.98)	0.064
Fentanyl	Yes (17)	HR	87 (77-105)	87 (72-100)	0.489
		SBP	112 (99-124)	109 (104-121)	0.571
		RespR	19 (18-21)	19 (17-22)	0.073
		SDNN	63.2 (50.9-79.1)	53.3 (32.1-75.9)	0.218
		RMSSD	41.9 (22.7-53.4)	20.5 (15.4-33.9)	0.033*
		pNN50	13.9 (3.9-30.2)	2.9 (0.5-12.5)	0.011*
		LFn	3.5 (1.7-6.2)	4.5 (2.1-10.2)	0.025*
		HFn	46.4 (30.6-64.1)	57.3 (36.0-63.9)	0.433
		B (LF/HF)	0.1 (0.04-0.1)	0.1 (0.1-0.2)	0.014*
		HFn+	0.96 (0.93-0.98)	0.96 (0.89-0.98)	0.021*
	No (30)	HR	87 (76.75-105.25)	87 (72-100.25)	0.097
		SBP	112 (99-124)	104 (96-107.5)	0.083
		RespR	19 (18-21)	18.5 (17-21.5)	0.228
		SDNN	70.1 (57.9-90.1)	53.6 (41.2-91.1)	0.039*
		RMSSD	58.3 (40.3-72.0)	29.3 (16.7-87.1)	0.027*
		pNN50	22.2 (15.8-37.0)	5.6 (0.9-28.3)	0.012*
		LFn	1.7 (1.5-3.6)	1.9 (1.4-4.1)	0.275
		HFn	43.1 (24.6-45.3)	38.2 (30.0-52.0)	0.509
		B (LF/HF)	0.1 (0.05-0.1)	0.1 (0.0-0.1)	0.446
		HFn+	0.98 (0.97-0.99)	0.97 (0.96-0.98)	0.136

Values are expressed as median (IQR-interquartile range); *Significant difference between measures before and after surgery ($p < 0.05$).

Table 3: HRV parameters according to Propofol, Sevoflurane and Fentanyl.

Fentanyl effect on HRV parameters was related to significant changes in RMSSD, SDNN, LFn and in balance (B).

In those cases in which this drug was not used, significant decreases were observed in all time domain components. 88.8% of the patients who were not submitted to fentanyl did lumbar epidural anesthesia.

Discussion

Over the last years, literature has highlighted the relevance of HRV on assessing ANS status as a mean of predicting post-operative complications, considering surgery and all its implications (pain, anesthetic drugs, emotional distress) as a cause of autonomic disruption with effects on systemic homeostasis [5,16-18]. The analysis of HRV can complement the reasoning for invasive monitoring and may hopefully guide preventive strategies for risk reduction [24-26]. Thus, the post-operative period is a period of increased cardiovascular and respiratory risk and a decreased HRV is recognized to be a more powerful predictor for mortality [5].

On children, little information exists regarding surgery effects on HRV, which means that research in this area is required. With this study, we sought to determine HRV changes among healthy children submitted to minor surgery and presents descriptive information about each HRV parameter.

It is known that HRV reflects the fluctuation in autonomic inputs to the heart. Diminished HRV occurs when there's both autonomic inactivity and excessive sympathetic inputs [2], showing an ANS imbalance that may be induced by increased stress or autonomic neuropathy [30]. Time domain parameters (SDNN, RMSSD and pNN50) strongly reflect parasympathetic modulation of sinus node [4] and, although there´s not a consensus among the scientific community about frequency domain parameters, most authors consider HF component as an expression of vagal activity influenced by respiration and LF component as a reflection of both cardiac sympathetic and parasympathetic activity with predominance of the sympathetic discharge [5]. Thus, LF/HF ratio represents a sympathovagal balance [5].

Regarding the results, with an overall analysis, it is possible to conclude that surgery influenced HRV values of the entire sample independently of other variables, as showed in Table 2. These findings suggest an increase in sympathetic control of the heart or a decrease in parasympathetic control of the heart. Probably, in younger children, surgery influences parasympathetic activity the most whereas, in the older children, it influences mostly the sympathetic activity as found in previous studies that suggest a decrease in the influence of parasympathetic activity that occurs with increasing age [8].

Normal ranges of respiratory rate in children are still under discussion. Fleming et al. [7] created new centiles of respiratory rate in children demonstrating a decline in respiratory rate from birth to early adolescence decreasing from a median of 44 breaths/minutes at birth to 26 breaths/minute at age of two. In our study only four children presented a respiratory rate over 24 breaths/minute (maximum RR of 28 breaths/minute). Since HF-HRV is defined in a spaning 0.15 to 0.4 Hz we calculated HFn+ to include the patients with RR >24 breaths/minute, but no significant differences were found from the HF-HRV.

Although sometimes conflicting, information in literature demonstrated age related changes in HRV due to ANS maturation [31,32]. Some authors describe a gradual decrease of the sympathetic activity in the first decade of life [3,31], while others describe an increase of parasympathetic activity in the same period of time,

reflected by increased values of all the time domain indices, followed by a gradual decrease [4, 32,33].

When comparing pre and post-surgical values between boys and girls, no significant differences were found in the same HRV parameters, which is consistent with previous studies that stated no differences in children HRV values according to gender [1,30].

Even though studies show a correlation between HRV and physical activity [1,34], in the present study, differences seen on HRV indices related to physical activity are probably biased by age because the group that practiced less than 2 h/week consists of younger children and the group that practiced more than 5 h/week is composed of the older participants.

Only the group in which surgery lasted from 30 to 60 min (Figure 1) revealed significant differences in time domain values, thus in parasympathetic modulation of ANS. One possible explanation could be the use of a lighter anesthesia used in short and less aggressive surgery with very low influence on ANS. There were only four cases in which surgery duration lasted more than 60 min (two adolescents), not enough cases to find any statistically difference.

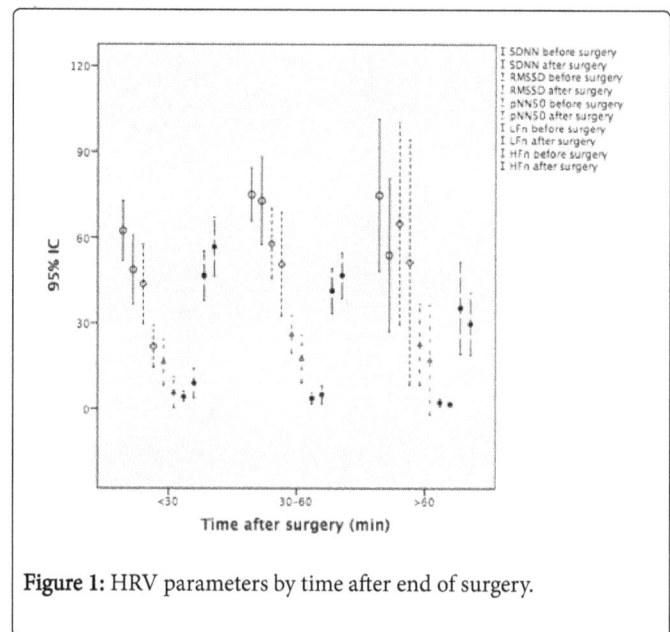

Figure 1: HRV parameters by time after end of surgery.

Results related to analysis of the time occurred from the end of the surgery until the measurement of HRV (Figure 2) showed a decreased parasympathetic activity in those patients whose HRV measurement was made in less than 30 min after surgery. A parasympathetic decrease and a sympathetic activity increase in those whose measurement was taken between 30 to 60 min after surgery was also found.

It is important to notice that, when measurements were taken after more than 60 min after surgery, no differences were found in HRV parameters. This can reflect a decreasing interference of surgery (and, possibly, the drugs used during the procedure) on ANS over time, with reestablishment of autonomic homeostasis. Despite the fact that our patients were only submitted to short duration anesthetic drugs, our study helps to support the time of 60 minutes as the minimum required period of standing in a post anesthesia care unit despite age or type of minor surgery.

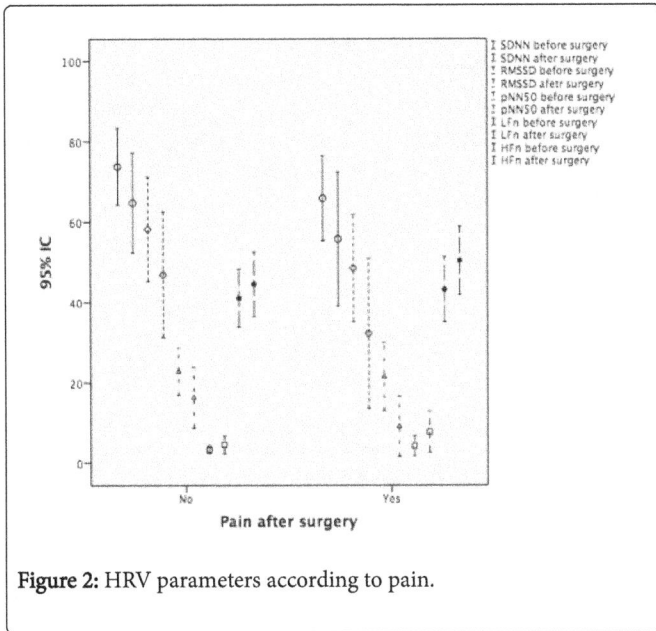

Figure 2: HRV parameters according to pain.

A diminished parasympathetic activity was seen on patients who have reported pain after surgery, as opposed to those who have not reported any pain (Figure 2). This result possibly leads to the establishment of a positive correlation between pain and parasympathetic inhibition and so a sympathetic dominance, also described in literature [35].

Anesthetics per se are known to affect ANS and HRV measurements. Despite this, during general anesthesia, anesthetic drugs may suppress autonomic activity oscillations and, depending on the combination of agents used, care must be taken when studying its influence on HRV [5,33]. Yet, inhalational anesthesia is known to negatively interfere with HRV indices [5].

HR decreases and SBP increases with age, this fact can explain why HR was lower and SBP higher, before and after surgery, in the cases submitted to propofol. Studies on propofol effect on HRV revealed a decrease in BP and HF proportional to the depth of anesthesia without any significant change on HR or LF, meaning that the cardiac parasympathetic nerve was inhibited to a higher degree than sympathetic nerve [5,36,37]. Other studies suggested propofol to induce cardiovascular depression by depressing sympathetic nervous activity [38].

In this study, results also showed an influence of propofol on the ANS activity. Patients who were submitted to propofol presented an increase of LF values and decrease of HF and HFn+ values after surgery. Reyes del Paso et al, suggested HRV power spectrum, including its LF component, is mainly determined by the parasympathetic system. These findings challenge the interpretation of the LF and LF/HF ratio as indices of sympathetic cardiac control and autonomic balance. According to this study findings we assume that our results suggests that propofol is an inhibitor of parasympathetic system that influenciate, in a higher proportion, the HF component. However, these results can have limited significance as propofol was only used in the older participants. In this population, induction of anesthesia with propofol was associated with a significant decrease in HR but not in SBP, as found in literature [36].

Sevoflurane was associated with decrease in BP or LF with little or no effect on the cardiac parasympathetic tone (5). The majority of our patients (93.6%) were submitted to sevoflurane so we cannot calculate the influence of this drug in our population. We found higher values of BP after surgery and no decrease of LF component. This finding could support the studies that suggest a mainly parasympathetic influence on LF component [38,39].

Few data on the effect of fentanyl on HRV are available [38]. Low dose fentanil led to sympathetic withdrawal and is believed to reduce LF power reflecting an increased parasympathetic tone [5]. We found that children who were on fentanyl showed a significant increase in LF and decrease in RMSSD and HFn+ component supporting the vagomimetic properties of this drug.

There are a number of studies that report a strong positive correlation between mean R-R interval and various time domain indices of HRV (e.g., the standard deviation of normal beats, SDNN) [40-42] such that HRV was greater during longer mean R-R intervals (slower heart rates) than at shorter mean R-R intervals (faster heart rates). Frequency domain analysis of HRV is similarly affected by mean heart rate. Sacha and Pluta [43] found that LF was directly related, while HF was indirectly related, to the average heart rate of the subject. As a consequence, they further report that LF/HF varied depending on heart rate, lower at slower and higher at faster heart rates. Thus, heart rate per se can influence LF/HF independent of changes cardiac autonomic nerve activity [39].

Respiratory parameters can also alter heart rate and R-R interval variability independent of changes in cardiac autonomic regulation (i.e., against a constant background level of automatic regulation) [44-48]. It is now well established that increases in respiratory frequency reduce the amplitude of heart rate oscillations [44,46,47] conversely, reductions in respiratory frequency increase HRV [44,46,47]. Thus, it is important to control breathing (paced or timed breathing) in order to interpret HRV data accurately. Brown and co-workers reported that respiratory parameters not only altered HF power but also strongly influenced the LF components of the R-R interval power spectrum, a component that previously was viewed to vary independently of changes in respiration [39].

Some studies suggest that opioids predominantly reduce LF power (reflecting an increased parasympathetic tone) and that general anesthesia with fentanyl leads to sympathetic withdrawal [49,50]. Our study showed an overall parasympathetic tone reduction on the patients submitted to minor surgery independently of receiving fentanyl or not. This can be explained by the use of epidural lombar anesthesia in 88.8% of patients not submitted to fentanyl. Tanaka et al. found that lumbar epidural anesthesia resulted in a significant increase in the low-frequency/HF ratio of HRV and unchanged spontaneous sequence baroreflex indices, suggesting sympathetic predominance [51].

With respect to sevoflurane impact on HRV parameters, although previous data suggests that it has little or even no effect on parasympathetic tone [52], no reliable conclusion can be made because almost all (but three cases) of the sample was submitted to sevoflurane during induction of anesthesia.

The interpretation of the results of this study naturally is subject to certain limitations. The main limitation is the measurement position. Although not very different concerning the degrees of inclination (45° before surgery and 30° after surgery) subjects were in a chair and sitting position before surgery and in a bed and supine position after surgery. Nepal et al. [39], found that a significant decreased in HRV parameters reflecting vagal activity and reciprocal increase in sympathetic activity in standing as compared to sitting and supine but there was no significant change in HRV in sitting as compared to supine.

Moreover, the small sample size compared with the diversity of the variables studied and the fact that the observed variables were not normally distributed is a strong impeditive to achieve more conclusions about some of the variables analyzed, particularly regarding multivariate analysis. No significant complications after surgery were found in our sample so any relation between ANS dysfunction and perioperative complications could be established.

Data in literature suggests that the measurement of HRV is a good tool to evaluate perioperative risk in patients with suspected autonomic dysfunction, select individuals who need further cardiac testing and optimize pre-operative status [5]. In this study, only healthy children with no surgical complications were studied and, still, they showed reduced HRV measurements. Further studies in children with suspected autonomic dysfunction or complicated surgery are necessary to better support the role of HRV monitoring on early prognosis prediction and risk stratification.

In addition, several other aspects that are known to influence HRV measurements were not taken into account, such as physical and emotional stress due to anticipation of the surgery, other drugs used during surgery, volemic status and changes in position [5]. Finally, because the studied population was composed of children and measurements were realized in the presence of other people, it was not always possible to have the desired and ideal quiet environment.

Conclusion

The measurement of HRV can be used as a helpful, non-invasive, bedside tool to evaluate the risk in patients who are going to be submitted to surgery. This study showed a decreased HRV in healthy children until one hour after being submitted to minor surgery in both time-domain and low frequency-domain parameters, reflecting a parasympathetic withdrawal and sympathetic predominance. When analyzing all patients no difference was found in HF domain and in balance.

Younger patients presented significant differences in HRV in time domain measures before and after surgery and older patients showed a difference in low frequency spectral component. In healthy children submitted to minor surgery no significant ANS dysfunction was found over 60 minutes after surgery. This data can support the time of 60 minutes as the required period for standing in post anesthesia care unit.

Nevertheless, it is important to notice that further investigation about this subject is required in order to a better comprehension of ANS behavior, particularly in the pediatric age group.

Acknowledgements

Authors would like to thank the director of Pediatric Surgery Department of Centro Hospitalar Sao Joao, José Estevão da Costa MD PhD, for giving permission to collect the data in his department.

Authors also acknowledge the support from Mortara Instr Inc., represented in Portugal by CardioSolutions, Lda. The first, third and sixth authors were partially supported by CMUP (UID/MAT/ 00144/2013), which is funded by FCT (Portugal) with national (MEC) and European structural funds through the programs FEDER, under the partnership agreement PT2020.

This study was partially supported by projects TEC2010-21703-C03-02 and TEC2013-42140-R from the Ministerio de Economia y Competitividad (MINECO) with European Regional Development Fund (FEDER), Spain, and by Grupo Consolidado BSICoS (T-96) from DGA (Aragon, Spain) and European Social Fund (EU).

Disclosures

No conflicts of interest declared.

References

1. Michels N, Clays E, De Buyzere M, Huybrechts I, Marild S, et al. (2013) Determinants and reference values of short-term heart rate variability in children. Eur J Appl Physiol 113: 1477-1488.

2. Malik M, Bigger JT, Camm AJ, Kleiger RE, Malliani A, et al. (1996) Heart rate variability: Standards of measurement, physiological interpretation, and clinical use. Task Force of the European Society of Cardiology and the North American Society of Pacing and Electrophysiology. Eur Heart J 17: 354-381.

3. Rajendra Acharya U, Paul Joseph K, Kannathal N, Lim CM, Suri JS (2006) Heart rate variability: a review. Med Biol Eng Comput 44: 1031-1051.

4. Silvetti MS, Drago F, Ragonese P (2001) Heart rate variability in healthy children and adolescents is partially related to age and gender. Int J Cardiol 81: 169-174.

5. Mazzeo AT, La Monaca E, Di Leo R, Vita G, Santamaria LB (2011) Heart rate variability: a diagnostic and prognostic tool in anesthesia and intensive care. Acta Anaesthesiol Scand 55: 797-811.

6. Reyes del Paso, Langewitz W, Mulder LJ, van Roon A, Duschek S (2013) The utility of low frequency heart rate variability as an index of sympathetic cardiac tone: A review with emphasis on a reanalysis of previous studies. Psychophysiology 50: 477-487.

7. Fleming S, Thompson M, Stevens R, Heneghan C, Pluddemann A, et al. (2011) Normal ranges of heart rate and respiratory rate in children from birth to 18 years of age: a systematic review of observational studies. Lancet 377: 1011-1018.

8. Chen W, Zhang XT, Guo CL, Zhang SJ, Zeng XW, et al. (2016) Comparison of heart rate changes with ictal tachycardia seizures in adults and children. Childs Nerv Syst 32: 689-695.

9. Akinci A, Celiker A, Baykal E, Tezic T (1993) Heart rate variability in diabetic children: sensitivity of the time- and frequency-domain methods. Pediatr Cardiol 14: 140-146.

10. Chessa M, Butera G, Lanza GA, Bossone E, Delogu A, et al. (2002) Role of heart rate variability in the early diagnosis of diabetic autonomic neuropathy in children. Herz 27: 785-790.

11. Ozgur S, Ceylan O, Senocak F, Orun UA, Dogan V, et al. (2014) An evaluation of heart rate variability and its modifying factors in children with type 1 diabetes. Cardiol Young 24: 872-879.

12. Henslee JA, Schechtman VL, Lee MY, Harper RM (1997) Developmental patterns of heart rate and variability in prematurely-born infants with apnea of prematurity. Early Hum Dev 47: 35-50.

13. Van Ravenswaaij-Arts C, Hopman J, Kollée L, Stoelinga G, Van Geijn H (1994) Spectral analysis of heart rate variability in spontaneously breathing very preterm infants. Acta Paediatr 83: 473-480.

14. Prietsch V, Knoepke U, Obladen M (1994) Continuous monitoring of heart rate variability in preterm infants. Early Hum Dev 37: 117-131.

15. Almeida R, Silva MJ, Rocha AP (2013) Exploring QT variability dependence from heart rate in coma and brain death on pediatric patients, in Computing in Cardiology Conference (CinC) 61-64.

16. Perticone F, Ceravolo R, Maio R, Cosco C, Mattioli PL (1990) Heart rate

variability and sudden infant death syndrome. Pacing Clin Electrophysiol 13: 2096-2099.

17. Antila KJ, Välimäki IA, Mäkelä M, Tuominen J, Wilson AJ, et al. (1990) Heart rate variability in infants subsequently suffering sudden infant death syndrome (SIDS). Early Hum Dev 22: 57-72.

18. Evans S, Seidman LC, Tsao JCI, Lung KC, Zeltzer LK, et al. (2013) Heart rate variability as a biomarker for autonomic nervous system response differences between children with chronic pain and healthy control children. J Pain Res 6: 449-457.

19. Laitio T, Jalonen J, Kuusela T, Scheinin H (2007) The role of heart rate variability in risk stratification for adverse postoperative cardiac events. Anesth Analg 105: 1548-1560.

20. Ushiyama T, Nakatsu T, Yamane S, Tokutake H, Wakabayashi H, et al. (2008) Heart rate variability for evaluating surgical stress and development of postoperative complications. Clin Exp Hypertens 30: 45-55.

21. Goldstein B, Ellenby MS (2000) Heart rate variability and critical illness: potential and problems. Crit Care Med 28: 3939-3940.

22. Bolea J, Almeida R, Laguna P, Sornmo L, Martínez JP (BioSigBrowser, biosignal processing interface (2009) Final Program and Abstract Book 9th International Conference on Information Technology and Applications in) BioSigBrowser, biosignal processing interface (2009) Final Program and Abstract Book 9th International Conference on Information Technology and Applications in Biomedicine, ITAB.

23. Martínez JP, Almeida R, Olmos S, Rocha AP, Laguna P (2004) A wavelet-based ECG delineator: evaluation on standard databases. IEEE Trans Biomed Eng 51: 570-581.

24. [Author not listed] (2007) Centers for Disease Control and Prevention and National Center for Health Statistics/CDC. CDC growth charts: United States 2002.

25. Tarvainen MP, Ranta-Aho PO, Karjalainen PA (2002) An advanced detrending method with application to HRV analysis. IEEE Trans Biomed Eng 49: 172-175.

26. Almeida R, Pueyo E, Martinez JP, Rocha AP, Olmos S, et al. (2003) A parametric model approach for quantification of short term QT variability uncorrelated with heart rate variability. Comput Cardiol 165-168.

27. Estafanous F, Brum J, Ribeiro M, Estafanous M, Starr N, et al. (1992) Analysis of heart rate variability to assess hemodynamic alterations following induction of anesthesia. Cardiothorac Vasc Anesth 6: 651-657.

28. Knugtten D, Trojan S, Weber M, Wolf M, Wappler F (2005) Pre-operative measurement of heart rate variability in diabetics: a method to estimate blood pressure stability during anesthesia induction. Anaesthesist 54: 44-49.

29. Hanss R, Renner J, Ilies C, Moikow L, Buell O, et al. (2008) Does heart rate variability predict hypotension and bradycardia after induction of general anaesthesia in high risk cardiovascular patients? Anaesthesia 63: 129-135.

30. Seppälä S, Laitinen T, Tarvainen MP, Tompuri T, Veijalainen A, et al. (2014) Normal values for heart rate variability parameters in children 6-8 years of age: the PANIC Study. Clin Physiol Funct Imaging 34: 290-296.

31. Finley JP, Nugent ST, Hellenbrand W (1987) Heart-rate variability in children. Spectral analysis of developmental changes between 5 and 24 years. Can J Physiol Pharmacol 65: 2048-2052.

32. Finley JP, Nugent ST (1995) Heart rate variability in infants, children and young adults. J Auton Nerv Syst 51: 103-108.

33. Shannon D, Carley D, Benson H (1987) Aging and modulation of heart rate. Am J Physiol 19: 1334-1341.

34. Gutin B, Howe C, Johnson MH, Humphries MC, Snieder H, et al. (2005) Heart rate variability in adolescents: relations to physical activity, fitness, and adiposity. Med Sci Sports Exerc 37: 1856-1863.

35. Hamunen K, Kontinen V, Hakala E, Talke P, Paloheimo M, et al. (2012) Effect of pain on autonomic nervous system indices derived from photoplethysmography in healthy vonlunteers. Br J Anaesth 108: 838-844.

36. Kanaya N, Hirata N, Kurosawa S, Nakayama M, Namiki A (2003) Differential effects of propofol and sevoflurane on heart rate variability. Anesthesiology 98: 34-40.

37. Win NN, Fukayama H, Kohase H, Umino M (2005) The different effects of intravenous propofol and midazolam sedation on hemodynamic and heart rate variability. Anesth Analg 101: 97-102, table of contents.

38. Unoki T, Grap MJ, Sessler CN, Best AM, Wetzel P, et al. (2009) Autonomic nervous system function and depth of sedation in adults receiving mechanical ventilation. Am J Crit Care 18: 42-50.

39. Nepal GB, Paudel BH (2012) Effect of posture on heart rate variability in school children. Nepal Med Coll J 14: 298-302.

40. Kleiger RE, Miller JP, Bigger JT Jr, Moss AJ (1987) Decreased heart rate variability and its association with increased mortality after acute myocardial infarction. Am J Cardiol 59: 256-262.

41. Van Hoogenhuyze D, Weinstein N, Martin GJ, Weiss JS, Schaad JW, et al. (1991) Reproducibility and relation to mean heart rate of heart rate variability in normal subjects and in patients with congestive heart failure secondary to coronary artery disease. Am J Cardiol 68: 1668-1676.

42. Bigger JT, Fleiss JL, Steinman RC, Rolnitzky LM, Kleiger RE, et al. (1992) Frequency domain measures of heart period variability and mortality after myocardial infarction. Circulation 85:164-171.

43. Sacha J, Pluta W (2005) Different methods of heart rate variability analysis reveal different correlations of heart rate variability spectrum with average heart rate. J Electrocardiol 38: 47-53.

44. Angelone A, Coulter NA Jr (1964) Respiratory Sinus Arrhythemia: A Frequency Dependent Phenomenon. J Appl Physiol 19: 479-482.

45. Davies CT, Neilson JM (1967) Sinus arrhythmia in man at rest. J Appl Physiol 22: 947-955.

46. Melcher AH (1976) On the repair potential of periodontal tissues. J Periodontol 47: 256-260.

47. Hirsch JA, Bishop B (1981) Respiratory sinus arrhythmia in humans: how breathing pattern modulates heart rate. Am J Physiol 241: H620-629.

48. Van De Borne P, Montano N, Narkiewicz K, Degaute JP, Malliani A, et al. (2001) Importance of ventilation in modulating interaction between sympathetic drive and cardiovascular variability. Am J Physiol Heart Circ Physiol 280: H722-729.

49. Billman G (2013) The LF/HF ratio does not accurately measure cardiac sympatho-vagal balance. In heart rate variability: clinical applications and interaction between HRV and heart rate. Front Physiol 4: 54-58.

50. Zickmann B, Hofmann HC, Pottkämper C, Knothe C, Boldt J, et al. (1996) Changes in heart rate variability during induction of anesthesia with fentanyl and midazolam. J Cardiothorac Vasc Anesth 10: 609-613.

51. Michaloudis D, Kochiadakis G, Georgopoulou G, Fraidakis O, Chlouverakis G, et al. (1998) The influence of premedication on heart rate variability. Anaesthesia 53: 446-453.

52. Tanaka M, Goyagi T, Kimura T, Nishikawa T (2004) The Effects of Cervical and Lumbar Epidural Anesthesia on Heart Rate Variability and Spontaneous Sequence Baroreflex Sensitivity. Anesth Analg 99: 924 -929.

28

History and Evolution of Anesthesia Education in United States

Mian Ahmad* and **Rayhan Tariq**

Department of Anesthesiology and Perioperative Medicine, Drexel University College of Medicine, Philadelphia, PA, USA

*Corresponding author: Mian Ahmad MD, Vice-Chair Education, Department of Anesthesiology and Perioperative Medicine, Drexel University College of Medicine, 245 N. 15th Street, MS 310, Philadelphia, PA 19102, USA, E-mail: mian.ahmad@drexelmed.edu

Abstract

Resident education is both, a science and an art. Quality and homogeneity of resident education has a considerable correlation with patient safety. This article appraises how formal training in anesthesiology was started in United States and how it has evolved over the years. A comprehensive literature search was performed to identify journal articles, periodicals and historic documents that detailed the development and progression of academic anesthesiology. Various Anesthesiology Departments were also consulted. In 1927 Dr. Waters established the first ever academic department of Anesthesiology at the University of Wisconsin, Madison. The graduates from that residency programs, the so called "Aqualumni" went on to establish residency programs throughout the country. In 1938 American Board of Anesthesiology was formed, elevating the level of anesthesiology to a distinct specialty. World War II and post war era was a period of rapid growth in anesthesiology in general and academic anesthesiology in particular. In late 1970's and early 80's American College of Graduate Medical Education (ACGME) closely regulated the anesthesiology residency programs by recommending minimum program requirements. Over the years the training model has transformed from a relatively heterogeneous one to a uniform outcome based model with focus on learning and teaching of 6 core competencies. This article explores how the anesthesiology education evolved throughout 20th century to its present form.

Keywords: Academic; Education; Residency; Internship; Anesthesiology history; Training; ABA; ACGME

Introduction

Today residency is considered to be the essential dimension that ensures the transformation of a graduating medical student into an independently practicing physician. The training model was not as clear in early days of medical education. Medicine had utilized the same apprentice based model that other trades were using to train the artisan of the next generation. An interested individual would get attached to a practicing physician, observe him dealing with patients and over time learn the knowledge and skills which enabled him to diagnose and treat conditions that patients presented with. Very slowly this model evolved into a structured and process based training. Anesthesia training however, never really followed that pattern. Initially, surgeons administered anesthetics to their patients and then directed nurses to do the same. Physicians interested in this branch of medicine had to teach themselves and soon felt the need to improve upon the technical and cerebral part of anesthetic administration.

This article is meant to review the differences between these early anesthetists and the physicians certified by American Board of Anesthesiology to be the anesthesiologists practicing this specialty of medicine today. Even more importantly, it is going to examine the content and structure of education as it has evolved overtime.

The Early Years: 1900-1920

Surgery has existed long before anesthesiology, but before anesthesia, surgery was a means of last resort. The notion of undergoing surgery was so painful that many would prefer to allow a disease to run its natural course than going under the knife. The greatest development in history of medicine no doubt is the ability to alleviate pain during surgery and essentially making modern surgical practice possible. Although the first public demonstration of General Anesthesia was in 1846 by a dentist at Massachusetts General Hospital, the growth of anesthesiology as a specialty was slow [1]. For most of the early 20th century Anesthesiology remained a neglected field because of the general perception that very little training was needed to administer anesthetics.

During most of the early part of the 20th century instructions in anesthesia were nonexistent and the specialty was being practiced only by a few self-taught individuals [2]. Among them was James T. Gwathmey who authored the first authoritative text on the subject in 1914. His book "Anesthesia" would remain a valuable educational resource over the next few decades [3]. He was the first president of the American Society of Anesthetists, later renamed American Society of Anesthesiologists (ASA) [4]. He, along with other regional anesthesiology societies emphasized the need to give organized instructions and training in Anesthesia.

In 1924, McMechan started the first journal in the specialty; Anesthesia and Analgesia [5]. Previously American Journal of Surgery used to publish quarterly supplements on anesthesia and analgesia. In 1940 Henry Ruth started Anesthesiology, the official journal of ASA. During these early years there was a gradual movement towards establishment of Anesthesia as distinct medical specialty that should be practiced by physicians. History of Anesthesiology residency training was interlinked with the push for specialty status for Anesthesiology in the late 1920's and 1930's.

A Transition from Nurse Anesthetists to Trained Physician Anesthetist

During the latter part of 19th century and the early part of 20th century anesthesia, usually in the form of ether, was mostly administered by surgical nurse or a medical student/intern. Fortunately the surgical procedures at that time were neither as lengthy nor as complicated so these practices seen as rather safe. However with the evolution of surgical techniques and introduction of new techniques in anesthesia including the use of breathing tube in trachea by Ivan Mcgill and the introduction of Neuraxial Blocks by James Corning, it was becoming apparent that anesthesiology was a specialty of its own and hence needed physicians that were specially trained to optimally deliver anesthesia [6]. Dr. Isabella Herb, chief anesthetist at Rush University was one of the first Individuals with an academic appointment in Anesthesiology. She advocated *"nurses when properly trained make very good anesthetizers but that their lack of medical training prevented them from being able to choose a particular anesthetic technique that would best suit the patient's and surgeon's needs* [7]. *Also nurses' minimal training in medicine and lack of training in research meant that they were not suited to carrying out research in anesthesia".*

Another contributing factor for this shift was the push from national and local Anesthesiology Societies. Gatch and other early ASA leaders emphasized the need to establish a standardized approach to train interns in Anesthesia [8].

Contributions of Dr. Isabella Herb

There was no formal training for anesthesia as a student or at postgraduate level. What little training was there was mostly through apprenticeship. At that time anesthesia training was essentially a short course of few weeks in which anesthetics agents and equipment was taught entirely in the OR. The physicians were being taught as technicians [9].

Wanting to rectify that while at Rush, Dr. Herb Developed a curriculum for teaching medical students comprised of pharmacology, physiology of Anesthesiology and selection of anesthetics [10]. Dr. Herb believed that this program was to be delivered by a physician who had expertise and training in delivery of anesthetics in that hospital, and not by surgeons [11]. She wrote, *"Unfortunately most anesthetists receive their meager instruction from surgeons during the operations, and it is a notorious fact that the majority of surgeons are poor anesthetists. From the fact that a man operates hundreds of times a year, it does not follow that he is proficient in the art of producing and maintaining anesthesia"* [7].

Although the curriculum was only for medical students and this was not a postgraduate training but it was first of its kind and it set course for further development of education in anesthesia.

Dr. Waters and the First Academic Residency Program in Anesthesiology

In 1927 Dr. Waters established the first ever academic residency program of Anesthesiology in University of Wisconsin, Madison. While Dr. Waters' division of anesthesia at the University of Wisconsin remained a section under the department of surgery until 1952, it truly was the foremost beacon of anesthesia education [12]. The graduates from this residency program who called themselves as the 'Aqualumini'

went on to establish residency programs all over the United States. Dr. Waters focused on education and research along with providing optimum patient care. He inculcated morbidity and mortality analysis and discussion (M&M) and literature review in the residency didactics. He hoped to train physicians in the art and science of anesthesia who would go on to train other physicians in the safe clinical practice of anesthesia [2].

The Aqualumini

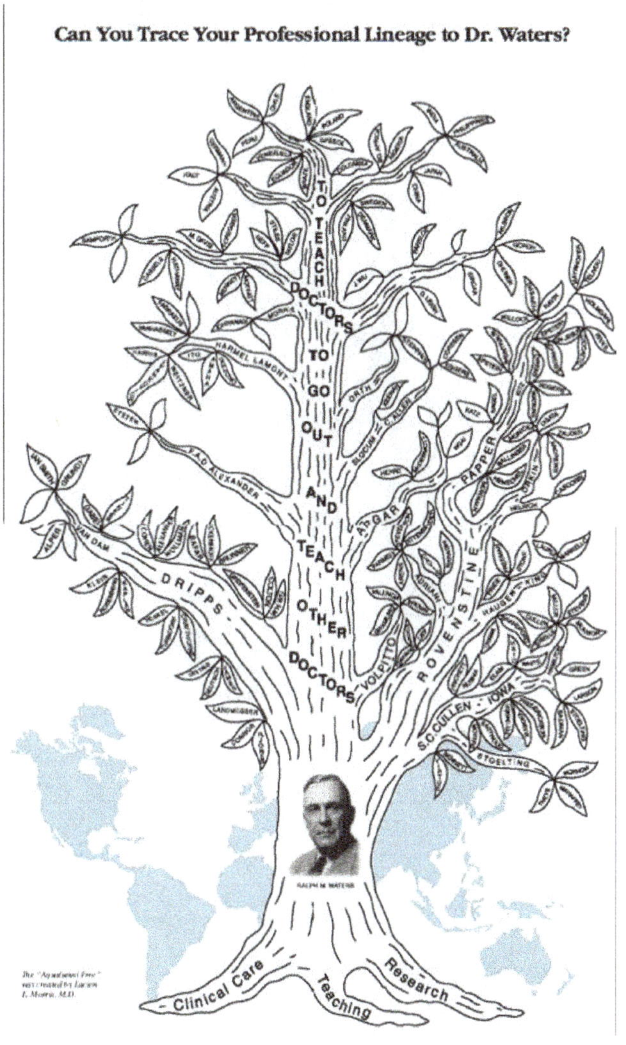

Figure 1: Aqualumni tree (Created by Lucien E. Morris, M.D., Founding Chair and Professor Emeritus, Department of Anesthesia, Medical College of Ohio, Toledo, Ohio.) [14]©, modified with Permission from American Society of Anesthesiology.

Individuals were attracted to anesthesiology from other specialties such as medicine, surgery and pharmacology. Among them is Emery Rovenstine who was Dr. Waters first and most distinguished disciple, he established the anesthesiology residency program at Bellevue/New York University (Figure 1). Among Rosenstein's notable residents were Stuart Cullen, Emanuel Papper, Virginia Apgar, Perry Volpitto, John Adriani, Louis Orkin, Sam Denson, Richard Ament, Gertie Marx, Martin Helrich, Sara Joffe, and Lewis Wright [13]. A genealogical review estimates that more than 80 departmental chairs out of the 120 Medical Schools in US have been of Waters' lineage (Table 1) [14].

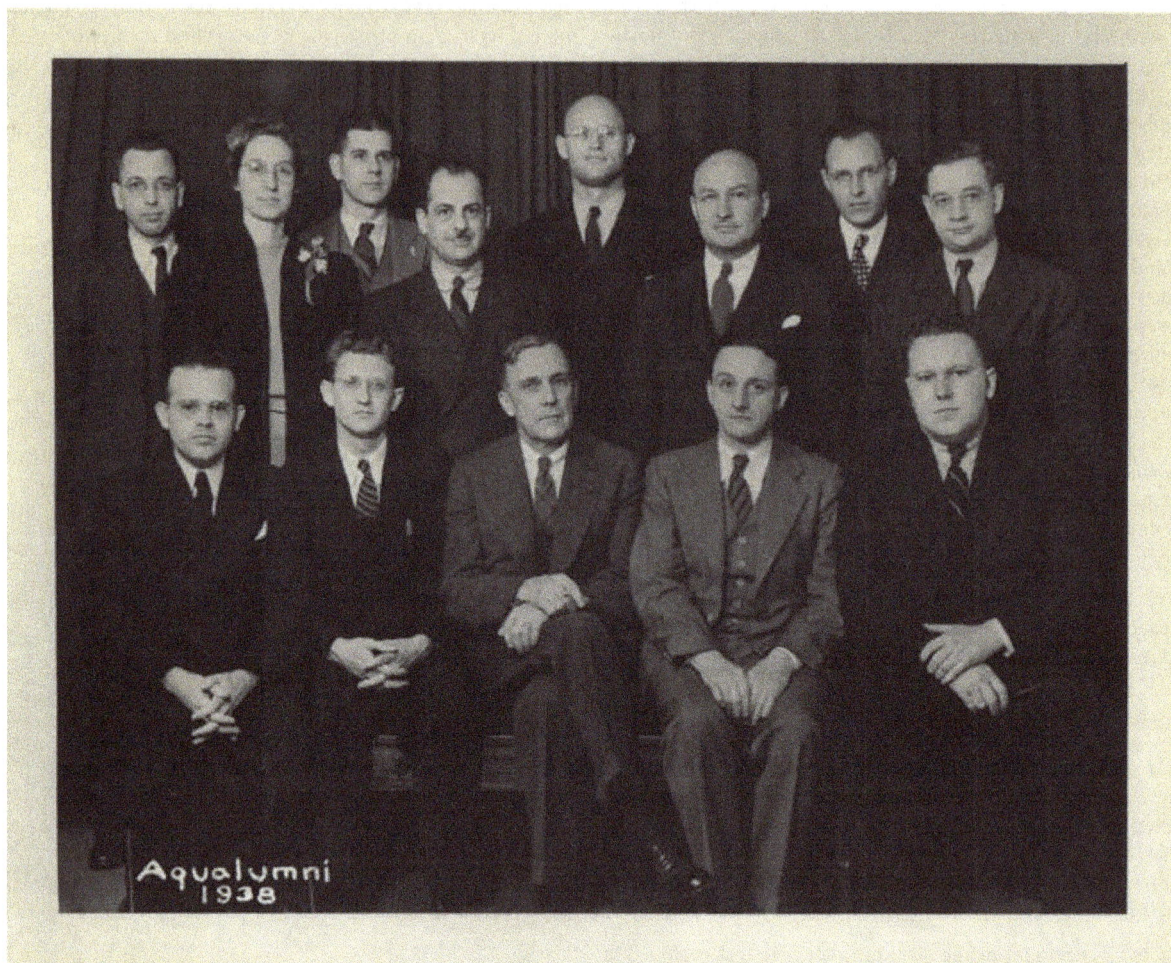

Figure 2: Aqualumini 1938 ©Mount Holyoke College. Archives and Special Collections, Virginia Apgar Papers (MS 0504).

Year Residency Program was Started	Institution/University	The First Chairman of the Department
1927	University of Wisconsin, Madison	Ralph Waters [2]
1929[a]	Hahnemann Medical College (now Drexel University College of Medicine)	Henry Swartley Ruth
1930 [12]	University of Oklahoma	John Alfred Moffitt
1935 [17]		
1935	New York University/Bellevue Hospital	Emery Rovenstine
1938[b]	University of Buffalo	John Evans
1939	Medical College of Georgia	Perry P. Volpitto [16,18]
1941[c]	UCSF	Stuart Cullen [19]
1941	Massachusetts General Hospital	Henry K. Beecher [20,21]
1943	University of Pennsylvania	Robert Dunning Dripps
1947 [22]	Ochsner Clinic Foundation, New Orleans, LA	George Grant
1949[d]	Columbia University	Emanuel Papper [2]

Table 1: Some of the earliest anesthesiology residency programs. [a]From Drexel University website http://drexel.edu/medicine/Academics/Residencies-and-Fellowships/Anesthesiology-Residency/; [b]From University of Buffalo website – Department History -http://www.smbs.buffalo.edu/anest/history.php (retrieved 8/25/2015); [c]From UCSF website – About Us http://anesthesia.ucsf.edu/extranet/about_us/index.php (retrieved 8/25/2015); [d]The Anesthesiology Service was first established as part of the Department of Surgery in 1937 under the direction of Dr. Virginia Apgar.

Dripps Started the Anesthesiology residency program at University of Pennsylvania; Cullen at UCSF; Emeul Papper established the anesthesiology department at Columbia University in 1949. Volpitto [15,16] established the first academic anesthesiology department in the south at medical college of Georgia, which he headed until 1972. The residency training program started slowly with the first resident in 1939 and the second one in 1941. From 1941-45, the majority of the male residents were recruited to a special wartime training program (Tables 1 and 2). John Lundy at Mayo Clinic started teaching anesthesiology as well as carrying out valuable research at that program. It was a chain reaction and soon enough residents graduating from above programs took the responsibility of propagating the knowledge of anesthesiology thorough out the country (Figures 2-4).

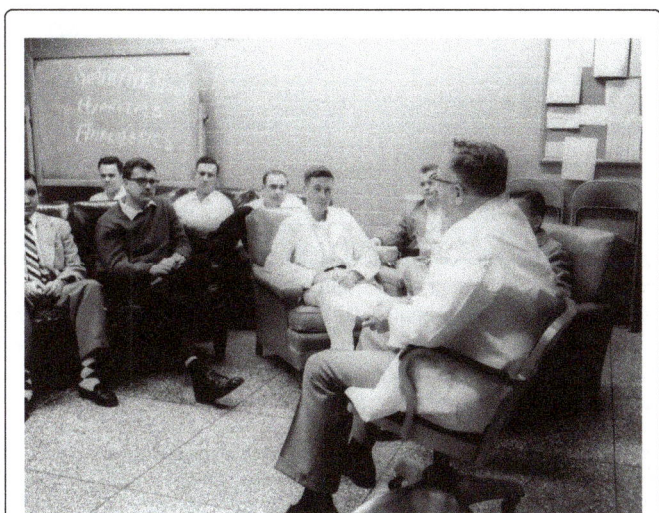

Figure 3: Dr. Volpitto teaching the Anesthesiology Residents[©], modified with Permission from Department of Anesthesiology and Perioperative Medicine, Medical College of Georgia, Georgia Regents University.

Year	Number of Residency Programs	Total number of Training Positions
1927	1	Data not available
1943	45	Data not available
1948	214	487
1949	214	650
1964	296	1,858 (of which 1,145 were filled)
1968	148	1,655
2010	132	5,556
2014[a]	133	5,686

Table 2: The growth of residency rrogram with years [23,24]. [a]From FREIDA Specialty training statistics (retrieved 8/28/2015).

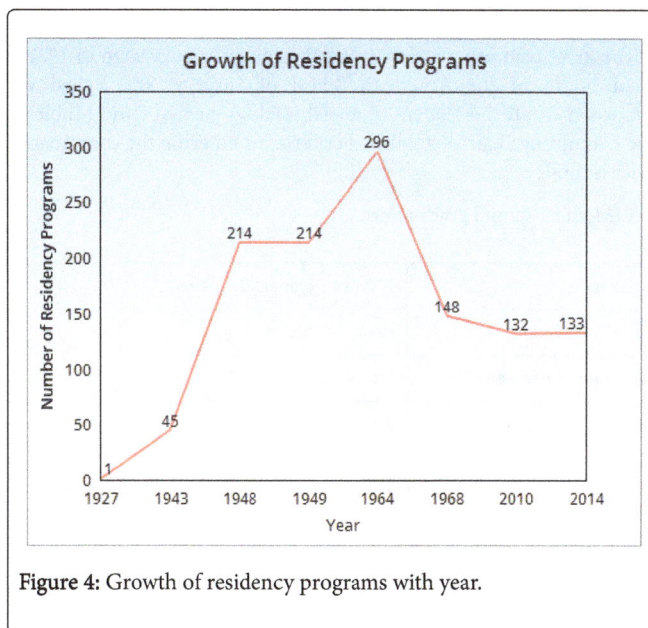

Figure 4: Growth of residency programs with year.

There was an increase in the number of residency programs after World War II which can be explained by the increased interest and increased demand for physician anesthesiologists.

The Influences of John Lundy

John Silas Lundy who is famed for the introduction of IV anesthetics in modern anesthetic practice [25] and the creation of first blood bank in the U.S. was the chair of anesthesia at Mayo Clinic from 1924-1959 [26,27]. Lundy's contribution to anesthesia however is not just the scientific advancement of knowledge but also the promotion of anesthesiology education. In 1925, John Lundy established the first anatomy laboratory at the Mayo Clinic where he taught regional Anesthesia techniques to surgery trainees [28]. He is accredited with creating the Anesthetists' Travel Club in 1929 in order to encourage flow of information between physicians practicing anesthesia. The participants, who were mostly in their thirties, discussed not only the clinical but also the basic research development relevant to anesthesiology. The Club met yearly till the start of World War II [29]. When the American Board of Anesthesiology (ABA) was formed in 1938 eight of the nine directors were members of the Travel Club. In 1941, in a large part due to his lobbying and political connections, the ABMS approved Anesthesia as a distinct specialty [30].

Development of ABA

It took more than a decade of meetings, conferences, and astute politics to convince public and professional organizations that this field merited specialty status. Finally an American Board of Anesthesiology (ABA) was formed as an affiliate of the American Board of Surgery (ABS) in 1937 and approved by American Board of Medical Specialties (ABMS) in 1938. The format of examination was changed to include MCQ within a decade and over time it was transformed to the current format. In 1941 it was approved as an independent primary Board (Table 3).

The First ABA Examination

The first "examining board in anesthesiology" was created in 1937 as a sub-board of the American Board of Surgery. The Board was composed of all the leaders of anesthesiology at that time (Table 5). The Examining Board established criteria for entering the examination process: [33].

1. Medical school graduation.

2. Completion of internship.

3. Two years of training, including 18 months of practical training in anesthesia.

4. Two years in the sole practice of anesthesia.

5. Membership in the AMA or a comparable approved national medical society.

President	Thomas Drysdale Buchanan[a]
Vice-President	Henry Ruth
Secretary-Treasurer	Paul Wood
Other Board Members	John Lundy, Emery Rovenstine, Harry Stewart, Ralph Tovell, Ralph Waters and Philip Wood-bridge.

Table 3: The first ABA committee [31], [a]Thomas Buchanan of the New York Medical Center-Bellevue Hospital was the recipient of ABA certificate number 1.

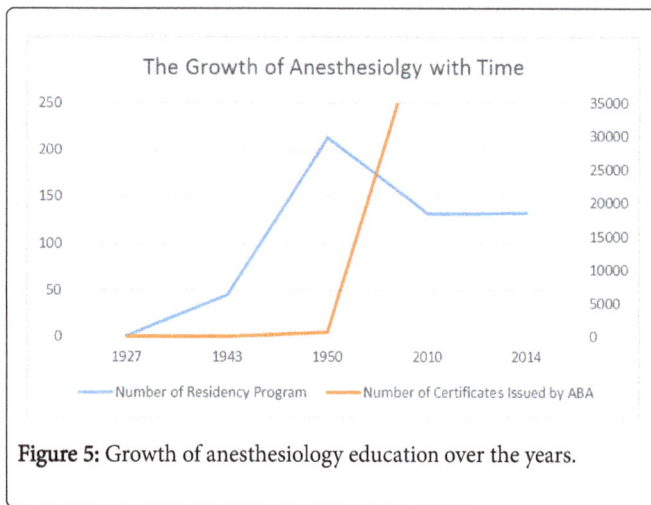

Figure 5: Growth of anesthesiology education over the years.

The process began slowly in the first year, when only 9 physicians were certified. Slowly gaining momentum, 272 anesthesiologists had been accredited by the end of World War II (Figure 5). Initially the Certificate was issued time indefinitely, but starting 2000 the candidates would be certified for a period of 10 years requiring re certification at the end of this period (Table 4).

Year	Number of Cumulative Certificates Issued by ABA
1939	9
1940	105
1950	706
1955	1,324
2015	>50,000

Table 4: Total number of certificates awarded by ABA [24,32].

Founders	Professors and Associate Professors previously elected to Fellowship in the ASA were to be certified without examination.
Group A	Those having practiced for 15 or more years were to appear before the Board and could be certified without examination.
Group B	Those practicing for 7.5 years or more or having administered anesthesia in at least 1500 major procedures could be certified following only an oral examination.
Group C	Those who met the 5 "criteria for entering the examination process" listed above and submitted 150 of their cases for evaluation were allowed to enter the full examination system.

Table 5: Categories for the first candidates for certification [33].

The Contribution of World War II to the Anesthesiology Education

World War II changed the course of American medicine significantly. The residency programs were depleted to meet the need of medical personnel of the U.S armed forces [9]. It was necessary to train more anesthetists (Medical anesthetists was the term used in early part of the 20th century for physicians whose primary responsibility was administration of anesthetics) to meet the war time need. A 12-week course was developed to train military physicians at academic institutions across the country. In addition, U.S. Surgeon General mandated all Army officers to take a 2-week course in Surgery and anesthesia, formerly only required of medical officers [31]. Ralph Tovell [34] (Chair of Anesthesiology, Hartford Hospital), was given the task to overlook this Anesthesiology training. Medical Officers, the so-called "90 day wonders" were taught anesthesia in a 12-week course at leading anesthesia departments such as those at Bellevue Hospital, Mayo Clinic, Hahnemann Medical College, and the University of Wisconsin General Hospital [35]. Recommended textbooks included Beecher's Physiology of Anesthesia (1938), Lundy's Clinical Anesthesia (1942), Gillespie's Endotracheal Anesthesia (1941), and Guedel's Inhalation Anesthesia (1937) and Fundamentals of Anesthesia (1942) which was regarded as "Bible for Physician-Anesthetists" at that time [36]. In Great Britain as opposed to the U.S., anesthesia was developed as a physician specialty and was comparatively more developed. This pioneer group of wartime anesthesiologists gained valuable skills and knowledge from their service in European theater of operations. These physician anesthetists proved their competency in the wartime and this led to a greater respect for anesthesia as a profession and it became apparent that this is a field that is more suited for physicians [37]. These veteran anesthesiologists brought back sophisticated Intravenous and regional anesthetics skills. After the war many of these veterans developed an interest in anesthesia and sought more thorough instructions in anesthesia. Many of these "90 day graduates" subsequently joined ASA and/or ABA [38]. Among the trainees was Virgil K. Stoelting, who would go on to become the first chair of anesthesiology at Indiana University. Anesthesiologists nationwide called for a movement to establish independent anesthesiology departments at academic institutions.

This led to creation of Association of University Anesthesiologists (AUA) with aim of promoting free and informal interchange of ideas, development of anesthesia teaching and research. Emeul Papper served as the first president and AUA, whose first meeting took place in Philadelphia, attended by the founding group of eight [39].

Post-World War Years and the Structuring of Graduate Medical Education

In 1955, the ABA required all the applicants to dedicate five years exclusively to the practice of anesthesiology. Also, the applicants were required to submit "case history abstracts of personally conducted anesthesia procedures" to ABA, a predecessor to the online case log system existing today. In addition to the written and oral exam, the ABA also incorporated the "survey exam", in which the applicants were observed in their own practice. The application fee for examination at that time was 125 US$ [32].

The Residency Review Committee (RRC) in Anesthesiology was formed in 1957, with members from both the ABA and American Medical Association. Initially the anesthesiology residency was 2 years but beginning in 1962 the RRC allowed programs to offer a 4-year course, with the extra year spent doing sub-specialty training or doing research. In 1964 ACGME adopted a more standardized approach to the number of years and recommended three-year residency [40]. During the same year doctors of osteopathic medicine were also deemed eligible for ABA certification [40].

In 1966 Citizen's Commission appointed by AMA found serious inadequacies in the current system of graduate medical education (GME) [41]. The commission noted an ineffectiveness of existing institutions of GME and persistence of apprenticeship in training. Citizen's Commission report can be regarded as a significant step forward in development of graduate medical education in general which also naturally effected anesthesiology residency programs. This report led to the formation of the Liaison Committee on Graduate Medical Education (LCGME) in 1972 as a result of collaboration between five concerned authorities namely; AMA, the ABMS, the American Hospital Association, the Association of American Medical Colleges, and the Council on Medical Specialty Societies. The mission of LCGME (later renamed as ACGME in 1981) was to improve healthcare by assessing and advancing the quality of resident physicians 'education through accreditation.

In the late 1970s' and early 1980s' LCGME extensively organized and laid out clear structural framework for anesthesiology residency programs. LCGME emphasized program structure, the amount and quality of formal teaching and promoted a balance between service and education. LCGME achieved this mandate by defining minimum requirements for anesthesiology programs, which became increasingly specific over the coming years. In 1980 the LCGME defined intern year for anesthesiology as the clinical base year which could be spent training in medicine, surgery, neurology, pediatrics or any combination of these with the approval of program director preferably at the same institution as the parent institution [42]. LCGME also recommended the curriculum for post graduate year 2 to 4 (termed as CA1- CA3), suggesting that at least one of the 24 months in CA1-CA2 be dedicated to "recovery room or specialized care unit". Over the recent years ACGME has recommended increased rotation in ICU, as well as mandatory rotation in Pain service. In 1993 [43] ACGME set criteria for the appointment of program director to anesthesiology residency program. ACGME also made recommendations for the qualifications of the faculty, ratio of faculty to number of residents, scholarly activity and resident record maintenance.

1980's was a transformative period for anesthesiology education. In addition to the structural reorganization of anesthesiology by ACGME, ABA also refined its examination process in order to reduce the variability in examination process [33]. During the same time, the Society for Education in Anesthesia (SEA) was formed with an aim of promotion of education in anesthesiology. Over the years, eventually these guidelines and efforts from ACGME, ABA, and anesthesiology societies transformed anesthesiology residency from the rather unstructured model of the past to the well-controlled learning environment of today.

The 80 Hour Work Week Restrictions

Following the death of Libby Zion, purported to be secondary to medical error caused by resident fatigue; Bell Commission recommended an 80 h per week restriction on resident duty hour in 1987. Progress however was slow and the 80 h per week was not officially adopted by ACGME until 2003. As a result of the 80 h work week restriction residents now spend approximately 15,000 h in training compared to 30,000 h before. It is imperative that the sophisticated training techniques should be incorporated into residents training in order to produce well trained anesthesiologist [44]. Interestingly however, Stedman noticed that at Ochsner anesthesiology residency program the work hour restriction caused no loss in total caseload (number of anesthetics administered per resident per year in 2006 was 411 vs. 304 in 1990). He attributed this to the increased OR efficiency and the increased number of cases residents performs in the newly formed regional anesthesia rotation [22].

The ACGME 80 h anesthesia resident work week did cause significant financial implication for Institutions which were used to having inexpensive labor in the form of anesthesia residents. Backeris et al. calculated the cost to replace residents with CRNA was between $236,000 to $581,876, assuming a 50 h resident work week, and $373,400 to $931,001, assuming an 80 h resident work week [45].

The Inoculation of Research in Anesthesia Education

One of the distinctions of an anesthesiologist from their nursing counterparts is the contribution they make to the development of the specialty by continuously trying to improve practice based on evidence. ACGME requires the faculty to create an environment of inquiry and for the programs to provide mechanisms and resources for the residents to conduct research and scholarly activity. There is constant emphasis on participation of the residents in scholarly activity. Residents are expected to learn skills to critically appraise the literature for its validity for future practice. There is however, a concern that there is not enough contribution to research in anesthesiology as compared to some of the peer specialties. Schwinn et al. [46] reported that while anesthesiologist make up 6% of the work force but they only received about 1% of NIH funding. There is a need to train more physician scientists. Incorporating research curriculum into resident education can help them be more academically productive [47-49]. A survey by Ahmad et al. showed that thirty-two percent of programs had a structured resident research education program. While the ACGME places a great deal of emphasis on the importance of research training in a residents' education, it seems that progress is slow in this aspect as well. It would probably require a change in the culture of academic anesthesiology to ensure the mandatory enhancement of resident research education [50]. Sakai et al. [51] observed how the implementation of research didactics including research lectures, research problem based learning discussions, and an elective research rotation translated into greater resident research involvement and publications. Similarly, Freundlich at al. [52] described how a month long research month proved to be a successful educational intervention at University of Michigan anesthesiology residency program. Recently as many as 35/131 (23%) of the approved ACGME residency programs have started offering a dedicated research track [53]. It seems likely that in coming years, anesthesiology departments will continue to devote more time and resources to ensure that anesthesiology residents are well trained in the research methodology; so they can continue to contribute to development of anesthesiology as a profession.

ACGME Core Competencies and Outcome Project

The traditional model of assessment in anesthesiology has been global clinical evaluation and standardized testing. There is a general notion that performance on standardized examinations can be used to predict clinical performance however this claim was not substantiated in any study and there was no direct correlation with actual clinical performance and standardized clinical measures for the same resident [54]. There has been a gradual evolution in anesthesiology education to nontraditional assessment methods that stimulate learning including self-assessment, peer review and simulation based learning.

Over the years the training model transformed from the traditional model to an outcome based model with focuses on learning and teaching of six core competencies [55,56]. These competencies as defined by ACGME are [57]:

1. **Patient Care:** that is compassionate, appropriate, and effective for treating health problems and promoting health;

2. **Medical Knowledge:** about established and evolving biomedical, clinical, and cognate (e.g., epidemiological and social-behavioral) sciences and the application of this knowledge to patient care;

3. **Practice-Based Learning and Improvement:** that involves investigation and evaluation of their own patient care, appraisal, and assimilation of scientific evidence, and improvements in patient care;

4. **Interpersonal and Communication Skills:** that result in effective information exchange and teaming with patients, their families, and other health professionals;

5. **Professionalism:** as manifested through a commitment to carrying out professional responsibilities, adherence to ethical principles, and sensitivity to a diverse patient population;

6. **Systems-Based Practice:** as manifested by actions that demonstrate an awareness of and responsiveness to the larger context and system of health care and the ability to effectively call on system resources to provide care that is of optimal value.

These six core competencies were introduced by ACGME in 1999 and gradually integrated into the residency curriculum in the 2000's. Schwengel et al. [58] described how they introduced Systems-Based Practice (SBP) and Practice-Based Learning and Improvement (PBLI) at John Hopkins Anesthesiology Residency Program. The CA-1 residents participate in a curriculum composed of lectures, interactive sessions and exercises designed to develop conceptual understanding of a wide range of topics, including fundamentals of safety and safe design, how to critically evaluate the literature and how to investigate defects. In the CA 2 and CA 3 years, residents work on an SBP improvement project.

The results of ACGME restructuring gradually became apparent. Variability in the quality of anesthesiology resident education decreased around the country. However, these ACGME minimum program requirements for anesthesiology curtailed the programs from innovation and added administrative burden to the program [59]. The National Interest in patient safety and outcomes measure lead ACGME to come up with The Outcome Project which mandated that residency programs teach six core competencies, create reliable tools to assess learning of the competencies, and use the data for program improvement. In 2014, ACGME implemented Next Accreditation System (NAS) for anesthesiology a program in which accreditation was to be based on educational outcomes in these competencies. It has been suggested that the New Accreditation System will allow better programs to innovate while allowing struggling programs to improve; all while decreasing the amount of administrative work done by the program director [60].

A key element of the NAS is the measurement and reporting of outcomes through the educational milestones. As the ACGME is moving toward continuous accreditation outcomes-based milestones which are specific for anesthesiology, are used for determining resident and fellow performance within the six ACGME Core Competencies [61]. These milestones result from a close collaboration among the ABA, the review committees, medical- specialty organizations, program-director associations, and residents.

The Development of Subspecialty Anesthesia

During 1960's interest increased in research and in sub-specialty anesthesiology training. A small number of anesthesiologists mostly at the larger academic centers would spend time focusing on, and doing research on particular cohort of patients. All these factors lead to advancements in knowledge of physiology and pharmacology with introduction of drugs such as fentanyl and ketamine. Similarly considerable scientific progress was made in critical care and the pediatric anesthesia. In 1959 Peter Safar established first multidisciplinary adult and pediatric ICU in the US at Baltimore City Hospital. In 1967 John Downes and Leonard Bachman established the first pediatric Intensive Care Unit (PICU) in US at Children's Hospital of Philadelphia [62].

Keeping up the development in subspecialty Anesthesiology, ABA mandated subspecialty rotations starting in 1980. In 1985 ABA began to issue certificate in Critical Care. In 1991 Pain Management (renamed Pain Medicine in 2002) was recognized as a subspecialty by ABA. And most recently in 2012 ABA approved an additional time-limited pediatric anesthesiology certificate. Currently the ACGME requires all residents to have a specified minimum recommended amount of subspecialty anesthesia rotations.

Combined Anesthesia Residencies

In 2009 American Board of Pediatrics and ABA announced combined training in pediatrics and anesthesiology. This program requires five, rather than six, years of training and allows physicians to be fully qualified and certified in both specialties [63]. As of 2014, there are 7 combined Anesthesiology/Pediatrics program training about 22 residents (FREIDA Online specialty training [https://freida.ama-assn.org/]). Interest in combined pediatrics-anesthesia training is growing among applicants [64].

The American Board of Internal Medicine (ABIM) and the ABA began a combined training program in Internal medicine and Anesthesiology in January 2012. As of 2016, there are 5 approved programs for combined residency training in Internal medicine and Anesthesiology [65].

Future of Anesthesiology Education-A Blended Educational Model

The advents in information technology in the past decades have also impacted anesthesiology education. Simulation has become an integral part of residency training. Simulation allows residents to experience clinical scenarios that are infrequent in daily practice, but critical to anesthesia practice such as anaphylaxis, airway fire or the use of bronchial blockers and double-lumen endotracheal tubes (ETT) for single lung isolation [66]. As of 2014 ACGME requires at least one simulation training session for residents every year.

With the 80 h work limit, educators are hard pressed to make anesthesiology training as enriching as possible. Educators are trying to find new and innovative ways to introduce technology in anesthesia education. Tanaka et al. [67] showed how the use of an iPad® in a two week anesthesiology rotation at Stanford University objectively increased residents' perception of overall teaching quality of the rotation. Educators are trying to shift to a blended educational model with podcasts, videos, online quizzes and other online educational modalities [68]. This has been somewhat difficult to achieve owing to the intrinsic nature of anesthesiology which requires face to face and hands-on training. There have been varying results on usefulness of different modalities and the effectiveness of these tools depends more on the learning style of the resident. However, it seems likely that with coming time anesthesiology training will evolve to utilize and incorporate more technological advances such as simulation training and e-learning. In conclusion, it is remarkable to see how a specialty that had its humble origins in a self-taught and practiced unstructured training has evolved into this well-planned and regulated educational system producing highly competent physicians that have been trained in all the domains that will help them succeed in providing high quality patient care as well as advance this discipline in the future.

References

1. Rushman GB, Davies NJH, Atkinson RS (1996) A Short History of Anaesthesia: The First 150 Years. Butterworth-Heinemann.

2. Bacon DR, Ament R (1995) Ralph Waters and the beginnings of academic anesthesiology in the United States: the Wisconsin Template. J Clin Anesth 7: 534–543.

3. Gwathmey JT (1914) Anesthesia. Appleton 1st ed.

4. Gwathmey JT (1913) The American Association of Anaesthetists. Ann Surg 58: 865–876.

5. Editorial Foreword (1922) Anesth Analg 1: 1.

6. Eckenhoff J (1966) Anesthesia from colonial times a history of anesthesia at the University of Pennsylvania. Montreal: Lippincott.

7. Herb IC (1911) Administration of General Anesthetics With Special Reference To Ether and Chloroform. JAMA J Am Med Assoc LVI: 1312–1315.

8. WD G (1911) Instructions of medical students and Hospital interns in Anesthesia. Am J Surg 30: 98–99.

9. ROVENSTINE EA, PAPPER EM (1947) Graduate education in anesthesiology. J Am Med Assoc 134: 1279–1283.

10. Strickland RA (1995) Isabella Coler Herb an early leader in anesthesiology. Anesth Analg 80: 600–605.

11. Herb IC (1921) Anesthesia in relation to medical schools and hospitals. Am J Surg 50–51.

12. Rao VS, Schroeder ME, Sim PP, Morris DC, Morris LE (2011) The University of Oklahoma: The First Independent Academic Anesthesia Department? Bull Anesth Hist 29: 40–48.

13. Wang B, Orkin CL, Sutin KM, Blanck, Thomas JJ (2003) The Contribution of Doctor Emory A. Rovenstine to Anesthesiology. Anesthesiology 99: A1271.

14. Morris LE, Ralph M (2001) Waters' Legacy: The Establishment of Academic Anesthesia Centers by the "Aqualumni." American Society of Anesthesiologists Newsletter. 21–24.

15. Steinhaus JE, Perry P, Volpitto (1999) The South's First Academic Anesthesiologist. Bull Anesth Hist 17: 1–8.

16. Bacon DR, Vachon CA (2002) Perry P Volpitto: Bringing the Waters Tradition South. Anesthesiology 96: A1161.

17. Bause GS (2011) The End of the Road for "Huron Road." J Am Soc Anesthesiol 115: 1062.

18. Steinhaus JE (1999) Perry P Volpitto, M.D. The South's First Academic Anesthesiologist. Bull Anesth Hist 17: 1–8.

19. Hamilton WK, Larson CP (1980) Stuart C. Cullen 1909-1979. Anesthesiology 52: 111–112.

20. Gravenstein JS (1998) Henry K. Beecher: The Introduction of Anesthesia into the University. Anesthesiology 88: 245–253.

21. Mizrahi I, Desai SP (2015) Establishment of the Department of Anaesthesia at Harvard Medical School-1969. J Clin Anesth 28: 47–55.

22. Stedman RB (2011) Core program education: tracking the progression toward excellence in an anesthesiology residency program over 60 years. Ochsner J 11: 43–51.

23. Approved Internships and Residencies in the United States 1949. J Am Med Assoc 140: 157–230.

24. Pardo M The Development of Education in Anesthesia in the United States. The Wondrous Story of Anesthesia pp: 483–496.

25. Lundy JS (1936) Intravenous anesthesia. Am J Surg 34: 559–570.

26. Joseph Rupreht, Lieburg MJV, Lee JA, W Erdmann (2012) Anaesthesia: Essays on Its History. pp: 42–44.

27. Nelson CW, Dr John S (1999) Lundy and the 75th anniversary of anesthesiology at Mayo. Mayo Clin Proc 1999. 74: 650.

28. Ellis TA, Narr BJ, Bacon DR (2004) Developing a specialty: J.S. Lundy's three major contributions to anesthesiology. J Clin Anesth 16: 226–229.

29. Lennon R, Lennon RL, Bacon DR (2009) The Anaesthetists' Travel Club: an example of professionalism. J Clin Anesth 21: 137–142.

30. Bacon DR, John S, Lundy, Ralph Waters, Paul Wood (1995) The founding of the American Board of Anesthesiology. Bull Anesth Hist 13: 1–5.

31. Rosenberg H, Axelrod JK (1993) Henry Ruth: pioneer of modern anesthesiology. Anesthesiology 78: 178–183.

32. Directory of Approved Internships and Residencies (1955). J Am Med Assoc 159: 251–377.

33. Eger II EI, Saidman LJ, Westhorpe RN (2014) The Wondrous Story of Anesthesia.

34. Little DM (1967) Ralph Moore Tovell 1901-1967. Anesthesiology 28: 307–308.

35. Parks CL, Schroeder ME (2013) Military anesthesia trainees in WWII at the University of Wisconsin: their training, careers, and contributions. Anesthesiology 118: 1019-1027.

36. Waisel DB (2001) The role of World War II and the European theater of operations in the development of anesthesiology as a physician specialty in the USA. Anesthesiology 94: 907-914.

37. Ruth HS (1945) Postwar Planning in Anesthesiology. J Am Soc Anesthesiol 6: 316-317.

38. Martin DP, Burkle CM, McGlinch BP, Warner ME, Sessler AD, et al. (2006) The Mayo Clinic World War II Short Course and Its Effect on Anesthesiology. J Am Soc Anesthesiol 105: 209-213.

39. Papper EM (1992) The origins of the Association of University Anesthesiologists. Anesth Analg 74: 436-453.

40. Directory of Approved Internships and Residencies 1964- Annual Report On Graduate Medical Education In The United States.

41. The graduate education of physicians: the report of the Citizens Commission on Graduate Medical Education: commissioned by the American Medical Association. Chicago: Council on Medical Education. American Medical Association 1966.

42. 1980/1981 Directory of Residency Training Programs ACCREDITED BY THE LIAISON COMMITTEE ON GRADUATE MEDICAL EDUCATION. Chicago, Illinois Available.

43. 1993-1994 Graduate Medical Education Directory-Accreditation Council for Graduate Medical Education. Chicago, Illinois: American Medical Association.

44. Ramsay M (2007) The new generation of graduating anesthesia residents: what is the impact on a major tertiary referral private practice medical center? Curr Opin Anaesthesiol 20: 568-571.

45. Backeris ME, Forte PJ, Beaman ST, Metro DG (2013) Financial Implications of Different Interpretations of ACGME Anesthesiology Program Requirements for Rotations in the Operating Room. J Grad Med Educ 5: 315-319.

46. Schwinn DA, Balser JR (2006) Anesthesiology physician scientists in academic medicine: a wake-up call. Anesthesiology 104: 170-178.

47. Moharari RS, Rahimi E, Najafi A, Khashayar P, Khajavi MR (2009) Teaching critical appraisal and statistics in anesthesia journal club. QJM 102: 139-141.

48. Mills LS, Steiner AZ, Rodman AM, Donnell CL, Steiner MJ (2011) Trainee participation in an annual research day is associated with future publications. Teach Learn Med 23: 62-67.

49. Vinci RJ, Bauchner H, Finkelstein J, Newby PK, Muret-Wagstaff S, et al. (2009) Research during pediatric residency training: outcome of a senior resident block rotation. Pediatrics 124: 1126-1134.

50. Ahmad S, Oliveira GS De, McCarthy RJ (2013) Status of anesthesiology resident research education in the United States: structured education programs increase resident research productivity. Anesth Analg 116: 205-210.

51. Sakai T, Emerick TD, Metro DG, Patel RM, Hirsch SC, et al. (2014) Facilitation of resident scholarly activity: strategy and outcome analyses using historical resident cohorts and a rank-to-match population. Anesthesiology 120: 111-119.

52. Freundlich RE, Newman JW, Tremper KK, Mhyre JM, Kheterpal S, et al. (2015) The impact of a dedicated research education month for anesthesiology residents. Anesthesiol Res Pract 2015: 623959.

53. Nagle PC (2011) Improving outcomes in anaesthesiology education on research. Best Pract Res Clin Anaesthesiol 25: 511-522.

54. Ferland JJ, Dorval J, Levasseur L (1987) Measuring higher cognitive levels by multiple choice questions: a myth? Med Educ 21: 109-113.

55. Mainiero MB, Lourenco AP (2011) The ACGME core competencies: changing the way we educate and evaluate residents. Med Health R I 94: 164-166.

56. Stephens MB (2010) ACGME core competencies: Who knows what and does it matter? Fam Med 42 :574.

57. Kavic MS (2002) Competency and the six core competencies. JSLS 6: 95-97.

58. Schwengel DA, Winters BD, Berkow LC, Mark L, Heitmiller ES, et al. (2011) A novel approach to implementation of quality and safety programmes in anaesthesiology. Best Pract Res Clin Anaesthesiol 25: 557-567.

59. Oliveira GS De, Almeida MD, Ahmad S, Fitzgerald PC, McCarthy RJ (2011) Anesthesiology residency program director burnout. J Clin Anesth 23: 176-182.

60. Nasca TJ, Philibert I, Brigham T, Flynn TC (2012) The next GME accreditation system-rationale and benefits. N Engl J Med 366: 1051-1056.

61. ACGME Anesthesiology Milestones (2015) The Accreditation Council for Graduate Medical Education and The American Board of Anesthesiology.

62. Mai CL, Coté CJ (2012) A history of pediatric anesthesia: a tale of pioneers and equipment. Paediatr Anaesth 22: 511-520.

63. Pediatrics-Anesthesiology Program (2009) The American Board of Pediatrics.

64. Sanford EL (2013) Pediatrics-anesthesia combined residency training: an applicant's perspective. Anesth Analg 116:1386-1388.

65. Internal Medicine & Anesthesiology. The American Board of Anesthesiology.

66. Lim G, McIvor WR (2015) Simulation-based Anesthesiology Education for Medical Students. Int Anesthesiol Clin 53: 1-22.

67. Tanaka PP, Hawrylyshyn KA, Macario A (2012) Use of tablet (iPad®) as a tool for teaching anesthesiology in an orthopedic rotation. Rev Bras Anestesiol 62: 214-222.

68. Kannan J, Kurup V (2012) Blended learning in anesthesia education: current state and future model. Curr Opin Anaesthesiol 25: 692-698.

29

Optimal Timing for the Initiation of Enteral Feeding in Neonates with Gastroschisis, Depending on Non-Invasive Doppler Ultrasound Evaluation of Hemodynamics in the Bowel Wall Arteries

OV Teplyakova[1*], EA Filippova[2], YL Podurovskaya[2], AV Pyregov[2], VV Zubkov[2], AA Burov[2], EI Dorofeeva[2] and MI Pykov[3]

[1]*Resuscitation and Intensive Care Department, Research Centre for Obstetrics, Gynecology and Perinatology, Ministry of Health of the Russian Federation, Moscow, Russia*

[2]*Research Centre of Obstetrics, Gynaecology, and Perinatology, Named after Academician V.I. Kulakov, Ministry of Health of the Russian Federation (MOH), Moscow, Russia*

[3]*Russian Medical Academy of Postgraduate Education, MOH, Moscow, Russia*

[*]**Corresponding author:** Teplyakova OV, Surgery, Resuscitation and Intensive Care Department, Research Centre for Obstetrics, Gynecology and Perinatology, Ministry of Health of the Russian Federation, 117997, Moscow, Russia, E-mail: olga.v.teplyakova@gmail.com

Abstract

Purpose: The objective of the study is to assess the clinical relevance of ultrasonography evaluation of hemodynamics in the bowel wall arteries for determining the optimal time of the initiation of enteral feeding in neonates with gastroschisis.

Patients and methods: The sample consisted of 28 newborns with gastroschisis. Doppler ultrasonography was used to evaluate hemodynamic patterns in the bowel wall arteries in the pre- and postop periods to determine the optimal time for the initiation of enteral nutrition. Swelling of the bowel wall and indefinite differentiation into layers were observed during the first 2-3 days upon gastroschisis surgery. The blood flow in the intestinal wall arteries was varying in different quadrants, demonstrating a mosaic pattern. Hyperemia, i.e. a dramatic blood flow increase, was documented. The peripheral resistance dropped with RI equal to 0.49-0.54, but there were also areas with definite RI increases up to 0.85. By days 5-6 of life, the intestinal wall still remained moderately thickened. The resistive index (RI) values for the intestinal wall arteries were approaching the norm, ranging from 0.58 to 0.72. By days 7-9 after birth, the bowel loops remained slightly thickened, but already gained a clear differentiation into layers. The peripheral resistance indices were within the normal limits, ranging from 0.62 to 0.67.

Results: In our study RI values based on Doppler evaluation of the intestinal wall hemodynamics were within 0.62-0.67.

Conclusions: The hemodynamic parameters were consistent with clinical characteristics of the normal passage of food through the digestive tract. Thus, a physician can rely on both clinical signs and ultrasonography data while monitoring the bowel function during pre- and postoperative periods to decide on the optimal time for the initiation of enteral feeding.

Keywords: Gastroschisis; Ultrasonography; Hemodynamics in the bowel wall arteries; Resistive index

Abbreviations and Acronyms: RI: Resistive Index.

Introduction

Gastroschisis is a malformation of the anterior abdominal wall with abdominal organs freely protruding due to a periomphalic full-thickness soft tissue defect (Figure 1). The number of newborns with gastroschisis is increasingly growing worldwide, varying from 1 per 1,500 to 1 per 5,000 live births.

Surgical correction techniques are robust and reliable, but perioperative management of gastroschisis cases remains challenging. Gastroschisis accounts for a large share of all surgically correctable congenital defects in neonatal surgery (Figure 2).

The objective of this study is to assess the relevance of ultrasound evaluation of microhemodynamics in the small bowel wall arteries for optimizing the time for the initiation of enteral nutrition in neonates with gastroschisis.

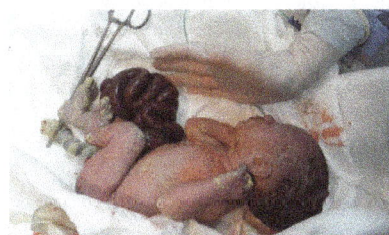

Figure 1: Newborn baby with gastroschisis.

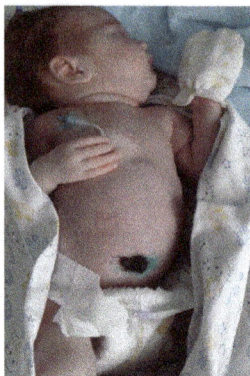

Figure 2: Newborn baby with gastroschisis at the age of 9 days

Background

According to available research data, gastroschisis is the most common congenital ventral wall defect [1-4]. Its average incidence of 1 per 5,000 live births increases 3-fold in young mothers aged less than 20 years: up to 1 case per 1,500 live births [5-8]. According to Castilla et al. in Mexico, its prevalence is higher than in Slovakia, and it tends to be higher in warm climates [8]. The number of newborns with gastroschisis is increasing worldwide [7-12], and gastroschisis accounts for a great share of all surgically correctable congenital defects in neonatal surgery.

Wide use of prenatal ultrasonography enables to detect or suspect fetal gastroschisis starting from 12-17 weeks of gestation. Several studies showed quite high accuracy of prenatal ultrasonography diagnosis of gastroschisis, reaching 90% [12-15]. However, despite early prenatal detection and preparedness of health personnel to handle such cases, the mortality among neonates with gastroschisis varies between 6.5% and 45% in some African and European countries, and reaches up to 95% in some regions, while in the world's reference hospitals, the mortality does not exceed 3-10% [8,16-24].

The greatest reduction in the mortality of neonates with gastroschisis is seen when surgical correction is provided in the same health facilities, i.e. in the maternity hospitals, without transportation to other health centres.

Gastroschisis case management is a challenge for neonatology, including neonatal surgery, resuscitation and intensive care. The growing gastrischisis rates have prompted the development of reliable and effective surgical correction techniques. Meanwhile, there is no uniform treatment protocol for newborns with gastroschisis in the perioperative period [25-27]. Specific challenges exist in pre-op management. In the post-op period, the most important task is to identify the optimal time for the initiation of enteral feeding.

Methods

Patient selection

This study included 28 children with diagnosed gastroschisis, admitted from December 2011 to June 2015 to the Surgical Intensive Care Department of the Research Centre of Obstetrics, Gynecology and Perinatology under the Ministry of Health of the Russian Federation. This number of patients reflects our hospital specialization in the treatment of children with gastroschisis. Pregnant women with prenatally diagnosed gastroschisis of fetus were admitted to our Center from all over Russia. All the children were diagnosed as gastroschisis cases prenatally at 13-14 weeks of gestation and were born through operative delivery. The Apgar score was 6.7 ± 1.3 points at 1 minute and 7.7 ± 1.3 points at 5 minutes. The sample included 15 boys and 13 girls. The gestational age was 37.5 ± 2.2 weeks. Their mean birth weight and length were 2,735 ± 137 g and 48.2 ± 2.3 cm respectively.

The following exclusion criteria were used in this study: Presence of such co-morbidities as intestinal atresia, sepsis, severe birth asphyxia, intraventricular hemorrhage of grade 3-4, or preceding mechanical ventilation, or preceding secondary plastic of the anterior abdominal wall due to the presence of abdomino-visceral disproportion. In all the cases, the parents gave their prior informed consent for ultrasonography examination of the neonates.

Clinical tests and examinations

All the neonates were subjected to thorough clinical and laboratory examinations and tests, including physical examination, monitoring of vital signs, blood count, urinalysis, blood chemistry, coagulation panel, ultrasonography examination of the abdominal cavity and retroperitoneal space.

Siemens ACUSON S2000 (Siemens, Germany, USA) with a 7-14 MHz linear transducer was used for ultrasound examinations. To measure intestinal loops and such parameters as the diameter of the bowel, wall thickness, wall differentiation into layers, presence of peristalsis, intraluminal content and free fluid in the inter-loops spaces, the gray-scale B-mode was used. Color Doppler flow imaging & mapping and pulsed wave Doppler were used for the evaluation of the bowel wall vessels. Maximum systolic velocity, blood flow volume (BFV) and resistive index (RI) were calculated based on the Doppler curve from the bowel wall vessels, vessels of mesenteric root and superior mesenteric artery.

No specific pharmaceuticals were used to prepare patients for ultrasonography examinations. All the neonates were breathing spontaneously after birth. The daily volume of preoperative infusion therapy was 150 ml/kg. A standard anesthesia (general intravenous anesthesia) was used during the surgery; surgical correction was provided within the first 3-4 h after birth in all the neonates. Parenteral nutrition was initiated on the first post-operative day and was followed with its expansion to the total parenteral nutrition (TPN) on post-operative days 4-5. Decompression of the stomach through a nasogastric tube on average lasted for 7 ± 1.3 days after surgery; the gastric volume reached 52 ± 6.2 ml per day. We do not use X-rays in children with gastroschisis because of its low informativeness to make a decision about the beginning of enteral feeding.

Results and Discussion

All the neonates with gastroschisis had incomplete intestinal rotation due to missing typical phases of intestinal rotation and fixation during the prenatal development, occurring outside the abdominal cavity of the fetus, as well as due to the absence of ligament of Treitz's, when the intestine and colon have a common mesentery on a narrow basis.

The malrotation is usually aggravated by compromised blood supply due to impaired vascular anatomy. In a healthy neonate, the superior mesenteric artery (SMA) forms a 40-50 degree angle with the abdominal aorta and travels in a straight-line manner (Figure 3). In gastroschisis cases, the SMA is not only tortuous, but arises from the abdominal aorta at an angle of 80-90 degrees (Figure 4). No doubt, such anatomical features impair the blood flow in the main trunk and in the branches, thus, habitual hemodynamic standards are not applicable to cases with abnormal vascular anatomy. Nevertheless, in gastroschisis cases, SMA hemodynamics was not significantly different from normal parameters, or significantly fluctuating-starting from the first hours of life and in the long-term, in contrast to hemodynamics in small arteries of the intestinal wall.

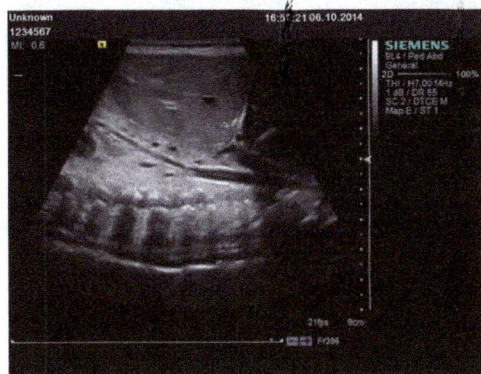

Figure 3: SMA trajectory echogram of a healthy neonate. Transabdominal examination, using a linear 14 MHz transducer. Longitudinal scanning detected the superior mesenteric artery, arising from the abdominal aorta in a typical locaton at 45-600 angle with a straight linear trajectory.

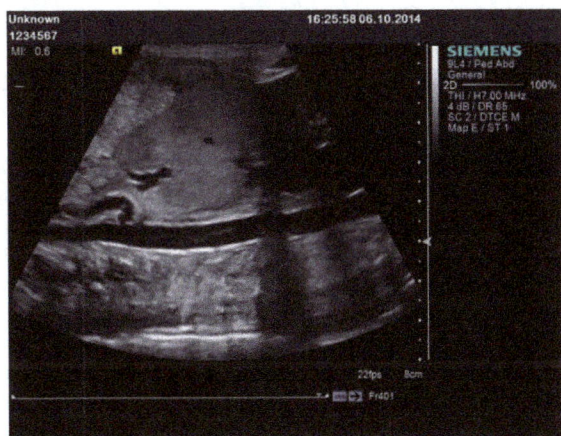

Figure 4: SMA trajectory echogram of a neonate with gastroschisis. In gastroschisis cases with incomplete intestinal rotation, longitudinal scanning detected higher origination of the superior mesenteric artery from the abdominal aorta at 80-900 angles with a coiled course.

Attempts to assess intra-op bowel wall micro-hemodynamics are reported in adult population and adolescents after failures with trans-abdominal approaches [28,29]. In addition, such measurements usually require using a contrast substance (dye), which is unacceptable in

neonatal practice [30-32]. In all reported studies, the authors evaluated the vascular reserve of large vessels, regretting that a direct assessment of small arteries was not possible without the use of a contrast medium [33,34]. Available publications also provide some information about dopplerographic criteria for evaluation of the intestinal wall in children with Crohn's disease [35-37]. However, the above-mentioned abnormal behavior of SMA in gastroschisis cases and specifics of hemodynamic patterns in neonates male all published data inapplicable to the current study.

However, in neonates with gastroschisis and bowel paresis, both Trans and intra-abdominal examinations are feasible with due regard to the structural defects of the abdominal wall. Such examinations usually provide identical data with a minimal bias.

The early postoperative period provides the best acoustic environment for US B-mode examination and detailed dopplerographic assessment (Figure 5), when peristalsis is partially or totally suppressed, intestinal wall is thickened, intraluminal gas-if present-is found in minimal amounts and free fluid is seen in the abdominal cavity.

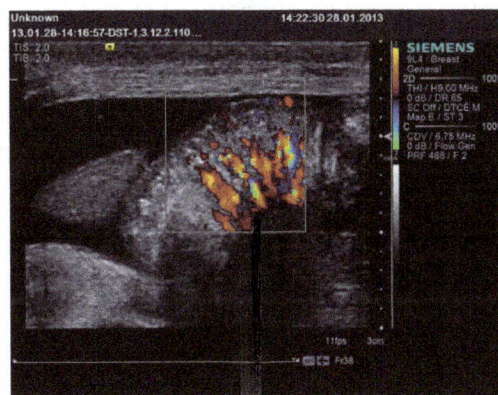

Figure 5: Echogram of the intestinal loop in a neonate with gastroschisis, day 2 postop. (B-mode, color Doppler mapping). Longitudinal linear B-mode scanning evaluates the peristalsis, diameter and intestinal wall thickness. Doppler imaging evaluates the blood flow patterns in the intestinal wall.

On the first 2-3 days after the operation, the bowel wall is swollen and thickened and differentiation into layers is unreadable in a newborn with gastroschisis. The bowel loops are deflated and sticking together or filled with a thick hypoechoic chyme and minor amount of intraluminal gas. The peristalsis is dramatically reduced or even not observed in some areas.

A considerable amount of free fluid is accumulated in all sloping areas of the abdominal cavity and in the inter-loop spaces. The blood flow in the intestinal wall is varying by quadrants, showing a mosaic pattern, and pronounced hyperemia (engorgement) of the bowel wall vessels.

The peripheral resistance parameters drop to 0.49 0.54 RI values, but there are also areas with noticeable RI increase up to 0.85 (Figure 6). At this stage, it is crucial to explore all segments of the bowel to ensure that no ischemic areas with a sharp decline or even absence of the blood flow should be missed.

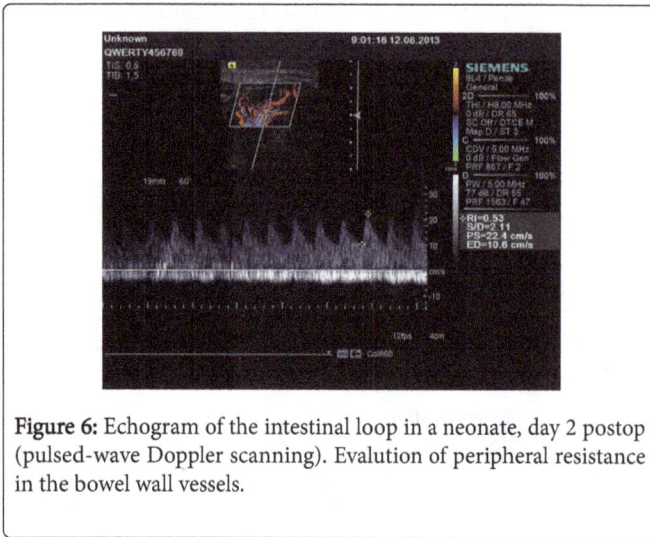

Figure 6: Echogram of the intestinal loop in a neonate, day 2 postop (pulsed-wave Doppler scanning). Evalution of peripheral resistance in the bowel wall vessels.

By days 5-6 after birth, the intestinal wall remains moderately thickened. The bowel loops look common, not distended. The intraluminal content is thick with moderate amount of gas.

Peristalsis is evident in all the segments. Small amounts of free fluid are still visible in the inter-loops spaces. The RI in bowel wall vessels is approaching the normal values, ranging between 0.58-0.72 (Figure 7).

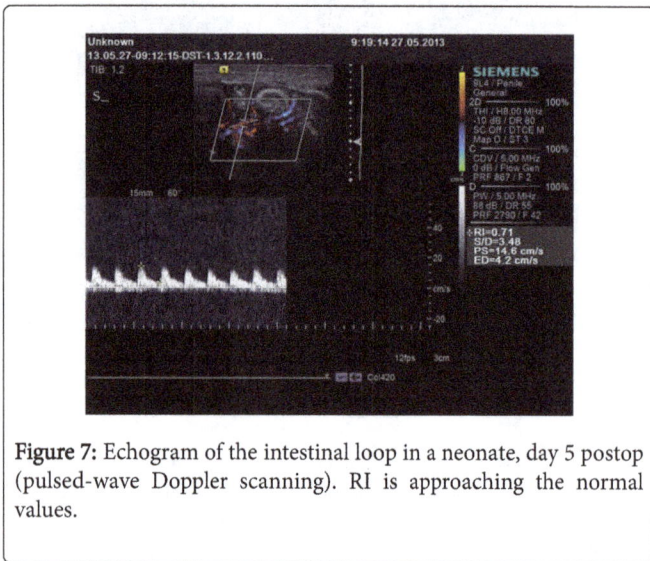

Figure 7: Echogram of the intestinal loop in a neonate, day 5 postop (pulsed-wave Doppler scanning). RI is approaching the normal values.

By days 7-9 after birth, the bowel loops are slightly thickened, with clear differentiation into layers. Peristalsis is present in all the segments.

The amount of intraluminal gas increased, interfering seriously with the assessment of the blood flow in the intestinal wall.

Traces of free liquid are seen in inter-loops spaces. Indicators of peripheral resistance are within normal ranges 0.62-0.67 (Figure 8) [37].

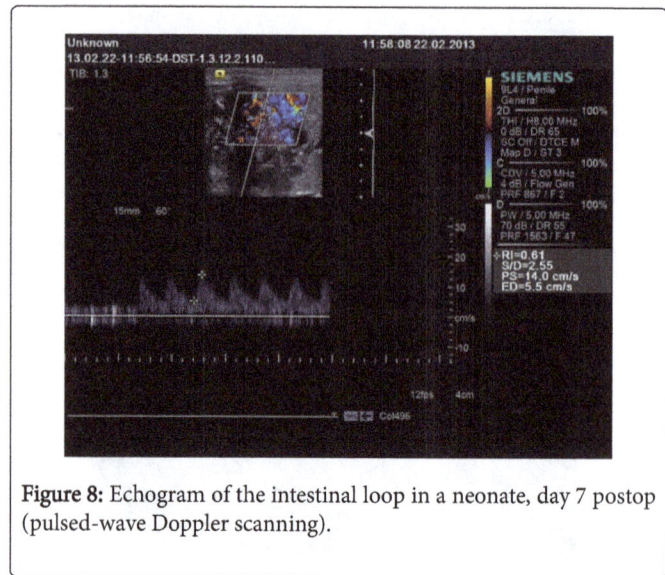

Figure 8: Echogram of the intestinal loop in a neonate, day 7 postop (pulsed-wave Doppler scanning).

Conclusions

Some issues remain unresolved in the nursing of newborns with gastroschisis despite the availability of well-established surgical correction techniques for this congenital malformation. Better outcomes are seen in settings where surgery is available in the maternity home, without the need to move the patient to another hospital, and with after-surgery monitoring provided before the patient is discharged.

Timely initiation of enteral nutrition is of great importance because favorable clinical outcomes and prospects for further adaptation of neonates with operated gastroschisis are largely dependent on adequate and timely enteral feeding.

The results of our study are consistent with reported data from Sjekavica et al. and Esteban et al. investigating the intestinal wall microhemodynamics in Crohn's disease [28,36,37]. The reported RI values based on Doppler evaluation of the intestinal wall hemodynamics during remission and in the control group were within 0.65-0.67 in these two studies. In our study, this range is somewhat broader: 0.62-0.67, which could be attributed to the functioning of such fetal communications in the neonatal period as the patent ductus arteriosus and ductus venosus Arantii. The results enable us to conclude that normalization of the intestinal wall blood flow should be viewed as the signal to initiate enteral feeding to avoid inappropriate burdens on the digestive tract. In our sample, enteral feeding was initiated in all the patients, on the average, in 8-9 days after surgery.

The hemodynamic parameters are consistent with the clinical characteristics, testifying to the normal passage of food through the digestive tract. Thus, a physician can rely on both clinical signs and ultrasonography data while monitoring the bowel function during pre- and postoperative periods to identify the optimal time for the initiation of enteral feeding.

Competing Interests

The authors declare that they have no competing interests.

Authors' Contributions

E.A. Filippova conceived the study and initiated its publication, performed abdominal ultrasonography and Doppler imaging in the neonates with gastroschisis at all the stages of the treatment, and provided pictures for the paper from her own archive.

O.V. Teplyakova and A.A. Burov were responsible for therapeutic management and stabilization of all the newborns with gastroschisis at the delivery room, for peri-op management and anesthetic support.

O.V. Teplyakova designed the study, coordinated it, and was responsible for statistical data processing and preparation of the text.

Yu.L. Podurovskaya and E.I. Dorofeeva provided the surgical treatment of the neonates with gastroschisis as well as nursing care upon completion of the intensive care. They participated in formatting the study design.

A.V. Pyregov led the work, supervised the study and revised the paper.

V.V. Zubkov led the work and supervised the study.

M.I. Pykov supervised the analysis.

All the authors read and approved the final version of the article.

References

1. Molik KA, Gingalewski CA, West KW, Rescorla FJ, Scherer LR, et al. (2001) Gastroschisis: a plea for risk categorization. J Pediatr Surg 36: 51-55.

2. Skarsgard E, Claydon J, Bouchard S, Kim PC, Lee SK, et al. (2008) Canadian Pediatric Surgical Network: a population-based pediatric surgery network and database for analyzing surgical birth defects. The first 100 cases of gastroschisis. J Pediatr Surg 43: 30-34.

3. Vu LT, Nobuhara KK, Laurent C, Shaw GM (2008) Increasing prevalence of gastroschisis: population-based study in California. J Pediatr 152: 807-811.

4. Keys C, Drewett M, Burge DM (2008) Gastroschisis: the cost of an epidemic. J Pediatr Surg 43: 654-657.

5. Baer RJ, Chambers CD, Jones KL, Shew SB, MacKenzie TC, et al. (2015) Maternal factors associated with the occurrence of gastroschisis. Am J Med Genet A 167: 1534-1541.

6. Loane M, Dolk H, Bradbury I, EUROCAT Working Group (2007) Increasing prevalence of gastroschisis in Europe 1980-2002: a phenomenon restricted to younger mothers? Paediatr Perinat Epidemiol 21: 363-369.

7. Grant NH, Dorling J, Thornton JG (2013) Elective preterm birth for fetal gastroschisis. Cochrane Database Syst Rev : CD009394.

8. Castilla E, Mastroiacovo P, Oriol IM (2008) Gastroschisis: international epidemiology and public health perspectives. Am J Med Genet C Semin Med Genet 148C: 162-179.

9. Tarca E, Ciongradi I, Aprodu SG (2015) Birth Weight, Compromised Bowel and Sepsis are the Main Variables Significantly Influencing Outcome in Gastroschisis. Chirurgia (Bucur) 110: 151-156.

10. Kilby MD (2006) The incidence of gastroschisis. BMJ 332: 250-251.

11. Di Tanna GL, Rosano A, Mastroiacovo P (2002) Prevalence of gastroschisis at birth: retrospective study. BMJ 325: 1389-1390.

12. Salihu HM1, Pierre-Louis BJ, Druschel CM, Kirby RS (2003) Omphalocele and gastroschisis in the State of New York, 1992-1999. Birth Defects Res A Clin Mol Teratol 67: 630-636.

13. Garne E, Loane M, Dolk H, De Vigan C, Scarano G, et al. (2005) Prenatal diagnosis of severe structural congenital malformations in Europe. Ultrasound Obstet Gynecol 25: 6-11.

14. Holland AJ, Walker K, Badawi N (2010) Gastroschisis: an update. Pediatr Surg Int 26: 871-878.

15. Pakdaman R, Woodward PJ, Kennedy A (2015) Complex abdominal wall defects: appearances at prenatal imaging. Radiographics 35: 636-649.

16. Bradnock TJ, Marven S, Owen A, Johnson P, Kurinczuk JJ (2011) Gastroschisis: one year outcomes from national cohort study. BMJ 343: d6749.

17. Baerg J, Kaban G, Tonita J, Pahwa P, Reid D (2003) Gastroschisis: A sixteen-year review. J Pediatr Surg 38: 771-774.

18. Gamba P, Midrio P2 (2014) Abdominal wall defects: prenatal diagnosis, newborn management, and long-term outcomes. Semin Pediatr Surg 23: 283-290.

19. Apfeld J, Wren S, Macheka N, Mbuwayesango B, Bruzoni M, et al. (2015) Infant, maternal, and geographic factors influencing gastroschisis related mortality in Zimbabwe. Surgery 158: 1475-1480.

20. Carvalho N, Helfer T, Serni P, Terasaka O, Boute T, et al. (2015) Postnatal outcomes of infants with gastroschisis: a 5-year follow-up in a tertiary referral center in Brazil. J Matern Fetal Neonatal Med 9: 1-5.

21. Wright NJ, Zani A, Ade-Ajayi N (2015) Epidemiology, management and outcome of gastroschisis in Sub-Saharan Africa: Results of an international survey. Afr J Paediatr Surg 12: 1-6.

22. Nembhard WN, Waller DK, Sever LE, Canfield MA (2001) Patterns of first-year survival among infants with selected congenital anomalies in Texas, 1995-1997. Teratology 64: 267-275.

23. Sekabira J, Hadley GP (2009) Gastroschisis: a third world perspective. Pediatr Surg Int 25: 327-329.

24. Feldkamp M, Carey J, Sadler T (2007) Development of gastroschisis: Review of hypotheses, a novel hypothesis, and implications for research Feldkamp. American Journal of Medical Genetics Part A 143A: 639-652.

25. Abdullah F, Arnold MA, Nabaweesi R, Fischer AC, Colombani PM, et al. (2007) Gastroschisis in the United States 1988-2003: analysis and risk categorization of 4344 patients. J Perinatol 27: 50-55.

26. Aldrink J, Caniano D, Nwomeh B (2012) Variability in gastroschisis management: a survey of North American pediatric surgery training programs. J Surg Res 176: 159-163.

27. Lusk L, Brown E, Overcash R, Grogan T, Keller R, et al. (2014) University of California Fetal Consortium. Multi-institutional practice patterns and outcomes in uncomplicated gastroschisis: a report from the University of California Fetal Consortium (UCfC). J Pediatr Surg 49: 1782-1786.

28. Esteban JM, Maldonado L, Sanchiz V, Minguez M, Benages A (2001) Activity of Crohn's disease assessed by colour Doppler ultrasound analysis of the affected loops. Eur Radiol 11: 1423-1428.

29. Yekeler E, Danalioglu A, Movasseghi B, Yilmaz S, Karaca C, et al. (2005) Crohn disease activity evaluated by Doppler ultrasonography of the superior mesenteric artery and the affected small-bowel segments. J Ultrasound Med 24: 59-65.

30. De Pascale A, Garofalo G, Perna M, Priola S, Fava C (2006) Contrast-enhanced ultrasonography in Crohn's disease. Radiol Med 111: 539-550.

31. Rapaccini GL, Pompili M, Orefice R, Covino M, Riccardi L, et al. (2004) Contrast-enhanced power doppler of the intestinal wall in the evaluation of patients with Crohn disease. Scand J Gastroenterol 39: 188-194.

32. Piscaglia F, Nolsoe C, Dietrich C, Cosgrove D, Gilja O, et al. (2011) The EFSUMB guidelines and recommendations on the clinical practice of contrast-enhanced ultrasound (CEUS): Update 2011 on nonhepatic applications. Ultraschall in Med 33: 33-59.

33. Huang BY, Warshauer DM (2003) Adult intussusception: diagnosis and clinical relevance. Radiol Clin North Am 41: 1137-1151.

34. Boyle MJ, Arkell LJ, Williams JT (1993) Ultrasonic diagnosis of adult intussusception. Am J Gastroenterol 88: 617-618.

35. Abuhamad A, Mari G, Cortina R, Croitoru D, Evans A (1997) Superior mesenteric artery Doppler velocimetry and ultrasonographic assessment

of fetal bowel in gastroschisis: a prospective longitudinal study. Am J Obstet Gynecol 176: 985-990.

36. Sjekavica I, Barbaric-Babic V, Šunjara V, Kralik M, Senecic-Cala I, et al. (2013) Resistance index in mural arteries of thickened bowel wall: predictive value for Crohn disease activity assessment in pediatric patients. Wien Klin Wochenschr 125: 254-260.

37. Sjekavica I, Barbaric-Babic V, Kralik M, Krznaric Z, Stern-Padovan R (2009) High resolution B-mode and Doppler ultrasound in diagnostic evaluation of Crohn's disease. Lijec Vjesn 131: 18-21.

30

Anesthetic and Analgesic Effect of Neostigmine when Added to Lidocaine in Intravenous Regional Anesthesia

Alaa Mohammed Atia* and Khaled Abdel-Baqy Abdel-Rahman

Department of Anesthesia and Intensive Care, Faculty of Medicine, Assiut University, Egypt

*Corresponding author: Alaa M Atia, Department of Anesthesia and Intensive Care, Faculty of Medicine, Assiut University, Egypt, E-mail: alaaguhina@yahoo.com

Abstract

Background: Intravenous regional anesthesia (IVRA) has various advantages during short surgical procedures in upper and lower limbs, but one of its disadvantages is minimal postoperative pain relief.

Aim of the study: To evaluate the anesthetic and analgesic effect of adding 1 mg neostigmine to 0.5% lidocaine in IVRA.

Patients and methods: This randomized double blind controlled clinical trial was carried out at Assiut University Hospital after the approval of its Ethical committee and after obtaining an informed consent from all the patients. Eighty ASA I or II patients who were scheduled for elective hand and forearm surgery were included. We excluded patients with chronic pain syndrome, Reynaud disease, sickle cell anemia, diabetes, pregnancy, lactation, drug allergy and psychological disorders. Patients were randomly assigned to control group who received 3 mg/kg 0.5% lidocaine plus 1 ml normal saline in 40 ml volume and neostigmine group who received 3 mg/kg 0.5% lidocaine plus 1 mg neostigmine in 40 ml volume. Patients were assessed for onset and recovery from the sensory and motor blocks, postoperative pain, analgesic request and incidence of complications. Results No statistically significant differences were observed between groups as regards demographic data, anesthetic or analgesic criteria or the incidence of complications .

Conclusion: Addition of 1 mg neostigmine to 0.5% lidocaine in IVRA has no anesthetic or analgesic effect, and there is no increase in the incidence of complications. There are no biological facts that support its use as adjuvant to local anesthetic agents in IVRA.

Keywords: Neostigmine; Lidocaine; Intravenous regional anesthesia; Analgesic effect; Anesthetic

Introduction

Intravenous regional anesthesia (IVRA) was first introduced by Karl August Bier in 1908 [1]. IVRA is considered as an easy technique with high success rate [2] and low cost suitable for short operative procedures in upper and lower limbs [3].

IVRA has also some disadvantages which include administration of high dose of local anesthetic, poor muscle relaxation, slow onset, tourniquet pain, nerve injuries, compartment syndrome, widespread petechial, skin discoloration and minimal postoperative pain relief [4,5]. Various adjuvant drugs have been evaluated in conjunction with LA to improve IVRA block with variable results [2].

Neostigmine is a typical cholinesterase inhibitor. It increases the level of acetylcholine (Ach) and indirectly stimulates both nicotinic and muscarinic receptors. In anesthesia neostigmine is a drug that has been used for reversal of residual neuromuscular block. Administration of neostigmine by intrathecal and epidural routes has been found to cause analgesia by inhibition of the breakdown of Ach in the spinal cord [6,7]. Some recent studies did not find significant effects in peripheral nerve blocks and IVRA [8,9].

This study was designed to evaluate the anesthetic and analgesic effects of adding 1 mg neostigmine to 0.5% lidocaine in IVRA.

Methods

This randomized double blind controlled clinical trial was carried out at Assiut University Hospital after approval of its Ethical committee and obtaining informed consents from all patients.

We included eighty unsedated ASA physical status I or II between 25 and 60 years of age who were scheduled for elective hand and forearm surgery with estimated time of surgery of less than 1 hour. We excluded patients with chronic pain syndrome, Reynaud disease, sickle cell anemia, diabetes, pregnancy, lactation, drug allergy and psychological disorders. Patients were randomly assigned using computer generated random numbers into one of two groups: The control group (group C, n=40) received 3 mg/kg 0.5% lidocaine plus 1 ml normal saline while the neostigmine group (group N, n=40), received 3 mg/kg 0.5% lidocaine plus 1 mg neostigmine. The study drugs were made to volume of 40 ml for both groups to avoid bias.

An intravenous line was placed into the dorsum of the hand to be operated upon for injection of the study drugs. A second IV line was placed into the other upper limb for fluids and emergency drugs administration. Patients were monitored with ECG, pulse oximetry and noninvasive blood pressure. Following exsanguination of the arm by its elevation for 1-3 minutes and wrapping Esmarch bandage, a pneumatic cuff was applied around the upper third of the arm and inflated to at least 100 mmHg above the patient's systolic pressure and the Esmarch bandage was removed, 40 ml of the study drug was then injected over one minute. When anesthesia was established, a second distal tourniquet was applied and inflated followed by release of the proximal one. At the end of surgery and after at least half an hour of intravenous local anesthetic injection the tourniquet was gradually deflated and all patients were transferred to the post anesthesia care unit. Intraoperative and postoperative bradycardia defined as heart rate <50 beat/min was treated with 0.5 mg intravenous atropine and intra- or postoperative hypotension defined as systolic arterial blood pressure <40% of the baseline was treated with intravenous fluids and/or intravenous 10 mg ephedrine.

Patients assessed their pain using visual analogue scale (on 10 points scale, 0-10) at half an hour interval. Patients whose pain score exceeds 3 were given 30 mg ketorolac and such was repeated on patient request. Intractable pain was managed with pethidine 100 mg IM. The onset of sensory block was assessed every minute with 22 gauge short beveled needle for pinprick and a piece of cotton for touch. The motor function was assessed by asking the patient to flex and extend his fingers and wrist. A complete motor block was defined as inability to move fingers voluntarily. The degree of tourniquet and hand pain was assessed using visual analogue scale (VAS). The duration of sensory and motor block after tourniquet release was determined by restoration of normal surface sensation and motor recovery as compared with the other sound limb. Any complication during surgery and after deflation of the tourniquet (such as nausea, vomiting, dyspnea, bradycardia, dizziness, or hypotension) was also recorded.

Statistical analysis

Data were expressed as mean ± SD unless otherwise indicated. Data were analyzed using fisher's exact t-tests and Mann Whitney test as appropriate. P-value <0.05 was considered statistically significant.

Results

Eighty patients were included in the study and were equally distributed among the two groups. There were no differences in the demographic data (age, weight, sex), duration of surgery and tourniquet time between both groups (Table 1). There was no significant difference in the onset of pinprick loss, touch loss and motor block between both groups (Table 2).

	Group C (n=40)	Group N (n=40)	P-value
Age (yr)	44.9 ± 13.3	45.3 ± 12.1	0.881
Sex (M/F)	32/8	28/12	0.439
Weight (kg)	76.4 ± 11.5	73.4 ± 13.1	0.281
ASA (I/II)	31/9	27/13	0.453
Surgical duration (min)	33.2 ± 8.4	35.9 ± 12.1	0.251
Tourniquet time (min)	47.7 ± 8.7	50.4 ± 12.1	0.254
Data were represented as mean ± SD unless otherwise indicated			

Table 1: Demographic and surgical data.

No significant differences were also observed in the pinprick, touch and motor block recovery after tourniquet deflation between both groups (Table 2).

At the time of admission in to the recovery room, we did not observe statistically significant difference in VAS score between both groups. Also no significant differences were observed between both groups as regards time to first analgesic request, the total dose of ketorolac used or the number of patients needing supplemental opioid (Table 3).

In addition, no significant differences in postoperative complications were observed between both groups (Table 4).

	Group C (n=40)	Group N (n=40)	P-value
Pinprick onset time (min)	7.3 ± 0.4	7.5 ± 0.4	0.128
Touch onset time (min)	10.2 ± 0.5	10.4 ± 0.7	0.235
Motor block onset time (min)	14.9 ± 1.5	15.1 ± 1.4	0.55
Pinprick recovery time (min)	4.0 ± 0.9	3.8 ± 1.0	0.287
Touch recovery time (min)	3.7 ± 1.2	3.4 ± 0.9	0.251
Motor block recovery time (min)	2.1 ± 0.6	1.9 ± 0.5	0.266
Data were represented as mean ± SD			

Table 2: Onset and recovery from sensory and motor block (min).

	Group C (n=40)	Group N (n=40)	P-value
VAS on admission to the recovery room	4.4 ± 1.4	4.1 ± 1.2	0.401
Time to 1st analgesic requirement (min)	25.3 ± 6.7	26.9 ± 7.3	0.334
Total ketorolac consumption(mg)	58.5 ± 23.5	61.5 ± 19.2	0.533
Patients in need of pethidine (No. (%))	5 (13%)	3 (8%)	0.712
Data were represented as mean ± SD and number (%)			

Table 3: VAS in the recovery room and the time of 1st analgesic requirement.

	Group C (n=40)	Group N (n=40)	P-value
Nausea	2 (5%)	5 (13%)	0.432
Vomiting	0 (0%)	2 (5%)	0.494
Dyspnea	0 (0%)	2 (5%)	0.494
Dizziness	5 (13%)	3 (8%)	0.712
Bradycardia	0 (0%)	1 (3%)	1
Hypotension	1 (3%)	2 (5%)	1

Table 4: Postoperative complications No. (%).

Discussion

The results of this study showed no significant differences between both groups in terms of gender, body weight, height, ASA status, type and duration of surgery and the tourniquet time. The study results also showed no statistically significant difference in both the onset of sensory and motor blocks; and the time to sensory and motor recovery in the two study groups.

Many studies on the analgesic efficacy of neostigmine in IVRA gave different results. Neostigmine has been used with different local anesthetic agents and in different doses. Turan et al. [10] in 2002 found that addition of 0.5 neostigmine to prilocaine causes shortened sensory and motor block onset, prolonged sensory and motor block recovery, improved quality of anesthesia and prolonged time to first analgesic request. The study by Turan et al. was in agreement with the results obtained by Marashi et al. [11] and Sethi et al. [12] in which 0.5 % lidocaine was used instead of prilocaine. Kang et al. [13] used ropivacaine and observed good outcome with 0.5 mg of neostigmine as an adjunct.

In contrary to our results, McCartney et al. [9] found no analgesic benefits of 1 mg neostigmine when added to 0.5% lidocaine. Kuyrukluyildiz et al. also did not find analgesic effect of neostigmine when compared to control group [14].

Evidences for analgesic effects of neostigmine are more with its intrathecal and epidural administration. The increased concentration of Ach binds to the muscarinic receptors [15] placed in the dorsal horn cells, substantia gelatinosa and lamina III and V of the spinal cord [16] and nicotinic receptors [17-19] placed in the descending noradrenergic fibers [18], dorsal root ganglion [20] and in microganglia [19]. The presence of cholinergic activity seems to be an important condition for neostigmine analgesic effect [21,22] which could be reversed by muscarinic receptor antagonists [23]. Although Day et al. [24] suggests that Ach receptors exists in peripheral nerve endings, it seems that strong evidences are lacking for this mechanism in the periphery.

The mechanism of action of IVRA itself is still unclear [25], some authors suggest nerve trunk as the main site of action of local anesthetics [26,27], while others suggest peripheral sites to be the main site of action [28,29]. In both cases, the presence of blood-nerve barrier at the innermost layer of perineurium and at the endothelial microvasculature [30] with its highly specialized characteristics as "barrier forming cells" [31] may prevent the transport of neostigmine (a quaternary ammonium compound) to the site of action with the main local anesthetic.

In conclusion, we found that addition of 1 mg neostigmine to 0.5% lidocaine in IVRA has no anesthetic or analgesic effect and there is no increase in the incidence of complications. We did not find any biological fact that supports the use of neostigmine as adjuvant to local anesthetic agents in IVRA.

References

1. Bier A (1908) A new method for local anaesthesia in the extremities. Ann Surg 48: 780.

2. Choyce A, Peng P (2002) A systematic review of adjuncts for intravenous regional anesthesia for surgical procedures. Can J Anaesth 49: 32-45.

3. Chan VW, Peng PWH, Kaszas Z, Middleton WJ, Muni R, et al. (2001) A comparative study of general anesthesia, intravenous regional anesthesia, and axillary block for outpatient hand surgery: clinical outcome and cost analysis. Anesth Analg 93: 1181-1184.

4. Brown EM, McGriff JT, Malinowski RW (1989) Intravenous regional anaesthesia (Bier block): review of 20 years' experience. Can J Anaesth 36: 307-310.

5. Guay J (2009) Adverse events associated with intravenous regional anesthesia (Bier block): a systematic review of complications. J Clin Anesth 21: 585-594.

6. Naguib M, Yaksh TL (1994) Antinociceptive Effects of Spinal Cholinesterase Inhibition and Isobolographic Analysis of the Interaction with a and az Receptor Systems. Anesthesiology 80: 1338-1348.

7. Lauretti GR, Reis MP, Prado WA, Klamt JG (1996) Dose-response study of intrathecal morphine versus intrathecal neostigmine, their combination, or placebo for postoperative analgesia in patients undergoing anterior and posterior vaginoplasty. Anesth Analg 82: 1182-1187.

8. Van Elstraete AC, Pastureau F, Lebrun T, Mehdaoui H (2001) Neostigmine added to lidocaine axillary plexus block for postoperative analgesia. Eur J Anaesthesiol 18: 257-260.

9. McCartney CJ, Brill S, Rawson R, Sanandaji K, Iagounova A, et al. (2003) No anesthetic or analgesic benefit of neostigmine 1 mg added to intravenous regional anesthesia with lidocaine 0.5% for hand surgery. Reg Anesth Pain Med 28: 414-417.

10. Turan A, Karamanlýoglu B, Memis D, Kaya G, Pamukçu Z (2002) Intravenous regional anesthesia using prilocaine and neostigmine. Anesth Analg 95: 1419-1422.

11. Marashi SM, Yazdanifard S, Shoeibi G, Bakhshandeh H, Yazdanifard P, et al. (2008) The analgesic effect of intravenous neostigmine and transdermal nitroglycerine added to lidocaine on intravenous regional anesthesia (Bier's block): a randomized, controlled study in hand surgery. International Journal of Pharmacology 4: 218-222.

12. Sethi D, Wason R (2010) Intravenous regional anesthesia using lidocaine and neostigmine for upper limb surgery. J Clin Anesth 22: 324-328.

13. Kang KS, Jung SH, Ahn KR, Kim CS, Kim JE, et al. (2004) The effects of neostigmine added to ropivacaine for intravenous regional anesthesia. Korean Journal of Anesthesiology 47: 649-654.

14. Kuyrukluyildiz U, Koltka N, Ozcekic AN, Sarar S, Celik M, et al. (2008) Addition of Dexmedetomidine or Neostigmine to Lidocaine for Intravenous Regional Anaesthesia: 379. Regional Anesthesia and Pain Medicine 33: e81.

15. Honda K, Harada A, Takano Y, Kamiya H (2000) Involvement of M3 muscarinic receptors of the spinal cord in formalin-induced nociception in mice. Brain Res 859: 38-44.

16. Wamsley JK, Lewis MS, Young WS 3rd, Kuhar MJ (1981) Autoradiographic localization of muscarinic cholinergic receptors in rat brainstem. J Neurosci 1: 176-191.

17. Duttaroy A, Gomeza J, Gan JW, Siddiqui N, Basile AS, et al. (2002) Evaluation of muscarinic agonist-induced analgesia in muscarinic acetylcholine receptor knockout mice. Mol Pharmacol 62: 1084-1093.

18. Vincler M, Eisenach JC (2004) Plasticity of spinal nicotinic acetylcholine receptors following spinal nerve ligation. Neuroscience research 48: 139-145.

19. Thomsen MS, Mikkelsen JD (2012) The α7 nicotinic acetylcholine receptor ligands methyllycaconitine, NS6740 and GTS-21 reduce lipopolysaccharide-induced TNF-a release from microglia. Journal of neuroimmunology 251: 65-72.

20. Genzen JR, Van Cleve W, McGehee DS (2001) Dorsal root ganglion neurons express multiple nicotinic acetylcholine receptor subtypes. Journal of Neurophysiology 86: 1773-1782.

21. Bouaziz H, Tong C, Eisenach JC (1995) Postoperative analgesia from intrathecal neostigmine in sheep. Anesthesia & Analgesia 80: 1140-1144.

22. Zhuo M, Gebhart GF (1991) Tonic cholinergic inhibition of spinal mechanical transmission. Pain 46: 211-222.

23. Naguib M, Yaksh TL (1997) Characterization of muscarinic receptor subtypes that mediate antinociception in the rat spinal cord. Anesthesia & Analgesia 85: 847-853.

24. Day NS, Berti-Mattera LN, Eichberg J (1991) Muscarinic cholinergic receptor-mediated phosphoinositide metabolism in peripheral nerve. J Neurochem 56: 1905-1913.

25. Brill S, Middleton W, Brill G, Fisher A (2004) Bier's block; 100 years old and still going strong! Acta Anaesthesiol Scand 48: 117-122.

26. Raj PP (1972) The site of action of intravenous regional anesthesia. Anesthesia & Analgesia 51: 776-786.

27. Risdall J (1997) A comparison of intercuff and single cuff techniques of intravenous regional anaesthesia using 0.5% prilocaine mixed with technetium 99m-labelled BRIDA. Anaesthesia 52: 842-848.

28. Haasio J, Hiippala S, Rosenberg PH (1989) Intravenous regional anaesthesia of the arm. Effect of the technique of exsanguination on the quality of anaesthesia and prilocaine plasma concentrations. Anaesthesia 44: 19-21.

29. Moore DC (1984) Bupivacaine toxicity and Bier block: the drug, the technique, or the anesthetist. Anesthesiology 61: 782.

30. Bell MA (1984) A descriptive study of the blood vessels of the sciatic nerve in the rat, man and other mammals. Brain 107: 871-898.

31. Sano Y, Shimizu F, Nakayama H, Abe M, Maeda T, et al. (2007) Endothelial cells constituting blood-nerve barrier have highly specialized cha racteristics as barrier-forming cells. Cell structure and function 32: 139-147.

31

A Comparative Study of Effect of Propofol, Etomidate and Propofol Plus Etomidate Induction on Hemodynamic Response to Endotracheal Intubation: A RCT

Kavita Meena[*], **Rajesh Meena, Sudhansu Sekhar Nayak, Shashi Prakash and Ajit Kumar**

Institute of Medical Sciences, Banaras Hindu University, Varanasi, Uttarpradesh, India

[*]**Corresponding author**: Kavita Meena, Institute of Medical Sciences, Banaras Hindu University, Varanasi, Uttarpradesh, India, E-mail: kvtamn68@gmail.com

Abstract

Objective: The primary objective of this study was to compare the efficacy of 3 different anesthesia induction approach (Inj. Propofol, Inj. Etomidate and Inj. propofol plus Inj Etomidate) in maintaining hemodynamic stability during induction and following endotracheal intubation in elective surgery.

Material and method: Ethical committee clearance taken, 90 patients aged 15 to 60 years of either sex and ASA physical status I or II scheduled for elective surgery under general anesthesia were taken for study. Written and informed consent was taken. The patients were randomly placed into three groups. Group I induced with Inj. Propofol (2.5 mg/kg) intravenous, Group II with Inj. Etomidate (0.3 mg/kg) intravenous and Group III with Inj. Propofol (1 mg/kg) plus Inj. Etomidate (0.2 mg/kg) intravenous. Heart rate (HR), systolic blood pressure (SBP), diastolic blood pressure (DBP), mean arterial blood pressure (MAP) and oxygen saturation (SPO_2) were noted at different time interval.

Results: Heart rate in all study groups decreases after induction and it was more in group I compared to group II and III (p<0.000) and after intubation HR increases in all three groups but this increase is greater in group II than other two groups. MAP among all three groups decreases after induction and it was more in group I than group II and III. Significant increase in MAP was seen at 1 min after intubation in all three groups but this increase was not sustained and returned to baseline in group II and III.

Conclusion: The combination of etomidate plus propofol has better hemodynamic stability than etomidate alone at 1 min after intubation, though etomidate was equally stable at other points of time. The combination proved to be significantly better than either propofol or etomidate alone.

Keywords: Propofol; Etomidate; Mean arterial pressure; Heart rate; Laryngoscopy

Introduction

In general anesthesia airway management and patient safety is the most important aspect of patient management. Endotracheal intubation is the gold standard and safest method for protecting the airway, delivering anesthetic gases and ensuring protection against aspiration [1,2]. Stress response during laryngoscopy and intubation leads to hemodynamic changes especially for patients who are under cardiac risk factors like hypertension and ischemic heart disease [3]. The unavoidable effects of laryngoscopy and tracheal intubation includes dysrhythmia, hypertension, myocardial ischemia, infarction, hypoxia, hypercapnea, laryngospasm, and bronchospasm, and some rare side effects such as increased intracranial pressure and increased intraocular pressure.

Since the introduction of general anesthesia, no ideal induction agent has yet been discovered in term of providing a stable hemodynamics during endotracheal intubation. Also there are very few published studies in the literature that have compared the physiological effect of various induction agents during laryngoscopy and intubation.

Propofol is one the commonly used drug for induction of general anesthesia. This is a short acting intravenous anesthetic agent. Recommended dose of propofol for induction is 1-2.5 mg/kg. Unwanted complication associated with this drug is hemodynamic instability and cardiovascular complications. Propofol can lead to bradycardia by increasing the production and release of nitrous oxide [4-6]. Also causes pain at injection site. Etomidate is a hypnotic agent which is cardiostable with no release of histamine. It is short acting drug, used for induction and maintenance of anesthesia [7]. The most important side effects of Etomidate are nausea and vomiting that may lead to aspiration in patients [8-10]. Intravenous Injection of Etomidate would cause a burning sensation. One of the most important, but rare side effects of this drug is the suppression of steroids production by reversible inhibition of 11betahydroxylase enzyme [10,11]. Induction of anesthesia by Etomidate would lead to a stable hemodynamic condition for performing laryngoscopy and endotracheal intubation [9,10,12].

In past many studies have been comparing different anesthetic induction agents, but studies regarding combination of propofol and etomidate are only few. These studies are focused on hemodynamic changes only during anesthesia induction and LMA insertion. The primary objective of this study was to compare the efficacy of 3 different approach of anesthesia induction (Inj. Propofol, Inj. Etomidate and Inj. propofol plus Inj. Etomidate) in maintaining hemodynamic stability during induction and following endotracheal intubation in elective surgery (Figure 1).

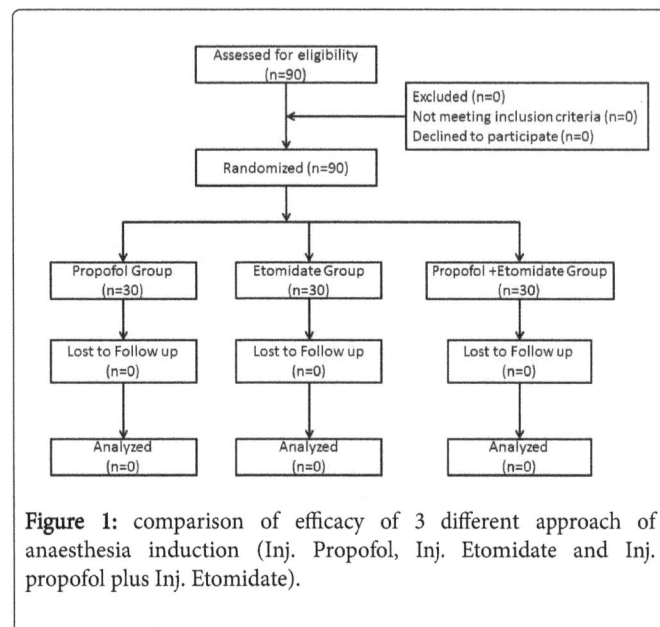

Figure 1: comparison of efficacy of 3 different approach of anaesthesia induction (Inj. Propofol, Inj. Etomidate and Inj. propofol plus Inj. Etomidate).

Material and Methods

This randomized double blind clinical trial was conducted at Department of Anesthesiology, Institute of Medical Sciences, Banaras Hindu University, Varanasi, India. Study period was from 2015-2016. After approval from institutional ethical committee, 90 patients aged between 15 to 60 years of either sex and ASA physical status I and II scheduled for elective surgery under general anesthesia were taken for study [13,14]. Written informed consent was taken from all patients. The patients were randomly divided into three groups. Randomization was done by computer generated random number tables.

- Group I Induction with Inj. Propofol (2.5 mg/kg) iv.
- Group II Induction with Inj. Etomidate (0.3 mg/kg) iv.
- Group III Induction with Inj. Propofol (1 mg/kg) plus Inj. Etomidate (0.2 mg/kg) iv. [15]

Patient having following criteria were excluded from the study

- Patient refusal.
- ASA physical status III and IV.
- Emergency surgery.
- Patient with history of hypersensitivity to Propofol /Etomidate.
- Mouth opening <2.5 cm.
- Patients with cardiovascular diseases like ischemic heart disease or hypertension.
- Bronchial asthma.
- Mallampati grade 3 and 4
- Existence of considerable pathology in pharynx / larynx.
- Patient with GERD.

Airway assessment like mouth opening, mallampati grading, dentition, neck flexion and extension of all patients was done. Baseline (preoperative) heart rate (HR), systolic blood pressure (SBP), diastolic blood pressure (DBP), mean arterial blood pressure (MAP) and oxygen saturation (SPO$_2$) were noted.

The patients were kept nil per orally for 8 hours prior to surgery. All patients were premedicated with tab. Alprozolam 0.25 mg, tab. Ranitidine 150 mg and tab. Metoclopramide 10 mg, at the night before surgery and in the morning. All patients received inj. glycopyrolate 0.2 mg IM 45 minutes before induction in the preoperative ward. On arrival at Operation Theater standard anesthesia monitors including electrocardiogram (ECG), non-invasive blood pressure (NIBP) and pulse oxymetry were attached and hemodynamic parameters were recorded. A 18 G intravanous (IV) canula was secured in left hand and ringer lactate infusion was started. Inj. midazolam 0.025 mg/kg IV and Inj. fentanyl 2 µg/kg IV was given 2 minutes before induction. For induction group I received inj. Propofol 2.5 mg/kg IV, group II received inj. Etomidate 0.3 mg/kg IV and group III received inj. Propofol 1 mg/kg plus inj. Etomidate 0.2 mg/kg IV. 15 All study drugs were prepared by an anesthesiologist who was blinded to the details of the study. Volume of medication and speed of injection (10 seconds) were equal in all three groups. After induction of anesthesia, hemodynamic variables were recorded. Later 60 seconds after of loss of consciousness, which was confirmed by inability to respond to verbal commands and loss of eyelash reflex. Inj. vecuronium (0.1 mg/kg) was given, Laryngoscopy and endotracheal intubation was done by experienced anesthesiologist. Duration of laryngoscopy was kept less than 10 seconds. Trachea was intubated with adequate size endotracheal tube. Proper placement of endotracheal tube was confirmed by capnography and bilateral auscaltation of chest. Following successful placement of ET tube anesthesia was maintained by isoflurane 1-1.5% and equal mixtures of oxygen-nitrous oxide (4 L/min) along with intermittent bolus of vecuronium as required throughout the surgery.

At the end of the surgery residual neuromuscular block was antagonized with inj. neostigmine (0.05 mg/kg) IV and inj. glycopyrolate (0.01 mg/kg) IV and extubation was performed when respiration was adequate and patient was able to obey verbal commands.

Heart rate, systolic blood pressure, diastolic blood pressure and mean arterial blood pressure and oxygen saturation were continuously monitored and recorded before induction, after induction and at 1 minute, 2 minute, 3 minute, 5 minute after intubation.

Power analysis

It is calculated according to previous studies, when MAP at the first minute of intubation is taken, as the main result in the event of at least 30 patients in each group, it was calculated that in respect of hemodynamic parameters, a 10% difference could be determined between the group at 80% power and 5% significance (α=0.05, β=0.80).

Statistical analysis

The obtained data were analyzed using SPSS 16; descriptive data was compared and presented as Mean ± SD for continuous variables and as no and percentage for nominal variable. The various categorical variables studied during observation period were compared using Chi-square test. The various hemodynamic variable parameters studied during observation period were compared using ANOVA test and inter group comparison of hemodynamic variable were made by post hoc test. The critical value of 'p' indicating the probability of significant difference was taken as <0.05 for comparison.

Results

Data of 90 patients were evaluated. There was no statistically significance difference was observed between the groups regarding patient characteristic and ASA score (Tables 1, 2A and 2B).

	Group I	Group II	Group III	p-value
Age (Y)	34.47 ± 6.72	33.90 ± 6.28	37.30 ± 9.39	0.178
BMI (kg/m)	22.46 ± 2.59	21.99 ± 1.95	22.77 ± 2.73	0.704
Gender (M/F)	14/16	15/15	20/10	0.241
Height (feet and inches)	5.41 ± 0.45	5.38 ± 0.41	5.42 ± 0.38	0.742

BMI: Body Mass Index; M/F: Male/Female; ASA: American Society of Anesthesiologist; Data presented as Mean ± SD or frequencies

Table 1: Patient's characteristics.

Baseline and pre-induction HR were comparable among all three groups with no statistical significant differences (p>0.05) Inter group comparison showed that there are significant differences (p<0.05) in heart rate among all three groups at time interval (after induction and 1, 2, 3 min after intubation). At 5min after intubation there are significant differences among groups except between group II and group III (Tables 3A and 3B).

Baseline and pre-induction SBP were comparable among all the three groups with no statistical significant differences (p>0.05). But SBP of three groups after induction and at 1, 2, 3, 5 minute after intubation were different both clinically and statistically, with p value <0.05.

Inter group comparison of SBP (mean ± SD) revealed significant differences among various groups at different points of time except that among group II and group III. Between group II and group III there was significant difference only at 1 min after intubation (Tables 4A and 4B).

Time Interval	Group I	Group II	Group III	f-value	p-value
Baseline HR	78.33 ± 6.572	76.40 ± 6.667	77.30 ± 5.466	0.686	0.562
HR pre induction	89.60 ± 5.975	88.03 ± 6.775	88.33 ± 5.785	0.355	0.786
HR after induction	69.43 ± 5.151	88.27 ± 7.249	82.63 ± 6.780	123.808	0.000
HR 1min after intubation	76.57 ± 4.539	99.30 ± 5.926	93.50 ± 6.648	274.713	0.000
HR 2mins after intubation	80.13 ± 4.747	96.37 ± 6.031	91.17 ± 6.747	112.567	0.000
HR 3mins after intubation	83.27 ± 4.863	94.40 ± 5.852	90.17 ± 6.018	43.931	0.000
HR 5mins after intubation	85.43 ± 4.337	92.50 ± 6.096	89.83 ± 5.670	15.984	0.000

Table 2A: Mean HR (Heart Rate) in (beats per minute).

Time Interval	Group I vs. II	Group I vs. III	Group II vs. III
Baseline HR	0.253	0.540	0.594
HR pre induction	0.355	0.455	0.859
HR after induction	0.000	0.000	0.001
HR 1min after intubation	0.000	0.000	0.000
HR 2mins after intubation	0.000	0.000	0.002
HR 3mins after intubation	0.000	0.000	0.016
HR 5mins after intubation	0.000	0.008	0.102

Table 2B: Group comparisons mean HR.

Time Interval	Group I	Group II	Group III	f-value	p-value
Baseline SBP	129.87 ± 6.146	127.83 ± 5.376	127.80 ± 7.208	0.876	0.456
SBP pre induction	125.50 ± 6.067	123.67 ± 5.839	124.97 ± 7.117	0.730	0.536
SBP after induction	100.53 ± 8.905	117.73 ± 5.705	118.40 ± 6.750	43.148	0.000
SBP 1min after intubation	111.77 ± 6.474	133.87 ± 5.758	130.57 ± 4.826	169.731	0.000
SBP 2mins after intubation	115.33 ± 7.906	129.10 ± 3.836	126.97 ± 3.891	79.327	0.000
SBP 3mins after intubation	121.73 ± 4.586	125.30 ± 4.473	125.20 ± 3.995	30.153	0.000
SBP 5mins after intubation	126.83 ± 3.270	122.47 ± 5.457	123.50 ± 4.431	20.563	0.000

Table 3A: SBP (systolic blood pressure) in (mmHg).

Baseline and pre-induction DBP were comparable among all the three groups with no statistical significant differences (p>0.05). But DBP of three groups after induction and at 1,2,3,5 minute after intubation were different both clinically and statistically, with p value <0.05.

Time Interval	Group I vs. II	Group I vs. III	Group II vs. III
Baseline SBP	0.198	0.191	0.983
SBP pre induction	0.251	0.738	0.415
SBP after induction	0.000	0.000	0.710
SBP 1min after intubation	0.000	0.000	0.035
SBP 2mins after intubation	0.000	0.000	0.120
SBP 3mins after intubation	0.002	0.002	0.929
SBP 5mins after intubation	0.000	0.006	0.384

Table 3B: Group comparison SBP.

Time Interval	Group I	Group II	Group III	f-value	p-value
Baseline DBP	75.80 ± 6.228	74.70 ± 4.757	75.23 ± 5.184	.336	.799
DBP pre induction	73.23 ± 6.447	72.17 ± 4.340	71.90 ± 5.498	0.377	0.770
DBP after induction	60.30 ± 4.236	68.00 ± 4.307	68.30 ± 5.338	22.357	0.000
DBP 1min after intubation	65.63 ± 3.728	77.00 ± 4.299	73.13 ± 4.183	76.835	0.000
DBP 2mins after intubation	67.37 ± 3.285	73.00 ± 3.833	72.27 ± 3.805	47.669	0.000
DBP 3mins after intubation	68.43 ± 3.191	72.37 ± 3.023	71.43 ± 3.598	35.550	0.000
DBP 5mins after intubation	72.40 ± 2.943	71.43 ± 2.269	70.27 ± 4.093	16.330	0.000

Table 4A: DBP (Diastolic Blood Pressure) in (mmHg).

Time Interval	Group I vs. II	Group I vs. III	Group II vs. III
Baseline DBP	0.427	0.682	0.700
DBP pre induction	0.428	0.322	0.843
DBP after induction	0.000	0.000	0.787
DBP 1min after intubation	0.000	0.000	0.005
DBP 2mins after intubation	0.000	0.000	0.580
DBP 3mins after intubation	0.000	0.004	0.357
DBP 5mins after intubation	0.305	0.025	0.216

Table 4B: Group comparison DBP (mmHg).

There were significant differences (p<0.05) in inter group comparison of DBP (mean ± SD) among the groups except group II and III. But there was significant difference between group II and III only at 1 min after intubation. At 5 min after intubation there were no significant differences between group I vs. II and group II vs. III (Tables 5A and 5B).

Baseline and pre-induction MAP were comparable among all the three groups with no statistical significant differences (p>0.05). But MAP of three groups after induction and at 1,2,3,5 minute after intubation were different both clinically and statistically, with p value <0.05. Inter group comparison of MAP (mean ± SD) revealed significant differences among various groups at different points of time except that among group II vs. group III. Between groups II vs. group III there was significant difference only at 1 min after intubation.

Discussion

Combinations of various anesthetic agents have been used; these combinations have created separate beneficial sedative, amnestic and hypnotic effect in anesthesia induction. With this method there has been evident reduction in anesthetic medication, significant reduction in side effect and cost [13,14].

Etomidae is one of the intravenous anesthetics used in anesthesia induction, either alone or in combination with other anesthestic drugs [16]. In a study by Hosseinzadeh et al. [15], comparing hemodynamic changes during placement of laryngeal mask airway (LMA) using propofol, etomidate and etomidate-propofol combination, after the administration of inj. fentanyl 2 mg/kg, group one was given inj. propofol 2.5 mg/kg, group two received inj etomidate 0.3 mg/kg and group three 1 mg/kg propofol+0.2 mg/kg etomidate. LMA placement was done after loss of eyelash reflex and no response to verbal command. The main finding of the study was that more stable hemodynamics was provided by combination of propofol and etomidate compared to propofol and etomidate and alone. Although the dose of both drugs are reduced in the combination of propofol and etomidate, it was reported that more stable hemodynamic state and better condition for LMA placement was provided.

Time Interval	Group I	Group II	Group III	f-value	p-value
Baseline Mean BP	93.70 ± 5.383	92.17 ± 4.379	91.73 ± 5.638	1.119	0.344
Mean BP pre induction	89.57 ± 4.783	88.57 ± 4.321	89.53 ± 5.686	.300	0.826
Mean BP after induction	73.71 ± 4.876	84.57 ± 4.192	85.00 ± 5.425	41.019	0.000
Mean BP 1min after intubation	81.67 ± 3.695	95.95 ± 4.082	92.77 ± 4.066	143.549	0.000
Mean BP 2mins after intubation	83.35 ± 3.927	91.70 ± 3.081	90.50 ± 3.555	88.266	0.000
Mean BP 3mins after intubation	86.20 ± 2.919	90.01 ± 2.484	89.35 ± 3.504	53.174	0.000
Mean BP 5mins after intubation	90.54 ± 2.453	88.44 ± 2.528	88.01 ± 3.830	28.420	0.000

Table 5A: Mean (Mean arterial BP) MAP (mmHg).

Time Interval	Group I vs. II	Group I vs. III	Group II vs. III
Baseline Mean BP	0.233	0.127	0.735
Mean BP pre induction	0.411	0.978	0.427
Mean BP after induction	0.000	0.000	0.715
Mean BP 1min after intubation	0.000	0.000	0.003
Mean BP 2mins after intubation	0.000	0.000	0.259
Mean BP 3mins	0.000	0.000	0.431
Mean BP 5mins after intubation	0.009	0.002	0.587

Table 5B: Group comparison mean (mean arterial BP).

In a study performed by Yağan Ö et al. [17], patients were randomly divided into three groups as group P (n=30, propofol 2.5 mg/kg), group E (n=30, etomidate 0.3 mg/kg) and group PE (n=30, propofol 1.25 mg/kg+etomidate 0.15 mg/kg). Measurement of the heart rate (HR) and mean arterial pressure values were defined as baseline, after the induction, before the intubation, immediately after the intubation and 1, 2, 3, 4, 5 and 10 minutes after the intubation. They found that Etomidate-propofol combination may be a valuable alternative when extremes of hypotensive and hypertensive responses due to propofol and etomidate are best to be avoided.

Another study reported that after anesthesia induction with etomidate (0.3 mg/kg) the ideal fentanyl dose was 5-10 mg/kg to prevent a hemodynamic response to laryngoscopy and intubation [18]. However, it can be predicted that use of such high dose of fentanyl may cause increased hypotension, nausea and vomiting.

In a study by Muriel et al. [19], a comparison was made of propofol (2 mg/kg), thiopental (5 mg/kg) and etomidate (0.3 mg/kg) in anesthesia induction. A statistically significant increase was determined in systolic and diastolic arterial pressure and HR in the etomidate and thiopental group after intubation and the highest rate of complication was reported in etomidate group.

Harris et al. [20] compared the hemodynamic response to tracheal intubation in 303 patients in whom anesthesia was induced with either thiopentone 4 mg/kg, etomidate 0.3 mg/kg or propofol 2.5 mg/kg with or without fentanyl 2 µg/kg. After propofol alone, there was a significant decrease in arterial blood pressure, which did not increase above control value after intubation. Significant increase in arterial pressure followed intubation in patients induced with thiopentone or etomidate alone. Increases in heart rate occurred with all agents after laryngoscopy and intubation. The use of fentanyl resulted in arterial pressure lower than those after the induction agent alone and in an attenuation, but not abolition, of responses to laryngoscopy and intubation. We got similar results in our study with significant decrease in arterial blood pressure, after induction with propofol which did not increase above baseline value after intubation, while, with etomidate, there was significant increase in arterial pressure following intubation. Also, increase in heart rate occurred with all agents after laryngoscopy and intubation

Schmidt et al. [21] found in their study that, hypotension caused by propofol is due to the reduction of heart's preload and afterload, which are not synchronized with heart's compensatory responses such as increased cardiac output and increased HR. This hemodynamic drop would be intensified by high doses of the drug and high speed injection of the drug. In our study we got similar results in group I i.e. after induction with propofol there was hypotension and not synchronized with increased HR.

Mehrdad et al. [22] conducted a study including patients of 18-45 years of age that were admitted for elective orthopedic surgeries. patients were divided in two groups, their cardiovascular responses including: systolic blood pressure (SBP), diastolic blood pressure (DBP), mean arterial pressure (MAP), heart rate (HR), and O_2 saturation (O_2 sat) were measured before the laryngoscopy, during the anesthesia induction with Etomidate (0.3 mg/kg) in group A and propofol (2-2.5 mg/kg) in group B and at 1, 3, 5, 10 min after the induction. They concluded that patients receiving Etomidate have more stable hemodynamic condition, if there would be no contraindications; it could be preferred over propofol for general anesthesia. Our study got similar results of better hemodynamic conditions with etomidate as compared to propofol.

In a study by Möller et al. [23] which used propofol and etomidate in general anesthesia induction accompanied by BIS monitoring, the MAP, cardiac index (CI) and systemic vascular resistance index (SVRI) values of 48 patients were compared. The hemodynamic data were found to be higher in the etomidate group up to 7 minutes after intubation. A significantly high level of hypotension incidence was found in the propofol group and a significantly high level of hypertension incidence in the etomidate group. Compared with etomidate, the use of propofol was determined to have caused less hypertension and tachycardia after intubation. In the current study, the MAP values after induction in the propofol group were significantly lower than those of the other two groups. Following intubation, the MAP and HR values of the etomidate group were statistically significantly higher than those of the other two groups. These results confirm with those in literature.

There was added advantage of combining Etomidate with propofol for attenuating intubation reflex as compared to Etomidate alone, and had obvious advantage than using Propofol or Thiopentone alone.

Not using BIS to measure the depth of anesthesia is a major limitation of our study. Another limitation is not measuring plasma cortisol and adrenocorticotropin hormone level. But it has been reported that adrenal suppression after single dose of etomidate is transient and clinically unimportant [24].

Conclusion

Induction with propofol alone is acceptable in patients with stable hemodynamics. However, propofol may cause hypotension in volume depleted patients. The combination of etomidate plus propofol has better hemodynamic stability than etomidate alone at 1 min after intubation, though etomidate was equally stable at other points of time. And, the combination proved to be significantly better than either propofol or etomidate alone.

References

1. Sakles JC, Laurin EG, Rantapaa AA, Panacek EA (1998) Airway management in the emergency department: a one-year study of 610 tracheal intubations. Ann Emerg Med 31: 325-332.

2. Stevenson AG, Graham CA, Hall R, Korsah P, McGuffie AC (2007) Tracheal intubation in the emergency department: the Scottish district hospital perspective. Emerg Med J 24: 394-397.

3. Montes FR, Giraldo JC, Betancur LA, Rincón JD, Rincón IE, et al. (2003) Endotracheal intubation with a lightwand or a laryngoscope results in similar hemodynamic variations in patients with coronary artery disease. Can J Anaesth 50: 824-828.

4. Riznyk L, FijaÅ‚kowska M, Przesmycki K (2005) Effects of thiopental and propofol on heart rate variability during fentanyl-based induction of general anesthesia. Pharmacol Rep 57: 128-134.

5. Basu S, Mutschler DK, Larsson AO, Kiiski R, Nordgren A, et al. (2001) Propofol (Diprivan-EDTA) counteracts oxidative injury and deterioration of the arterial oxygen tension during experimental septic shock. Resuscitation 50: 341-348.

6. Kelicen P, Ismailoglu UB, Erdemli O, Sahin-Erdemli I (1997) The effect of propofol and thiopentone on impairment by reactive oxygen species of endothelium-dependent relaxation in rat aortic rings. Eur J Anaesthesiol 14: 310-315.

7. Cuthbertson BH, Sprung CL, Annane D, Chevret S, Garfield M, et al. (2009) The effects of etomidate on adrenal responsiveness and mortality in patients with septic shock. Intensive Care Med 35: 1868-1876.

8. Eames WO, Rooke GA, Wu RS, Bishop MJ (1996) Comparison of the effects of etomidate, propofol, and thiopental on respiratory resistance after tracheal intubation. Anesthesiology 84: 1307-1311.

9. Sarkar M, Laussen PC, Zurakowski D, Shukla A, Kussman B, et al. (2005) Hemodynamic responses to etomidate on induction of anesthesia in pediatric patients. Anesth Analg 101: 645-650, table of contents.

10. Zed PJ, Mabasa VH, Slavik RS, Abu-Laban RB (2006) Etomidate for rapid sequence intubation in the emergency department: is adrenal suppression a concern? CJEM 8: 347-350.

11. Lipiner-Friedman D, Sprung CL, Laterre PF, Weiss Y, Goodman SV, et al. (2007) Adrenal function in sepsis: the retrospective Corticus cohort study. Crit Care Med 35: 1012-1018.

12. Kalogridaki M, Souvatzis X, Mavrakis HE, Kanoupakis EM, Panteli A, et al. (2011) Anaesthesia for cardioversion: a prospective randomised comparison of propofol and etomidate combined with fentanyl. Hellenic J Cardiol 52: 483-488.

13. Morgan M, Lumley J, Whitwam JG (1977) Respiratory effects of etomidate. Br J Anaesth 49: 233-236.

14. Anderson L, Robb H (1998) A comparison of midazolam co-induction with propofol predosing for induction of anaesthesia. Anaesthesia 53: 1117-1120.

15. Hosseinzadeh H, Golzari SE, Torabi E, Dehdilani M (2013) Hemodynamic Changes following Anesthesia Induction and LMA Insertion with Propofol, Etomidate, and Propofol + Etomidate. J Cardiovasc Thorac Res 5: 109-112.

16. Morgan M, Lumley J, Whitwam JG (1977) Respiratory effects of etomidate.Br J Anaesth 49: 233-236.

17. Yagan O, Tas N, Kucuk A, Hanci V, Yurtlu BS (2015) Haemodynamic Responses to Tracheal Intubation Using Propofol, Etomidate and Etomidate-Propofol Combination in Anaesthesia Induction.J Cardiovasc Thorac Res 7: 134-140.

18. Weiss-Bloom LJ, Reich DL (1992) Haemodynamic responses to tracheal intubation following etomidate and fentanyl for anaesthetic induction. Can J Anaesth 39: 780-785.

19. Muriel C, Santos J, Espinel C (1991) Comparative study of propofol with thiopental and etomidate in anesthetic induction. Rev Esp Anestesiol Reanim 38: 301-304.

20. Harris CE, Murray AM, Anderson JM, Grounds RM, Morgan M (1988) Effects of thiopentone, etomidate and propofol on the haemodynamic response to tracheal intubation. Anaesthesia 43 Suppl: 32-36.

21. Schmidt C, Roosens C, Struys M, Deryck YL, Van Nooten G, et al. (1999) Contractility in humans after coronary artery surgery. Anesthesiology 91: 58-70.

22. Masoudifar M, Beheshtian E (2013) Comparison of cardiovascular response to laryngoscopy and tracheal intubation after induction of anesthesia by Propofol and Etomidate. J Res Med Sci 18: 870-874.

23. Möller Petrun A, Kamenik M (2013) Bispectral index-guided induction of general anaesthesia in patients undergoing major abdominal surgery using propofol or etomidate: a double-blind, randomized, clinical trial. Br J Anaesth 110: 388-396.

24. Sawano Y, Miyazaki M, Shimada H, Kadoi Y (2013) Optimal fentanyl dosage for attenuating systemic hemodynamic changes, hormone release and cardiac output changes during the induction of anesthesia in patients with and without hypertension: a prospective, randomized, double-blinded study. J Anesth 27: 505-511.

A Cross-Sectional Study Evaluating the GuardianCPV™ Supraglottic Airway Device in a Clinical Setting

Michael Hua-Gen Li*, **Howard Ho-Fung Tang, Celestine Johnny Bouniu and Jun Keat Chan**

Department of Anesthesia and Perioperative Medicine, The Northern Hospital, Australia

*Corresponding author: Michael Hua-Gen Li, Department of Anesthesia and Perioperative Medicine, The Northern Hospital, 185 Cooper St, Epping, VIC 3076, Australia, Email: Michael.Huagen.Li@gmail.com

Abstract

Objective: The GuardianCPV™ is a new second-generation supraglottic airway device (SAD), for which there is currently limited information on efficacy or safety. Our aim is to clarify further the efficacy of the Guardian, and to assess any potential predictors for success or failure of insertion.

Methods: We conducted a cross-sectional pilot study over a two-month period, recruiting 67 operative cases (33 males; 34 females; weight 81.1 ± 23.0 kg) at the Northern Hospital (TNH), Victoria, Australia, that used the Guardian airway in an elective setting. For each case, the operator of the airway reported, via a voluntary questionnaire, several factors of interest: (1) the overall success rate (primary outcome); (2) ease of insertion; (3) cuff seal pressure (CSP); (4) need for repositioning of the SAD; and (5) patient, airway, operator and technique-related predictors, including past experience with the Guardian (as determined by number of times previously used) and insertion technique.

Results: The overall success rate was 78%. There was a positive association between prior experience with the Guardian and subsequent success rates (p=0.049). Successful insertion was associated with greater ease with insertion (p=0.012), and greater CSPs (p<0.0001). The most popular insertion technique was sideways-and-rotate. No other patient, airway or technique-related factors had any significant impact on success rates with the Guardian.

Conclusion: The Guardian SAD demonstrated similar efficacy to other SADs as reported in the literature. Prior familiarization with a new airway device is a key determinant in its successful use.

Keywords: Airway management; Laryngeal mask

Abbreviations: CSP: Cuff Seal Pressure; OLP: Oropharyngeal Leak Pressure; SAD: Supraglottic Airway Device; TNH: The Northern Hospital.

Background

The Guardian CPV™ ("Guardian") is a second-generation supraglottic airway device (SAD) developed in 2011 by Ultimate Medical (Richmond, Australia). There is currently limited information on the safety and efficacy of this particular model. Other popular second-generation SADs (LMA Supreme™, i-gel®, Proseal LMA™) typically achieve success rates of 71 to 100% [1-9]. At the time that this study was performed, there was only one known study in the literature that specifically assessed the Guardian, comparing it with the Supreme [10]. According to that study, efficacy was equivalent between both models, with equivalent insertion success rates on first attempt (100%), and slightly superior oropharyngeal leak pressure (OLP) for the Guardian compared to the Supreme.

The purpose of this study is to further characterize the efficacy of the Guardian in a tertiary hospital setting, and to identify factors that may contribute to its success or failure. We hypothesized that the success rate of insertion for the Guardian is comparable to those of other SADs reported in the literature.

Materials and Methods

Sample collection

We conducted a prospective pilot study of adult operative cases from the Northern Hospital (TNH), Epping, Australia, that used the Guardian, from 1st May 2013 to 31st July 2013. Anesthetists and medical trainees were approached and recruited for the study on a voluntary basis. For each case, the characteristics and outcomes were reported via a questionnaire (Table 1) by the individual who performed the SAD insertion (i.e. the "operator"). In all cases, the Guardian was used electively and not as rescue device. The study was approved by the Northern Health Human Research Ethics Committee via the low-risk pathway. All cases were de-identified prior to statistical analysis. The existing literature for the Guardian LMA reports 100% success rate. [10,11] Using G*Power [12], a sample size of at least 50 was needed to identify a statistically-significant difference (one-tailed, α=0.05, β=0.80) from an expected success rate of 95% to an actual success rate of 80%.

Evaluation of outcomes

The primary outcome of interest was the rate of successful insertion for the Guardian. Success in this context was defined as the ability to ventilate through, and the continued use of, the Guardian airway without need for replacement with an alternative device, and regardless of the number of attempts. Other outcomes assessed were the total number of insertion attempts; ease of insertion; cuff seal pressure (CSP); and need for physical repositioning of the SAD in the airway.

The ease of insertion was evaluated via an ordinal scale, from one to five in ascending order of difficulty (Table 1)-a score of one was equivalent to the device slipping in without effort; a score of three meant that the insertion required additional assistance from other theatre staff; and a score of five meant complete failure of insertion.

The cuff seal pressure (CSP) was defined as the maximum pressure that the anesthetist could apply via positive pressure ventilation, with the adjustable pressure limiting valve closed, before a leak was detected. The CSP was used as a surrogate measure for oropharyngeal leak pressure (OLP), due to limitations in the precise measurement of OLP in the acute theatre setting. Again, CSP was evaluated as an ordinal variable on a scale from one to five. A score of one denoted a pressure above 30 cmH_2O; a score of two for pressures from greater than 22.5 to 30 cmH_2O; a score of three for pressures from 15 to 22.5 cmH_2O; a score of four for pressures less than 15 cmH_2O but with achievable ventilation; and a score of five for cases where ventilation was not possible at all.

From the collated data we then estimated the proportion of all cases where "clinically-positive" outcomes were obtained. These positive outcomes were explicitly defined as follows: (1) number of insertion attempts was less than three; (2) the score for ease of insertion was less than three; (3) the CSP was greater than 15 cmH_2O (i.e. CSP score was less than four); and (4) no SAD repositioning was required.

Property	Options	Scoring
Patient-related		
Sex	Male	-
	Female	
Weight, in kg	-	-
Airway-related		
Mallampati score	-	1
		2
		3
		4
Thyromental score (and distance, in cm)	<6 cm	1
	6 to 8 cm	2
	>8 cm	3
Teeth	Full set	1
	Partial set	2
	Edentulous	3
SAD size	3	1
	4	2
	5	3
Operator-related		
Operator level	Resident/intern	1

	Registrar	2
	Consultant	3
Previous use of Guardian SAD	0 to 4	1
	5 to 10	2
	>10	3
Outcomes		
Ease of insertion score	Slips in with ease	1
	Slips in with difficulty, but able to manage on own	2
	Requiring some help from other staff	3
	Requiring significant help from other staff	4
	Unable to insert	5
Number of attempts at insertion	1	1
	2	2
	≥ 3	3
Degree of cuff inflation	Cuff fully deflated	1
	Cuff partially inflated	2
	Cuff fully inflated	3
Insertion technique	Pen grip	-
	Finger guided	
	Sideways and rotate	
	Upside down and rotate	
	Laryngoscope/Bougie	
Additional maneuvers to position properly (over and above usual SAD insertion techniques)	Extra mouth opening	-
	Extra jaw thrust	
	Extra head extension	
Cuff seal with CuffPilot in green zone	Seals at >30 cmH2O	1
	Seals at >22.5 to 30 cmH2O	2
	Seals at 15 to 22.5 cmH2O	3
	Seals at <15 cmH2O, but with achievable ventilation	4
	Unable to ventilate despite good positioning	5
Need for SAD repositioning during case	Yes, and reason for repositioning	
	No	
SAD=Supraglottic Airway Device		

Table 1: Structure of Questionnaire.

Evaluation of predictors

For each case we recorded a number of other parameters defined as "predictors". These were categorized into patient, airway, operator, and technique-related predictors (Table 1). Patient-related predictors were patient sex and weight. Airway-related predictors were the Mallampati score (scored from one to four); thyromental distance (scored as an ordinal variable, with score of one meaning less than 6cm, score of two meaning 6 to 8 cm, and score of three meaning greater than 8 cm); dentition status (full set, partial set, or edentulous); and the size of the SAD used for the case (sizes 3, 4 and 5). Operator-related predictors were level of medical training (resident, registrar, or consultant) and prior experience with the Guardian (scored from one to three, with one meaning 0 to 4 times of prior Guardian use, two meaning 5 to 10 times, and three meaning greater than 10 times). Technique-related predictors were the level of cuff inflation (fully deflated, partially inflated, or fully inflated), insertion technique (sideways and rotate; pen-grip; upside-down and rotate; finger-guided; and multiple techniques), and extra airway maneuvers (jaw thrust; head extension; mouth opening; and multiple maneuvers).

Association between predictors and outcomes

We then assessed for any association between each predictor and success of insertion. We also looked at possible relationships between successful insertion and positive outcomes. These assessments were performed via Chi-square tests for categorical predictors, Kendall tau-c tests for ordinal predictors, and logistic regression for continuous predictors. Where appropriate, Spearman correlation was performed between predictors to look for confounding effects.

Statistical analysis

All statistical tests were performed using Predictive Analytics Software Statistics 22 (IBM Corporation, New York, 2013) and Microsoft Excel 2013 (Microsoft Corporation, Redmond, 2012). Graphs were plotted using GraphPad Prism 5 (GraphPad Software, La Jolla, 2007). In most cases, a result was considered significant if $p<0.05$ by two-tailed test. The exception was the use of a one-tailed test in comparing our observed success rate to an a priori success rate of 95%; we were only clinically interested if success rate was lower than this figure (see Sample collection).

Results

Outcomes

For this study we were able to collect a total of 67 cases. The general characteristics of this sample are described in Table 2, while the results for the outcomes of interest are described in Table 3. The overall success rate was 78%, which is significantly lower than an assumed a priori success rate of 95% ($p<0.0001$, one-tailed binomial test). The proportion of all cases where the number of insertion attempts was less than three was 89%. Also 66% of cases had an ease of insertion score less than three; 84% of cases had a CSP score of less than four (i.e. CSP greater than 15 cmH_2O); and 85% of cases did not require any SAD repositioning.

Property	Sample size	Value
Sex	67	33 male (49%)

		34 female (51%)
Weight in kg; mean (SD)	61	81.1 (23.0)
Mallampati score[a]; median (IQR)	50	2 (1 to 2)
Thyromental score[a]; median (IQR)	51	2 (2 to 2)
SAD size; median (IQR)	66	4 (3 to 4)
Dentition status	51	39 full set (76%)
		8 partial set (16%)
		4 edentulous (8%)
Level of training of operator performing SAD insertion	65	8 by resident (12%)
		21 by junior registrar (32%)
		7 by senior registrar (11%)
		29 by consultant (45%)
Previous experience with GuardianCPV	67	13 with 0-4 trials (19%)
		14 with 5-10 trials (21%)
		39 with >10 trials (58%)

SD=Standard Deviation; SAD=Supraglottic Airway Device; [a]Mallampati score: 1=complete visibility of uvula; 2=incomplete visibility of the uvula; 3=visibility of soft and hard palate only; 4=visibility of hard palate only; Thyromental score: distance between thyroid notch and mentum (chin); 1=<6 cm; 2=6 to 8 cm; 3=>8 cm; Mallampati and thyromental scores are used by anaesthetists to judge airway dimensions and intubation difficulty.

Table 2: General characteristics of analyzed sample.

Outcome	Sample size	Value	Association with overall success
Overall success	67	52 (78%)	
Insertion attempts, median (IQR)	66	1 (1 to 2)	p=0.001
Insertion attempts <3	66	59 (89%)	p=0.032
Ease of insertion scorea, median (IQR)	67	2 (2 to 3)	p=0.01
Ease of insertion score <3	67	44 (66%)	p=0.003
CSPb score, median (IQR)	60	2 (1 to 3)	p<0.0001
CSP score <4	60	50 (83%)	p<0.0001
No SAD repositioning required	64	54 (84%)	p<0.0001

aEase of insertion score: 1=device slipping in without effort; 3=required additional assistance; 5=complete failure of insertion; bCSP=cuff seal pressure; CSP score: 1=>30 cmH_2O; 2=22.5 to 30 cmH_2O; 3=15 to 22.5 cmH_2O; 4=<15 cmH_2O but ventilation achievable; 5=no ventilation possible

Table 3: Outcomes of interest and relationship with success.

Successful insertion was significantly associated with fewer attempts at insertion, (p=0.001); easier insertion (p=0.012); higher CSPs (p<0.0001); and reduced need for SAD repositioning (p<0.0001).

Predictors of success

Statistical tests were performed to individually assess each predictor and its relationship with the success of each case; the results of these are summarized in Table 4.

Predictors	Association with overall success
Patient-related	
Patient sex	p=0.72
Patient weight	p=0.28
Airway-related	
Mallampati score	p=0.72
Thyromental distance score	p=0.38
Dentition status	p=0.06
SAD size	p=0.87
Operator-related	
Prior experience with the Guardian	p=0.049*
Training level of Guardian operator	p=0.18
Technique-related	
Degree of cuff inflation	p=0.18
Insertion technique	p=0.12
Type of extra airway maneuver used	p=0.11
SAD=Supraglottic Airway Device	

Table 4: Predictors of interest, and relationship with success.

Chi-square tests did not identify any significant relationship between success rate and patient sex (p=0.72) or weight (p=0.28). Neither was there any significant relationship between success rates and airway-related parameters, such as Mallampati score (p=0.72), thyromental distance (p=0.38) and SAD size (p=0.87). A mild trend was noted with dentition status (p=0.06): greater chances of success were observed with fewer teeth (100% for edentulous patients, *vs.* 71% for patients with full sets).

Previous operator experience with the Guardian was associated with greater chances of success (p=0.049). An 87% success rate was observed amongst those with an experience score of 3 (>10 times prior use of the Guardian), *vs.* 62% with experience score 1 (0-4 times prior experience). Also, Spearman correlation revealed a weak negative trend between experience with the Guardian and ease of insertion ($\rho(67)$=-0.265, p=0.030); those who had more experience appeared to give lower (i.e. better) scores for ease of insertion. There was no significant association between operator training level and success rate (p=0.18).

In terms of the level of cuff inflation (recorded n=63), 25 cases (40%) were fully deflated, 36 cases (57%) were partially inflated, and 2 cases (3%) were fully inflated. There was no significant relationship between degree of cuff inflation and success rate (p=0.18). Spearman correlation did not find any relationship between cuff seal pressure and degree of cuff inflation ($\rho(61)$=-0.028, p=0.832).

With regards to insertion technique (recorded n=67), the most popular techniques in descending order were sideways and rotate (52%); pen grip (25%); upside-down and rotate (10%); and finger-guided (6%); multiple techniques were used in the remaining 7% of cases. A Chi-square test did not identify any relationship between technique used and success rate (p=0.12). Overall, when used singularly, most of the techniques appeared to demonstrate a success rate of 75 to 88%; upside-down and rotate had a 100% success rate, but sample size was small (n=7).

In relation to extra airway maneuvers, 41% of cases did not require the use of any type of maneuver, while 59% required use of at least one maneuver (n=39). Of these 39 cases, the most popular maneuvers in descending order were jaw thrust (48%), head extension (13%), and mouth opening (10%); multiple maneuvers were used in the remaining 30% of cases. Chi-square testing did not identify any relationship between maneuver used and success rate (p=0.11).

Discussion

Context of this study

In general, the clinical evaluation of SADs is complicated by a number of practical limitations; the relative infrequency of difficult airways and airway complications often necessitates high-powered, multicentre studies [13], and the subsequent cost and difficulty renders such trials an unattractive option. Lately non-inferiority trials of airways devices have been employed [14]; these found that most popular second-generation SADs (i.e. LMA Supreme, i-gel, and Proseal LMA) yielded comparable or slightly superior results to the older SADs (i.e. LMA Classic) [15-19]. This may be due to features that distinguish second-generation SADs from first-generation, including improved pharyngeal and oesophageal sealing, and the presence of gastric drains and integral bite blocks. Second-generation SADs feature the separation of the gastrointestinal and respiratory tracts, which theoretically provides additional protection against aspiration [20]. Although the UK NAP4 Study currently recommends the use of second-generation SADs over older SADs [20], it is still not yet clear whether all second-generation SADs, particularly the Guardian, have the same performance overall. The ever-increasing market for airway devices poses the challenge of ensuring that each device is rigorously validated before widespread use.

At the time of conducting this study in 2013, there was only one previous study evaluating the efficacy of the Guardian, with a further study published after the completion of our study. Tiefenthaler et al. found that both Guardian and Supreme yielded 100% successful insertion rates (n=60 each) with trained anesthetists, and that the Guardian offered slightly superior OLP to the Supreme (31 *vs.* 27 cmH$_2$O, p<0.0001) [10]. Some limitations of this study include all patients being female and paralyzed, and all insertions having been performed by one of two consultant anesthetists experienced in the use of both models. The subsequent 2015 study by Pajiyar et al. showed 95% success rates of Guardian insertion with an insignificant difference to rates of Proseal insertion (n=40 each, p>0.05) with slightly superior OLP (32 *vs.* 29 cmH$_2$O, p<0.05) [11]. Limitations of this subsequent study were similar, with all patients being female and paralyzed. A number of other devices have been similarly trailed on patients undergoing surgery (Table 5). Our study contributes new data from a real-life application of this device in a tertiary teaching hospital.

	Compared Devices	First attempt success rate	P value	Oropharyngeal leak pressure (cmH$_2$O)	P value
Tiefenthaler et al.	Supreme	100%	N/A	27	p<0.0001
	Guardian	100%		31	
Pajiyar et al.	Proseal	97.50%	p>0.05	29	P<0.05
	Guardian	95%		32	
Belena et al.	Supreme	96.70%	p<0.01	26.8	p<0.01
	Proseal	71.20%		30.7	
Lee et al.	Supreme	94%	p>0.05	27.9	p<0.01
	Proseal	91%		31.7	
Eschertzhuber et al.	Supreme	95%	p>0.05	21-28	p<0.0001
	Proseal	92%		29-34	
Ragazzi et al.	Supreme	77%	p<0.05	29	p<0.01
	i-gel	54%		23	
Chew et al.	Supreme	97.80%	p>0.05	25.6	p<0.001
	i-gel	93%		20.7	
Teoh et al.	Supreme	94%	p>0.05	26.4	p>0.05
	i-gel	96%		25	

Table 5: Comparison with other supraglottic airway devices.

Outcomes with the guardian

Our study found that the success rate achieved at TNH with the Guardian (78%) was lower than that documented in Tiefenthaler et al. (100%) [10] and significantly lower than a reasonable rate of 95%; it was otherwise more comparable with other success rates observed for other second-generation SADs, such as the Supreme [1-3,5,6,9], the previous SAD model employed at TNH. Success with the Guardian was associated with perceived ease of insertion, higher seal pressures, and reduced need for SAD repositioning. Greater than 80% of all cases had positive outcomes with insertion attempts, CSPs, and repositioning requirements. However, ease of insertion remained a problem (66% positive outcome). Our operators subjectively described difficulty passing the tip through the oropharynx, due to the extra length and rigidity of the cuff. All this suggests difficulty with Guardian insertion as a key problem for the staff at TNH.

Experience was a key predictor for success with the guardian

Analysis identified a significant relationship between prior experience with the Guardian and subsequent successful insertion (p=0.049). Those with more experience with Guardian (experience score 3, i.e. greater than 10 times prior use of the Guardian) appeared to achieve higher success rates (87%). This appears to suggest a "learning effect", and that further training and familiarization with the Guardian may ameliorate some of the difficulties experienced by the staff. This is somewhat supported by the statistically-significant correlation between experience and perceived ease of insertion-those who had more experience appeared to find the Guardian easier to

insert. It is likely that the differences in outcome between this study and Tiefenthaler et al. differ due to the increased heterogeneity in population and operator experience in our study.

Trends in insertion techniques with the guardian

Our study identified that the most popular insertion technique for TNH staff was sideways-and-rotate. This was in contrast to the technique reported in Tiefenthaler et al. where both operators in the paper exclusively used a finger-guided technique [10]. The original manufacturer, Ultimate Medical, also recommended using the finger-guided technique for their product (AM Keogh, personal communication). This difference in technique may have had some bearing on overall success rates, although our analysis did not show any significant association between insertion technique and success rates.

Other examined factors did not factor significantly into success with the guardian

Other patient, airway, and technique-related factors did not appear to have any significant impact on success with the Guardian. We did note that edentulous cases tended to have somewhat higher success rates compared to cases with full teeth sets.

Context of questionnaire

The impracticalities of fully studying, in a well-controlled randomized manner, the safety and efficacy of a new device recently introduced in the hospital setting makes it challenging to be done [21], especially routinely. Limited published literature or ones that have potential conflicts of interests, in the form of device manufacturer funding etc., make it difficult for both the hospital and clinicians to determine the suitability of the device for their setting [21,22]. Our study takes into account the heterogeneity of patient population in a tertiary hospital setting with various levels of experiences of the operators, compared to the existing papers. The questionnaire was designed to be broad in order to suitably address these issues, as well as to be able to identify as many factors that may prove of significance for further follow-up or future studies. Key findings from this study can serve as a launching pad or be a study pilot that can assist in more exhaustively investigating factors of interest or significance.

Limitations

This pilot study has successfully identified several limitations, which will contribute to constructing an improved framework for the follow-up study. The non-compulsory nature of case recruitment introduced an element of volunteer bias. Case reporting in the questionnaires, though performed soon after recruitment, was still retroactive and therefore subject to recall bias. The small sample size (n=67), sufficient in identifying significant differences in overall success rates, may have been underpowered to identify subtle relationships between predictors and outcomes. For this particular pilot study, cases with multiple insertion attempts featured the same operator, with the experience level as reported; however, in realistic clinical situations, this is unlikely to be always the case, as an operator who encounters difficulty will likely seek assistance from other more experienced staff. It would be of particular interest to document help-seeking for future studies, as this will reduce selection bias associated with non-reporting of failure amongst junior and less-experienced operators. Finally, it may be useful to seek information on anesthetic procedure in future studies, given that this may also affect ease of insertion of SADs.

Due to practical limitations within this study, much of the data collected had to be re-organized as categorical or ordinal variables, rather than continuous variables. For instance, thyromental distance and CSP had to be converted to ordinal data due to the limited accuracy of measuring implements in theatre. With these limitations in mind, a follow-up study would benefit from the inclusion of a comparison device with an adequately powered sample size and revised questionnaire.

Conclusions

In conclusion, our pilot study demonstrated that the Guardian SAD was comparable in efficacy to other SADs, although not as effective as previously reported by Tiefenthaler. There were perceived difficulties in inserting the Guardian, but there was some evidence that further training and acclimatization to the device could reduce difficulty and increase success rates. Our study paves the way for a follow-up study of this SAD model. The questionnaire had been designed to be suitably broad which had successfully identified key factors of both interest and significance that should aid in streamlining further follow-up studies regarding the Guardian SAD. Ideally, proper auditing and familiarization with new airway devices should take place prior to mass uptake in the clinical setting. However, given that this may prove impractical in the hospital setting, a questionnaire designed similar to ours may assist in identifying safety and efficacy rates of new devices. We should note this study has influenced, in part, to the clinical decision to replace the Guardian SAD with another that had been proven more successful.

Competing interests

All authors have no conflicts of interest to disclose.

Funding

We have no sources of funding to declare.

Authors' contributions

MHL performed data collection and was involved in drafting of the paper. HFT performed statistical analyses and was involved in drafting of the paper. CJB was involved drafting of the paper. JKC was involved in conceptual design and supervision of the project. All authors read and approved the manuscript.

Acknowledgements

We have no acknowledgements to declare.

References

1. Belena JM, Nunez M, Anta D, Carnero M, Gracia JL, et al. (2013) Comparison of Laryngeal Mask Airway Supreme and Laryngeal Mask Airway Proseal with respect to oropharyngeal leak pressure during laparoscopic cholecystectomy: a randomised controlled trial. Eur J Anaesthesiol 30:119-123.

2. Chew EE, Hashim NH, Wang CY (2010) Randomised comparison of the LMA Supreme with the I-Gel in spontaneously breathing anaesthetised adult patients. Anaesth Intensive Care 38: 1018-1022.

3. Eschertzhuber S, Brimacombe J, Hohlrieder M, Keller C (2009) The laryngeal mask airway Supreme--a single use laryngeal mask airway with an oesophageal vent. A randomised, cross-over study with the laryngeal mask airway ProSeal in paralysed, anaesthetised patients. Anaesthesia 64: 79-83.

4. Lee AK, Tey JB, Lim Y, Sia AT (2009) Comparison of the single-use LMA supreme with the reusable ProSeal LMA for anaesthesia in gynaecological laparoscopic surgery. Anaesth Intensive Care 37: 815-819.

5. Ragazzi R, Finessi L, Farinelli I, Alvisi R, Volta CA (2012) LMA Supreme vs. i-gel--a comparison of insertion success in novices. Anaesthesia 67: 384-388.

6. Russo S, Cremer S, Galli T, Eich C, Brauer A, et al. (2012) Randomized comparison of the i-gelTM, the LMA SupremeTM, and the Laryngeal Tube Suction-D using clinical and fibreoptic assessments in elective patients. BMC Anesthesiology 12:18.

7. Teoh WH, Lee KM, Suhitharan T, Yahaya Z, Teo MM, et al. (2010) Comparison of the LMA Supreme vs the i-gel in paralysed patients undergoing gynaecological laparoscopic surgery with controlled ventilation. Anaesthesia 65: 1173-1179.

8. Tham HM, Tan SM, Woon KL, Zhao YD (2010) A comparison of the Supreme laryngeal mask airway with the Proseal laryngeal mask airway in anesthetized paralyzed adult patients: a randomized crossover study Can J Anaesth 57: 672-678.

9. Theiler LG, Kleine-Brueggeney M, Kaiser D, Urwyler N, Luyet C, et al. (2009) Crossover comparison of the laryngeal mask supreme and the i-gel in simulated difficult airway scenario in anesthetized patients. Anesthesiology 111: 55-62.

10. Tiefenthaler W, Eschertzhuber S, Brimacombe J, Fricke E, Keller C, et al. (2013) A randomised, non-crossover study of the GuardianCPV Laryngeal Mask versus the LMA Supreme in paralysed, anaesthetised female patients. Anaesthesia 68: 600-604.

11. Pajiyar AK, Wen Z, Wang H, Ma L, Miao L (2015) Comparisons of clinical performance of Guardian laryngeal mask with laryngeal mask airway ProSeal. BMC Anesthesiol 15: 69.

12. Faul F, Erdfelder E, Buchner A, Lang AG (2007) G*Power 3: A flexible statistical power analysis program for the social, behavioral, and biomedical sciences. Behaviour Research Methods 39: 175-191.

13. Isono S, Greif R, Mort TC (2011) Airway research: the current status and future directions. Anaesthesia 66 Suppl 2: 3-10.

14. Pandit JJ, Popat MT, Cook TM, Wilkes AR, Groom P, et al. (2011) The Difficult Airway Society 'ADEPT' Guidance on selecting airway devices: the basis of a strategy for equipment evaluation. Anaesthesia 66: 726-737.

15. Ali A, Canturk S, Turkmen A, Turgut N, Altan A (2009) Comparison of the laryngeal mask airway Supreme and laryngeal mask airway Classic in adults. Eur J Anaesthesiol 26: 1010-1014.

16. Brimacombe J, Keller C, Boehler M, Puhringer F (2001) Positive pressure ventilation with the ProSeal versus classic laryngeal mask airway: a randomized, crossover study of healthy female patients. Anesth analg 93: 1351-1353.

17. Cook TM, Nolan JP, Verghese C, Strube PJ, Lees M, et al. (2002) Randomized crossover comparison of the ProSeal with the classic laryngeal mask airway in unparalysed anaesthetized patients. Br J Anaesth 88: 527-533.

18. Coulson A, Brimacombe J, Keller C, Wiseman L, Ingham T, et al. (2003) A Comparison of the ProSeal and Classic Laryngeal Mask Airways for Airway Management by Inexperienced Personnel After Manikin-only Training. Anaesth Intensive Care 31: 286-289.

19. Lu PP, Brimacombe J, Yang C, Shyr M (2002) ProSeal versus the Classic laryngeal mask airway for positive pressure ventilation during laparoscopic cholecystectomy. Br J Anaesth 88: 824-827.

20. Cook T (2011) Supraglottic airway devices. In: Major complications of airway management in the United Kingdom. The Royal College of Anaesthetists 2011: 86-95.

21. Ventola CL (2008) Challenges in evaluating and standardizing medical devices in health care facilities. P T 33: 348-359.

22. Baim DS, Donovan A, Smith J, Briefs N, Geoffrion R, et al. (2007) Medical device development: Managing conflicts of interest encountered by physicians. Catheter Cardiovasc Interv 69: 655-664.

A Comparative Evaluation of General Anesthesia versus Spinal Anesthesia Combined with Paravertebral Block for Renal Surgeries: A Randomized Prospective Study

Ahmed Eldaba and Sabry Mohamed Amin*

Department of Anesthesiology and Surgical Intensive Care, Faculty of Medicine, Tanta University, Egypt

***Corresponding author:** Sabry Mohamed Amin, Department of Anesthesiology and Surgical Intensive Care, Faculty of Medicine, Tanta University, Egypt, E-mail: sabry_amin@yahoo.com

Abstract

Background: General anesthesia with endotracheal intubation has remained the most common technique used for open renal surgeries because of the abnormal body position and its ability to control the diaphragmatic movement during the surgery. Combined spinal and thoracic paravertebral block (TPVB) can be used as alternative technique for open renal surgery, where spinal anesthesia provides fast and reliable to start the surgery and the duration of anesthesia can be extended with a catheter in the paravertebral space.

Aim of the work: To compare general anesthesia versus combined spinal/paravertebral block in patients undergoing open renal surgeries

Patients and methods: The patients were classified according to anesthetic technique into two groups as follow: Group I: include 50 patients received combined spinal/ paravertebral block. Group II: include 50 patients received general anesthesia. Measurements: -HR and MABP - Surgeon satisfaction - Patient satisfaction - Postoperative analgesia -The time to first dose of analgesia- Side effects such as nausea and vomiting, and shivering were noted.

Results: The MABP and HR were increased significantly in group II after intubation while it maintained stable in group I. The Time to first analgesic request was statistically significant longer in group I than group II. No significant differences were found as regards to surgeon's satisfaction between both groups. The patient's satisfaction was better in group I. The incidences of side effects were higher in group II than group I.

Conclusion: Combined spinal and paravertebral block can be safely and effectively used in patients undergoing open renal surgeries.

Keywords: Open renal surgery; General anesthesia; Spinal anesthesia; Paravertebral block

Introduction

Anesthesia for renal surgeries requires certain characteristics include the ability to maintain hemodynamic stability, patients immobility, diaphragmatic control, satisfactory intraoperative and postoperative analgesia, and lower incidence of side effects such as nausea, vomiting, and shivering [1]. General anesthesia with endotracheal intubation remained the most common technique used for open renal surgeries because of the abnormal body position; ensure immobility of the patients and its ability to control the diaphragmatic movement during the operation [2].

A higher incidence of side-effects with general anesthesia leaves bad experience and make general anesthesia unwanted by the patients [3].

Regional anesthesia can be safely used for renal surgeries and associated with stable hemodynamic, decrease blood loss and blood transfusion with prolonged postoperative analgesia and fewer side effects, so, regional anesthesia better alternative to general anesthesia [1,2,4].

A paravertebral block (PVB) results in unilateral somatic and sympathetic nerve block. The PVB produces a dense afferent block that abolishes somatosensory evoked responses also it blocks the impulse pass through the thoracic sympathetic chain which explain the pre-emptive effect of this technique [5,6].

However, the disadvantages of paravertebral anesthesia include the following, technical failure, local anesthetic toxicity, bilateral block, pneumothorax. Hypotension, vascular puncture, it is more challenging to teach because it requires stereotactic thinking and needle maneuvering. A certain "mechanical" mind or sense of geometry is necessary to master it [7].

The hypothesis of the present study:

1-Combined spinal/paravertebral block is better than general anesthesia as regards to hemodynamics, patient's and surgeon's satisfaction.

2-Combined spinal/paravertebral block is associated with better postoperative analgesia.

3-Postoperative side effects (shivering, nausea and vomiting) are more with general anesthesia.

Aim of the Work

Our study was carried out to compare combined spinal/paravertebral block versus general anesthesia in patients undergoing open renal surgeries as regards to, hemodynamic parameters, surgeon's, and patient's satisfaction, postoperative analgesia and side effects.

The primary outcome was the intraoperative hemodynamic changes, patients and surgeon's satisfaction, and complication. While anesthesia time, operative time, postoperative pain scores and time to fist rescue analgesia were the secondary outcome.

Patients and Methods

Our study was carried out on one hundred adult patients ASA I&II aged 18- 60 years undergoing open renal surgeries after approval of the ethical committee and obtaining written informed consent from each patient. All patients' data were confidential with secret codes and was used for the current study only. Any unexpected risk appears during the course of the study was cleared to the patients and the ethical committee on time and the proper measures were taken to minimize or overcome these risks. The approval code of ethical committee is 2904/11/14. The study duration was 12 months.

Open renal surgeries include pyeloplasty, pyelotomy, pyelolithotomy, nephrolithotomy and nephrectomy.

Exclusion criteria

Patients' refusal to share in the study, coagulopathy, patients' on anticoagulant or thrombolytic therapy and hemodynamic instability is the exclusion criteria (Figure 1).

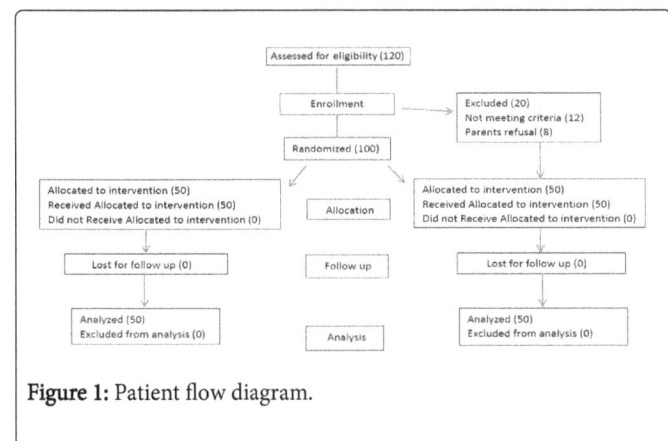

Figure 1: Patient flow diagram.

Preoperative preparation

All patients were underwent preoperative assessment by history taking, physical examination and laboratory investigations which include complete blood count, liver function, renal function, prothrombin time, INR, ECG, blood group and chest x-ray.

Premedication

All patients received 150 mg ranitidine and 10 mg of metoclopramide one hour before anesthesia.

Patients were fasted for 8 hours before the time of operation. On arrival to operating room an intravenous line was inserted. All patients were preloaded with 10 ml/kg ringers solution and were attached to monitor displaying the following: ECG, HR, NIBP, and O_2 saturation and urinary catheter for urine output monitoring. $ETCO_2$ was used in group II only.

The patients were randomly classified using sealed envelope technique into two equal groups according to anesthetic technique as follow:

Group I: Include 50 patients received combined spinal/paravertebral block.

Group II: Include 50 patients received general anesthesia.

Anesthetic technique in group I

PVB was performed while the patients in sitting position, shoulders and head relaxed and leaning forward.

The skin was cleaned with an antiseptic solution, the subcutaneous tissues and paravertebral muscles are infiltrated with 3 ml of Lidocaine 2%. An 18 G Touhy needle was advanced perpendicularly to the skin at T8-T9 level. After the transverse process is contacted, the needle is withdrawn to the skin level and redirected superiorly or inferiorly to "walk off" the transverse process, walking off the inferior aspect of the transverse process is recommended to reduce the risk of intra-pleural placement of the needle. Thoracic PVB space was identified by loss of resistance to air, epidural catheter was inserted 3-4 cm inside the space and 10 ml of 0.5% bupivacaine was injected in the paravertebral space.

After securing the paravertebral catheter, Spinal anesthesia was performed with 25 gauge spinal needle at L3-L4 by injecting 2.5 ml of heavy bupivacaine 0.5% into subarachnoid space.

The sensory level was checked with pin prick method while motor block was assessed with modified Bromage scale (0=no block, 1=inability to raise the extended leg, 2=inability to flex the knee and 3=inability to flex the knee and foot).

The rectus abdominis muscle (RAM) score was used to assess the degree of abdominal muscle relaxation [8].

RAM score ranged from 0 to 5 (0=full motor activity while 5=full abdominal muscle relaxation) score 3 was required for the surgery (Table 7).

The RAM-test was performed as follows: The patient was allowed to lie in the supine position and legs extended. The patient was asked to rise slowly from the supine to a sitting position and the degree of block was assessed.

Patients were placed in kidney (lateral) position after complete establishment of sensory and motor block and received ringer's solution at 5 ml/kg/h.

The patients in this group received a bolus dose of dexmedetomidine (Precedex®, Meditera, 200 µg/2 mL) 0.5 ug/kg over 10 minutes followed by continuous infusion 0.2-0.5 ug/kg/h to maintain sedation between 3-4 by Ramsay sedation score during the surgical procedure.

Ramsay sedation scale

- Patient is anxious and agitated or restless, or both
- Patient is co-operative, oriented, and tranquil
- Patient responds to commands only

- Patient exhibits brisk response to light glabellar tap or loud auditory stimulus
- Patient exhibits a sluggish response to light glabellar tap or loud auditory stimulus
- Patient exhibits no response

The paravertebral catheter was kept in place for 48 hours postoperatively for administration of local anesthetic to control the postoperative pain.

Anesthetic technique in group II

The patients in this group received general anesthesia which induced by fentanyl 2 ug/kg, propofol 2 mg/kg and cisatracurium 0.15 mg/kg. The lungs were ventilated manually for three minutes then endotracheal tube was inserted and secured. Anesthesia was maintained with isoflurane 1% in oxygen. The tidal volume 6-8 ml/kg and respiratory rate 12-14/minutes and were adjusted to achieve SpO_2 $\geq$ 95% and end-tidal CO_2 between 32 and 35 mmHg. Top up doses of fentanyl and cisatracurium were given as needed.

The patients were placed in kidney position where the operative site was placed upper most and received ringers solution at 5 ml/kg/h.

During skin closure, intravenous (IV) infusion of diclofenac sodium (150 mg diluted in 100 Ml of normal saline) and 1gm of paracetamol were given and 100 mg of pethedine was given intramuscular for post-operative analgesia.

After completion of surgery, inhalational anesthesia was stopped and muscle relaxant was reversed with atropine and neostagmine and the patient allowed breathing spontaneously. The ETT was removed when the patients fulfilled the criteria of extubation (spontaneous eye opening, purposeful movement, intact reflex).

After completion of surgery the patients in both groups were transferred to postanesthesia care unit for 24 h and the hemodynamic and side effects were observed.

Hypotension was defined as decease in MABP 25% below baseline and was treated by blouse fluid 250 ml of ringer's solution and 6 mg of ephedrine. Bradycardia was defined heart rate 60 beats/minutes or less and was treated by 0.5 mg of atropine.

Metoclopramide 0.15 mg/kg and dexamethasone 0.15 mg/kg were administered for prophylaxis of postoperative nausea and vomiting (PONV) before the end of surgery. Ondansetron 0.1 mg/kg was administered for treatment of PONV.

Randomization

The randomization was performed using sealed numbered envelopes indicating the group of each patient. A blind nurse who did not participate in patients follow up read the number and made group assignments.

The process of inclusion in the study went on until the required number of patients was reached.

Measurements

- Demographic data.
- HR and MABP as base line and every 5 minutes till end of surgery.

- Surgeon's satisfaction criteria with the anesthesia technique include the surgical field bleeding, immobility of the patient, and degree of muscle relaxation.
- Patient's satisfaction criteria with the anesthesia procedure include any pain, or discomfort during surgery and in the post-operative period and acceptance in the future.
- Postoperative analgesia

The pain intensity was assessed by a person who was blind to study by using VAS scale graded from 0 to 10 (0=no pain, 10=the worst possible pain) in the following time 2 hours, 4 hours, 6 hours, 8 hours, 12 hours, 18 and 24 h hours after recovery.

Postoperative analgesia was given to all patients depending on pain score. If the value was less than 5, intravenous paracetamol 1 gm was given, if the value was more than 5, tramadol 1 mg/kg was given intravenously and recorded. The time to first dose of analgesia and total amount of tramadol used were recorded in all patients.

- Postoperative side-effects such as nausea and vomiting, and shivering were noted.
- Anesthesia time was measured from start of anesthesia to extubation in group II or end of surgery in group I.
- Operative time was measured from skin incision to skin closure.

Quality of surgical field (by the operating surgeon every 30 minutes): with a predefined scale adapted from that of Dolman et al. [9].

1=Minimal bleeding: not a surgical nuisance.

2=Mild bleeding: but does not affect dissection.

3=Moderate bleeding: slightly compromises dissection.

4=Severe bleeding: significantly compromises dissection.

5=Massive bleeding: prevent dissection.

The rectus abdominis muscle (RAM) score was used to assess the degree of abdominal muscle relaxation [8].

Patients were discharged postoperatively when they had no or mild pain (VAS<3), were able to tolerate clear fluids and soft food and had no bleeding and or nausea or vomiting.

Statistical analysis

The sample size required for the study was determined based on the primary outcome measure. A power analysis suggested that a sample size of 48 patients should be adequate to detect a 20% reduction in blood pressure and heart rate with a power of 0.8 (alpha=0.05). However, to avoid potential errors, 50 patients were included in the study.

The statistical analysis was done using SPSS Version 20 for Macintosh.

Comparisons of demographic data, time of surgery, anesthesia time were done by Student's t-test. Two way analysis of variance for repeated measurements was used for heart rate and blood pressure comparison. Mann–Whitney–U test was used for nonparametric measurements including pain score. Values are reported as mean ± SD. P values <0.05 were considered significant.

Results

This study was carried out on 100 patients divided into two groups, 50 in each group. The groups were comparable as regards to demographic data including age, weight, and duration of surgery. The duration of anesthesia was significantly longer in group II than group I (Table 1).

Characters	Group I (N=50)	Group II (N=50)	P
Age (years)	48.7 ± 5.4	52.8 ± 7.5	0.75
Weight (kg)	68.5 ± 8.7	72.6 ± 7.8	0.62
Height (cm)	170.6 ± 10.4	168.4 ± 8.5	0.53
BMI (kg/m-2)	28.4 ± 3.4	26.4 ± 3.4	0.73
Mallampati score	I-III	I-III	0.69
Duration of surgery (h)	3.34 ± 3.5	3.35 ± 3.4	0.74
Duration of anesthesia (h)	3.45 ± 3.8	3.55 ± 4.5	0.03
ASA (I/II)	40/10	38/12	0.61
Male/Female	35/15	36/14	0.78
Time to first analgesic request (h)	12.4 ± 8.55	2.5 ± 1.43	0.001

Values are means ± SD (standard deviation); N=Numbers of the patients; BMI=Body Mass Index

Table 1: Demographic data, duration of surgery, duration of anesthesia, a time to first analgesia.

There were no differences in the baseline heart rates and mean arterial blood pressure in the patients in both groups.

The HR and MABP were increased significantly in group II 5 minutes, 10 minutes, and 30 minutes after intubation and while it maintained stable in group I (Tables 2 and 3).

HR	Group I (N=50)	Group II (N=50)	P value
Base line	84.6 ± 5.62	85.5 ± 7.74	0.45
T1	82.7 ± 8.56	96.5 ± 5.4	0.032
T2	84.7 ± 6.86	92.6 ± 8.65	0.042
T3	84.5 ± 7.55	94.5 ± 6.62	0.035
T4	80.5 ± 6.65	82.8 ± 8.45	0.32
T5	82.7 ± 7.45	84.7 ± 9.54	0.42
T6	84.5 ± 6.65	82.6 ± 8.65	0.54
At end of operation	86.4 ± 7.86	84.5 ± 9.75	0.65

T1=5 minutes after induction; T2=10 minutes after induction; T3=30 minutes after induction; T4=60 minutes after induction; T5=90 minutes after induction; T6=120 minutes after induction

Table 2: Heart rate (beat/minute) changes in both groups.

Pain score after 2 hours was statistically insignificant between both groups (P>0.05), while pain score at 4 hours, 6 hours, 8 hours, and 12 hours in group I was significantly less when compared to group II (p<0.05) (Table 4).

Pain score at 18 h and 24 hours postoperatively was comparable between both groups p>0.05 (Table 4).

MABP	Group I (N=50)	Group II (N=50)	P value
Base line	75.63 ± 9.45	74.54 ± 8.65	0.84
T1	84.6 ± 9.55	92.52 ± 8.45	0.043
T2	86.4 ± 9.65	100.6 ± 10.5	0.032
T3	80.7 ± 9.45	92.4 ± 7.55	0.02
T4	84.6 ± 9.55	88.5 ± 8.76	0. 35
T5	80.7 ± 8.55	86.4 ± 9.86	0. 22
T6	82.5 ± 7.65	86.6 ± 6.55	0. 37
At end of operation	86.23 ± 9.54	90.45 ± 8.55	0. 45

T1=5 minutes after induction; T2=10 minutes after induction; T3=30 minutes after induction; T4=60 minutes after induction; T5=90 minutes after induction; T6=120 minutes after induction

Table 3: MABP (mmHg) changes in both groups.

Time	Group I (N=50)	Group II (N=50)	P value
2 h	0.85 ± 0.73	0.95 ± 0.86	0.65
4 h	0.95 ± 0.87	4.65 ± 0.95	0.001
6 h	2.50 ± 0.61	5.25 + 0.89	0.004
8 h	2.30 ± 0.37	5.90 ± 0.79	0.001
12 h	3.2 ± 0.83	5.55 ± 1.06	0.02
18 h	3.35 ± 0.9	4.40 ± 0.65	0.33
24 h	3.35 ± 0.6	3.45 ± 0.62	0.43

Table 4: Visual analogue scale in both groups.

The Time to first analgesic request was statistically significant longer in group I than group II (Table 1).

The surgeon satisfaction's criteria were comparable between both groups as regards to (degree of muscle relaxation, immobility of the patients and bleeding) and were accepted in the 95% of the patients in group1and 96% in group II (Table 5).

Features	Group I (N=50)	Group II (N=50)	P value
bleeding	48 (96%)	46 (92%)	0.25
muscle relaxation	47 (94%)	48 (96%)	0.74
immobility of the patient	48 (96%)	50 (100%)	0.62
Overall	95%	96%	0.73

Table 5: Surgeon's satisfaction.

The patient's satisfaction criteria were better in group I than group II (Table 6).

The incidences of postoperative side effects were higher in group II than group I as regards to coughing/laryngospasm, sore throat, nausea and vomiting and shivering (Table 8).

Features	Group I (N=50)	Group II (N=50)	P value
Pain relief [n (%)]	48 (96%)	46 (92%)	0.042
Comfort [n (%)]	48 (96%)	46 (92%)	0.03
Overall satisfaction [n (%)]	48(96%)	46 (92%)	0.04
Accept the same anesthesia	48 (96%)	46(92%)	0.02

Table 6: Patient's satisfaction. N= Numbers of the patients.

Muscle power (%)	RAM score	criteria
100	0	Able to rise from supine to sitting position with hands behind head
80	1	Can sit only with arms extended
60	2	Can lift only head and scapulae off bed
40	3	Can lift only shoulders off bed
20	4	An increase in abdominal muscle tension can be felt during effort; no other response
0	5	Full abdominal muscle relaxation

Table 7: Rectus abdominis muscle score. RAM: Rectus Abdominis Muscle.

Characters	Group I (N=50)	Group II (N=50)	P value
Coughing	0%	6 (12%)	0.001
Laryngospasm	0%	6 (12%)	0.001
Sore throat	0%	1 (2%)	0.001
Nausea and vomiting	2 (4%)	10 (20)	0.033
Shivering	3 (6%)	12 (24%)	0.023

Table 8: The incidence of postoperative adverse events. N= Numbers of the patients.

Discussion

Our study demonstrated that, combined spinal/ paravertebral block anesthesia provides good surgical condition with stable hemodynamic, prolonged postoperative analgesia and fewer side effects when compared to general anesthesia group.

While surgeon's satisfaction was comparable in both groups the patient's satisfaction criteria was better in group I than group II.

Our result could be explained by the fact that, the administration of two different anesthesia by different routes on the same patient resulted in improved quality, effectiveness and less side effects.

Combined Spinal /paravertebral anesthesia was chosen in our study; because spinal anesthesia provides fast, reliable anesthesia and good muscle relaxation to start the surgery and the duration of anesthesia can be prolonged with a catheter in the paravertebral space. The Combined Spinal /paravertebral block have many advantages which include, small doses of local anesthetic is used, adequate motor block, and excellent analgesia, no airway manipulation, intact reflexes, and no risk of aspiration.

In the present study, The HR and MABP showed significant increase in group II after intubation which can be explained by the stress response to laryngoscopy and intubation. While the hemodynamic parameters remained almost stable in group I.

Injection of local anesthetic into the paravertebral space results in unilateral block of somatic and sympathetic nerve which lead to anesthesia which resemble unilateral epidural block which associated with stable hemodynamic and less hypotension and bradycardia.

Abdallah et al. [10] and Nakano et al. [11] found the HR and MABP were increased in patients received general anesthesia than in patients underwent regional block which support our findings.

Also, Moawad et al. [12] concluded that, single injection PVB resulted in greater hemodynamic stability than epidural analgesia in patients undergoing renal surgery.

Moreover, Pintaric et al. [13] concluded that, Thoracic paravertebral blockade resulted in more stable hemodynamics and equivalent analgesia when compared to thoracic epidural analgesia.

While the operative time was comparable between both groups the duration of anesthesia was significantly longer in general anesthesia group when compared to combined spinal/paravertebral group.

We keep in mind that, there are many factors affect the operative time and anesthesia time which include, the skill of anesthesiologist and surgeon, and the nature of surgery and type of anesthesia used. Although in our study, operative time is similar in both the groups. This difference is mainly due to anesthesia time which could be explained by the time taken for reversal of muscle relaxant and extubation in the general anesthesia group.

The time to first analgesic request was shorter in general anesthesia group than spinal/paravertebral group and this difference was statistically significant (p<0.05).

Our finding was in agreement with other studies [14-18] which demonstrated that paravertebral block was associated with prolonged postoperative analgesia.

Additionally, Kumar et al. [19] found that the PVB was associated with prolonged postoperative analgesia extended up to 24 hours after surgery and single dose of tramadol was used in the second postoperative day in 48% of the patients.

The exact mechanism of prolonged analgesia of paravertebral block (PVB) was unknown but it may be due to the unique property of producing dense afferent blockade combined with complete block of transmission within the sympathetic chain may be factors that are associated with the extended duration of PVB. Also PVB produces a direct action of the local anesthetic on the spinal nerve, lateral extension along with the intercostal nerves and medial extension into the epidural space through the intervertebral foramina [6].

As regards to surgeon's satisfaction in our study we found no significant differences between both groups.

As our study Haberal et al. [20] did not observe any significant difference in the levels of surgeon's satisfaction during the perioperative period in patients undergoing Living-donor nephrectomy under combined spinal-epidural anesthesia.

Also Karacalar et al. [21] found no difference in the surgeon's satisfaction in patients undergoing percutaneous nephrolithotripsy under Spinal-epidural anesthesia or general anesthesia.

The patient's satisfaction was better in group I and this could be explained by less postoperative nausea and vomiting with prolonged analgesia compared to group II in which the patients received more opioid to control postoperative pain which associated with increased incidence of postoperative nausea and vomiting.

In agreement of the present study, Tangpaitoon et al. [22] found that better patients satisfaction, in patients received regional anesthesia compared to general anesthesia.

Moreover, Bajwa et al. [23] found in their study the surgeon's satisfaction scores were comparable in both groups while patient's satisfaction scores were better in regional anesthesia.

In contrast to our study Singhal et al. [24] found that there was no statistical difference between the general anesthesia group and regional anesthesia group in terms of surgeon and patients satisfaction in patients undergoing total abdominal hysterectomy.

The incidence of side-effects in our study such as nausea and vomiting and shivering were statistically significant higher in general anesthesia group which may be due to use of opioid for intraoperative and postoperative analgesia was linked to nausea and vomiting, while the inhalational anesthetics, unhumidified anesthetic gases, and infusion of unwarmed fluids used during surgery explain the increase in the incidence of shivering in general anesthesia group.

The limitations of the present study, include the following; no control group, we did not measure the amount of blood loss, the scale used for assess the quality of surgical site bleeding was subjective, we did not use ultrasound for paravertebral block, and the general anesthesia group not received regional block.

Conclusion

Combined spinal/ paravertebral block can be safely and effectively used in patients undergoing open renal surgeries, as it provides stable hemodynamic, prolonged postoperative analgesia with better surgeon and patients' satisfaction and fewer side effects.

References

1. Sener M, Torgay A, Akpek E, Colak T, Karakayali H, et al. (2004) Regional versus general anesthesia for donor nephrectomy: Effects on graft function. Transplant Proc 36: 2954-2958.

2. Hadimioglu N, Ertug Z, Bigat Z, Yilmaz M, Yegin A (2005) A randomized study comparing combined spinal epidural or general anesthesia for renal transplant surgery. Transplant Proc 37: 2020-2022.

3. Dogan R, Erbek S, Gonencer HH, Erbek HS, Isbilen C, et al. (2010) Comparison of local anaesthesia with dexmedetomidine sedation and general anaesthesia during septoplasty. Eur J Anaesthesiol 27: 960-964.

4. Akpek E, Kayhan Z, Kaya H, Candan S, Haberal M (1999) Epidural anesthesia for renal transplantation: A preliminary report. Transplant Proc 31: 3149-50.

5. Richardson J, Jones J, Atkinson R (1998) The effect of thoracic paravertebral blockade on intercostal somatosensory evoked potentials. Anesth Analg 87: 373-376.

6. Lönnqvist PA (2005) Pre-emptive analgesia with thoracic paravertebral blockade? Br J Anaesth 95: 727-728.

7. New York School of Regional Anesthesia (2009) Continuous Thoracic Paravertebral Block.

8. Kopacz DJ, Allen HW, Thompson GE (2000) A comparison of epidural levobupivacaine 0.75% with racemic bupivacaine for lower abdominal surgery. Anesth Analg 90: 642-648.

9. Dolman RM, Bentley KC, Head TW, English M (2000) The effect of hypotensive anesthesia on blood loss and operative time during Le Forte osteotomies. J Oral Maxillofac Surg 58: 834–839.

10. Abdallah MW, Elzayyat NS, Abdelhaq MM, Gado AA (2014) comparative study of general anesthesia versus combined spinal–epidural anesthesia on the fetus in cesarean section. Egyptian Journal of Anaesthesia 30: 155-160.

11. Nakano M, Matsuzaki M, Narita S, Watanabe J, Morikawa H, et al. (2005) Comparison of radical retropubic prostatectomy under combined lumbar spinal and epidural anesthesia with that under combined general and epidural anesthesia. Nihon Hinyokika Gakkai Zasshi 96: 11-16.

12. Moawad HE, Mousa SA, El-Hefnawy AS (2013) Single-dose paravertebral blockade versus epidural blockade for pain relief after open renal surgery: A prospective randomized study. Saudi J Anaesth 7: 61-67.

13. Pintaric T, Potocnik I, Hadzic A, Stupnik T, Pintaric M, et al. (2011) Comparison of Continuous Thoracic Epidural With Paravertebral Block on Perioperative Analgesia and Hemodynamic Stability in Patients Having Open Lung Surgery. Reg Anesth Pain Med 36: 256-260.

14. Naja ZM, Raf M, El-Rajab M, Daoud N, Ziade FM et al. (2006) A comparison of nerve stimulator guided paravertebral block and ilio-inguinal nerve block for analgesia after inguinal herniorrhaphy in children. Anaesthesia 61: 1064-1068.

15. Naja ZM, Raf M, El Rajab M, Ziade FM, Al Tannir MA, et al. (2005) Nerve stimulator-guided paravertebral blockade combined with sevoflurane sedation vs. general anesthesia with systemic analgesia for postherniorrhaphy pain relief in children. Anesthesiology 103: 600-605.

16. Naja MZ, Ziade MF, Lönnqvist PA (2003) Nerve-stimulator guided paravertebral blockade vs. general anaesthesia for breast surgery: a prospective randomized trial. Eur J Anaesthesiol 20: 897-903.

17. Naja MZ, Ziade MF, Lo"nnqvist PA (2004) General anaesthesia combined with bilateral paravertebral blockade (T5-6) vs. general anaesthesia for laparoscopic cholecystectomy: a prospective, randomized clinical trial. Eur J Anaesthesiol 21: 489-495.

18. Jamieson BD, Mariano ER (2007) Thoracic and lumbar paravertebral blocks for outpatient lithotripsy. J Clin Anesth 19: 149-151.

19. Kumar N, Arora S, Singh R, Jain S (2014) Lower Thoracic Paravertebral Block as an Adjuvant to General Anesthesia for Renal/ Ureteric Surgeries- A Case Series. Analg Resusc: Curr Res 3: 3.

20. Haberal M, Emiroglu R, Arslan G, Apek E, Karakayali H, et al. (2002) Living-donor nephrectomy under combined spinal-epidural anesthesia. Transplant Proc 34: 2448-2449.

21. Karacalar S, Bilen CY, Sarihasan B, Sarikaya S (2009) Spinal-epidural anesthesia versus general anesthesia in the management of percutaneous nephrolithotripsy. J Endourol 23: 1591-1597.

22. Tangpaitoon T, Nisoog C, Lojanapiwat B (2012) Efficacy and safety of percutaneous nephrolithotomy: A prospective and randomized study comparing regional epidural anesthesia with general anaesthesia. Int Braz J Urol 38: 504-511.

23. Bajwa SJ, Kaur J, Singh A (2014) A comparative evaluation of epidural and general anaesthetic technique for renal surgeries: A randomised prospective study. Indian J Anaesth 58: 410-415.

24. Singhal S, Johar S, Kaur K, Sangwan A (2015) Combined Spinal-Epidural Anaesthesia and General Anaesthesia For Total Abdominal Hysterectomy- A Comparative Study. Indian Journal of Applied Research 5: 81-85.

Permissions

All chapters in this book were first published in JCT, by OMICS International; hereby published with permission under the Creative Commons Attribution License or equivalent. Every chapter published in this book has been scrutinized by our experts. Their significance has been extensively debated. The topics covered herein carry significant findings which will fuel the growth of the discipline. They may even be implemented as practical applications or may be referred to as a beginning point for another development.

The contributors of this book come from diverse backgrounds, making this book a truly international effort. This book will bring forth new frontiers with its revolutionizing research information and detailed analysis of the nascent developments around the world.

We would like to thank all the contributing authors for lending their expertise to make the book truly unique. They have played a crucial role in the development of this book. Without their invaluable contributions this book wouldn't have been possible. They have made vital efforts to compile up to date information on the varied aspects of this subject to make this book a valuable addition to the collection of many professionals and students.

This book was conceptualized with the vision of imparting up-to-date information and advanced data in this field. To ensure the same, a matchless editorial board was set up. Every individual on the board went through rigorous rounds of assessment to prove their worth. After which they invested a large part of their time researching and compiling the most relevant data for our readers.

The editorial board has been involved in producing this book since its inception. They have spent rigorous hours researching and exploring the diverse topics which have resulted in the successful publishing of this book. They have passed on their knowledge of decades through this book. To expedite this challenging task, the publisher supported the team at every step. A small team of assistant editors was also appointed to further simplify the editing procedure and attain best results for the readers.

Apart from the editorial board, the designing team has also invested a significant amount of their time in understanding the subject and creating the most relevant covers. They scrutinized every image to scout for the most suitable representation of the subject and create an appropriate cover for the book.

The publishing team has been an ardent support to the editorial, designing and production team. Their endless efforts to recruit the best for this project, has resulted in the accomplishment of this book. They are a veteran in the field of academics and their pool of knowledge is as vast as their experience in printing. Their expertise and guidance has proved useful at every step. Their uncompromising quality standards have made this book an exceptional effort. Their encouragement from time to time has been an inspiration for everyone.

The publisher and the editorial board hope that this book will prove to be a valuable piece of knowledge for researchers, students, practitioners and scholars across the globe.

List of Contributors

Robert L Thurer
Gauss Surgical Inc., Los Altos, CA, USA

Jose Muniz Castro
Department of General Surgery, Houston Methodist Hospital, Houston, TX, USA

Mazyar Javidroozi
Englewood Hospital and Medical Center, Englewood, NJ, USA

Kimberly Burton and Nicole P Bernal
University of California, Irvine School of Medicine, Irvine, CA, USA

Krzysztof Laudanski, Rose Wei and Linda Korley
Hospital of University of Pennsylvania, Philadelphia, USA

Aysun Caglar Torun
Department of Oral and Maxillofacail Surgery, Faculty of Dentistry, Ondokuz Mayis University, Samsun, Turkey

Frikh Mohammed, Abdelhay Lemnouer and Mostafa Elouennass
Department of Bacteriology, Faculty of Medicine and Pharmacy, Military Hospital of Instruction Mohammed V, University Mohammed V, Rabat, Morocco
Group of Research and Study for Antibiotic Resistance and Bacterial Infections, University Mohammed V Rabat, Morocco

Nabil Alem
Department of Bacteriology, Faculty of Medicine and Pharmacy, Military Hospital of Instruction Mohammed V, University Mohammed V, Rabat, Morocco

Adil Maleb
Faculty of Medicine Oujda, University Mohammed First, Morocco

Mukesh Tripathi
Department of Anesthesiology, All India Institute of Medical Sciences, Rishikesh, India
Department of Anesthesiology, Sanjay Gandhi Postgraduate Institute of Medical Sciences, Lucknow, India

Sanjay Kumar
Department of Anesthesiology, Sanjay Gandhi Postgraduate Institute of Medical Sciences, Lucknow, India

Nilay Tripathi
Internist, Department of Medicine, King George's Medical University, Lucknow, India

Mamta Pandey
Department of Emergency Medicine, Sanjay Gandhi Postgraduate Institute of Medical Sciences, Lucknow, India

Catarina Barbosa Petiz
Instituto Ciências Biomédicas Abel Salazar, Universidade do Porto, Porto, Portugal

Humberto S Machado
Instituto Ciências Biomédicas Abel Salazar, Universidade do Porto, Porto, Portugal
Serviço de Anestesiologia, Centro Hospitlar Universitário do Porto, Porto, Portugal
Centro de Investigação Clínica em Anestesiologia, Centro Hospitalar Universitário do Porto, Porto, Portugal

Alaa M Atia and Khaled A Abdel-Rahman
Anesthesia Department, Faculty of Medicine, Assiut University, Egypt

Ahmed Medhat Ahmed Mokhtar Mehanna
Lecturer of General Surgery, Ain Shams University, Egypt

Atteia Gad Ibrahim
Lecturer of Anesthesia, Tanta University, Egypt

Mona Mohamed Mogahed, Atteia Gad Anwar, Rabab Mohamed Mohamed, Wessam Mohamed Nassar and Mohamed Ali Abdullah
Faculty of Medicine, Tanta University, Egypt

Seyed Mohammad Mireskandari, Kasra Karvandian, Yashar Iranpour, Sanaz Shabani, Afshin Jafarzadeh, Shahram Samadi, Jalil Makarem, Negar Eftekhar
Department of Anesthesiology & Critical Care, Imam khomeini Hospital Complex, Tehran University of Medical Sciences, Tehran, Iran

Jayran Zebardast
Department of Electronic Learning in Medical Education, Statistics Expert, Deputy of Universality affairs, Imam Khomeini Hospital, Tehran University, of medical sciences, Tehran, Iran

Aslan Bilge, Arıkan Müge, Gedikli Ahmet, Kısa Karakaya Burcu and Moraloğlu Özlem
Zekai Tahir Burak Education and Research Hospital, Turkey

Madhu Mala, Prabha Parthasarathy and Raghavendra Rao
Department of Anaesthesiology, Bangalore Medical College, Karnataka, India

Sabry Mohamed Amin, Mohamed Gamal Elmawy and Rabab Mohamed Mohamed Ahmed Eldaba
Departments of Anesthesiology and Surgical Intensive Care, Faculty of Medicine, Tanta University, Egypt

Tomo Hayase, Shunsuke Tachibana and Michiaki Yamakage
Department of Anesthesiology, Sapporo Medical University School of Medicine, Sapporo, Japan

Andreas Liedler, Benedikt Sattler, Ingo Zorn, Christian Fohringer, Sabine Ottenschlager, Herbert Steininger and Christoph Hormann
Department of Anesthesiology and Intensive Care Medicine, University Hospital St Polten, Austria

Rajesh Meena, Sandeep Loha, Arun Raj Pandey, Kavita Meena, Anil Kumar Paswan, Lalita Chaudhary and Shashi Prakash
Department of Anaesthesiology, BHU, India

Reena Nayar and Jui Lagoo
Department of Anesthesiology, St Johns Medical College Hospital, Bangalore, India

Chandra Kala
Department of Pediatrics, St Johns Medical College, Bangalore, India

Mohamed F Mostafa and Ragaa Herdan
Department of Anesthesia, Faculty of Medicine, Assiut University, Egypt

Mohammed Yahia Farrag Aly
Department of Surgery, Faculty of Medicine, Assiut University, Egypt

Azza Abo Elfadle
Department of Clinical Pathology, Assiut University Hospital, Assiut, Egypt

Amit Lehavi, Vitaliy Borissovski, Avishay Zisser and Yeshayahu (Shai) Katz
Department of Anesthesiology, Rambam Healthcare Campus, Haifa, Israel

Semagn Mekonnen
Department of Anesthesiology, Dilla University, Dilla, Ethiopia

Kokeb Desta
Department of Anesthesiology, Debre Birhan University, Debre Birhan, Ethiopia

Bassant M Abdelhamid
Lecturer of anesthesia, Cairo University, Egypt

Inas Elshzly and Sahar Badawy
Professor of anesthesia Cairo University, Egypt

Ayman Yossef
Assistant Lecturer of Anesthesia, Cairo University, Egypt

Carolina Tintim and Humberto S Machado
Largo Professor Abel Salazar, Centro Hospitlar do Porto, Serviço de Anestesiologia, Portugal

Fei Liu, Hai B Song and Jin Liu
Department of Anesthesiology, West China Hospital, Sichuan University, Chengdu, Sichuan 610041, People's Republic of China

Fu S Lin
College of Medicine, Sichuan University, Chengdu, Sichuan 610041, People's Republic of China

Yong G Peng
Department of Anesthesiology, College of Medicine, University of Florida, Gainesville, Florida, USA

Li Liu
School of Computing, National University of Singapore, 117417, Singapore

Massimiliano Meineri
Department of Anesthesia and Pain Management, Toronto General Hospital, University Health Network, 200 Elizabeth Street EN 3-442, Toronto, ON, M5G 2C4, Canada

Natesh Prabu, Alok Kumar Bharti, Ghanshyam Yadav, Vaibhav Pandey, Yashpal Singh, Anil Paswan, Bikram Kumar Gupta and Dinesh Kumar Singh
Institute of Medical Sciences, Banaras Hindu University, Varanasi, India

Levantesi Laura, Oggiano Marco, Fiorini Federico, Sessa Flaminio, Congedo Elisabetta and De Cosmo Germano
Institute of Anaesthesiology and Intensive Care, Catholic University of Sacred Heart, Rome, Italy

De Waure Chiara
Department of Public Health, Catholic University of Sacred Heart, Rome, Italy

Marta Joao Silva
Faculdade de Medicina da Universidade do Porto (FMUP), Portugal
Unidade de Cuidados Intensivos Pediatricos, Centro Hospitalar São João, Porto, Portugal
CMUP-Centro de Matemática da Universidade do Porto, Departamento de Matemática da FCUP, Universidade do Porto, Porto, Portugal

Raquel Pinheiro
Faculdade de Medicina da Universidade do Porto (FMUP), Portugal

Rute Almeida
CMUP-Centro de Matemática da Universidade do Porto, Departamento de Matemática da FCUP, Universidade do Porto, Porto, Portugal
Faculdade de Ciências da Universidade do Porto (FCUP), Portugal
BSICoS Group, Aragon Institute for Engineering Research (I3A), IIS Aragón, Universidad de Zaragoza and CIBER-Bioingeniría, Biomateriales y Nanomedicina, Communications Technology Group (GTC), Zaragoza University, Spain

Francisco Cunha
Centro da Criança e do Adolescente, Hospital Cuf Porto, Porto, Portugal
Center for Health Technology and Services Research (CINTESIS), Portugal

Augusto Ribeiro
Unidade de Cuidados Intensivos Pediatricos, Centro Hospitalar São João, Porto, Portugal

Ana Paula Rocha
CMUP-Centro de Matemática da Universidade do Porto, Departamento de Matemática da FCUP, Universidade do Porto, Porto, Portugal

Faculdade de Ciências da Universidade do Porto (FCUP), Portugal

Hercília Guimaraes
Faculdade de Medicina da Universidade do Porto (FMUP), Portugal
Unidade de Cuidados Intensivos Neonatais, Centro Hospitalar São João, Porto, Portugal

Mian Ahmad and Rayhan Tariq
Department of Anesthesiology and Perioperative Medicine, Drexel University College of Medicine, Philadelphia, PA, USA

OV Teplyakova
Resuscitation and Intensive Care Department, Research Centre for Obstetrics, Gynecology and Perinatology, Ministry of Health of the Russian Federation, Moscow, Russia

EA Filippova, YL Podurovskaya, AV Pyregov, VV Zubkov, AA Burov and EI Dorofeeva
Research Centre of Obstetrics, Gynaecology, and Perinatology, Named after Academician V.I. Kulakov, Ministry of Health of the Russian Federation (MOH), Moscow, Russia

MI Pykov
Russian Medical Academy of Postgraduate Education, MOH, Moscow, Russia

Alaa Mohammed Atia and Khaled Abdel-Baqy Abdel-Rahman
Department of Anesthesia and Intensive Care, Faculty of Medicine, Assiut University, Egypt

Kavita Meena, Rajesh Meena, Sudhansu Sekhar Nayak, Shashi Prakash and Ajit Kumar
Institute of Medical Sciences, Banaras Hindu University, Varanasi, Uttarpradesh, India

Michael Hua-Gen Li, Howard Ho-Fung Tang, Celestine Johnny Bouniu and Jun Keat Chan
Department of Anesthesia and Perioperative Medicine, The Northern Hospital, Australia

Index

A

Abdominal Surgery, 36-37, 39-41, 75, 134-137, 146, 149, 152, 188

Acute Appendicitis, 42-43

Anaesthetics Local, 83

Analgesia, 8-9, 11, 24, 36-37, 40-42, 45, 54, 57, 59-71, 75, 83-84, 87-95, 100-103, 106, 109-112, 124-126, 128-132, 134-137, 140, 146, 149, 164, 179, 182, 196-201

Anesthesia, 8-11, 16, 22-25, 36-46, 53-59, 61-63, 69-72, 74-78, 82, 84, 86-89, 93, 95-114, 120-126, 131, 135, 137, 143, 145, 151-155, 158, 160-172, 179-184, 186-189, 196-201

Antimicrobial Resistance, 21

Apgar Score, 59, 61, 103, 106-107, 117-118, 120-124, 174

Arthroscopic, 83, 85, 87, 125-126, 130

Autonomic Nervous System, 154-155, 163

B

Blood Loss, 1-7, 9, 37, 69, 74-76, 150-153, 196, 201

Brachial Plexus, 83, 87-90, 93-94, 96, 100-102, 129-131

Bupivacaine, 9, 11, 36-37, 39-40, 42, 45, 56, 58-59, 61, 63, 67-68, 86-90, 93-96, 100-102, 118, 125-126, 130, 148-149, 182, 197, 201

C

Cancer, 8-12, 40, 67, 132, 134-136, 138-141, 151

Capnography, 22, 25, 70, 184

Cardiopulmonary Resuscitation, 13, 16

Cardiovascular System-responses, 150

Children, 24, 46, 69-70, 72, 74-76, 106, 108, 111-112, 116, 148, 154-158, 160-163, 170, 174-175, 201

Cognitive Dysfunction, 77, 82

Colonic, 132-141, 148

Colorectal, 11-12, 40, 132-141, 149, 153

Curare Cleft, 22, 24-25

Curare Crest, 22, 24

D

Dentistry, 13-16

Dexamethasone, 43, 71, 83-89, 125-126, 129-131, 198

Dexmedetomedine, 95

Digestive, 132, 173, 176

E

Effect On Neonates, 103

Emergence Agitation, 108-113

Endovascular Coiling, 26-28, 31, 34-35

Epidural, 8-9, 11, 36-42, 55-57, 61, 68, 100, 102-104, 107, 123-125, 129, 132, 138, 140, 161, 163, 179, 181, 197, 201

Esmolol, 31, 69-71, 73-76

Experience, 6, 13, 15-16, 29, 34, 52, 57, 63, 66-67, 76, 83, 136-137, 140-142, 144-145, 171, 181, 189, 191-194, 196

F

Fentanyl, 11, 22-23, 36-40, 42-43, 45, 56, 59, 61, 70, 73-76, 84, 101-102, 104, 109, 112-113, 129, 131, 134, 147, 157-161, 163, 170, 184, 186-188, 198

Fluid Therapy, 135, 150

G

Gastrectomy, 112, 132-137, 139-141

Gastrointestinal, 6, 63, 132-137, 140, 192

General Anesthesia, 8-9, 11, 16, 22-25, 36-40, 43, 46, 55, 58, 69-70, 74, 77, 82, 84, 87, 93, 95, 97, 103-109, 111-113, 118, 120-124, 135, 151, 161, 181, 188, 196-198, 200-201

H

Healthy, 55, 140, 154-155, 160, 162-163, 174-175, 195

Heart Rate Variability, 94, 154, 162-163, 188

Hemodilution, 1, 76

Hippocampus, 77-78, 80-82

Hypotensive Anesthesia, 69, 74-76, 201

I

Infusion Therapy, 47, 49-51

Inguinal Hernia Repair, 43, 55, 58, 149

Isat, 26-29, 32-35

K

Ketamine; Lidocaine, 47

Knee Surgeries, 125

L

Labor, 59, 61, 169

Laparoscopic Appendicitis, 42

Laparoscopy, 42-43, 46, 112, 134

Lumbar Plexus Block, 125-126

M

Magnesium, 53, 87, 95-102, 137-138

Monitoring, 6, 22-25, 31, 37, 48, 63-64, 71, 74, 104, 108-109, 112, 116, 134-135, 142, 150-154, 160, 162, 173-174, 176, 187, 197

Multimodal Analgesia, 62-63, 65-67, 136, 140, 146, 148-149

N

Nasal Surgery, 69-70, 72, 74-75

Neonate, 103-104, 106-107, 117, 123, 174-176

Neurologic Adaptive Capacity Score, 117, 121-123

Neuropathic Pain, 47, 52-54, 63

Neurosurgical Clipping, 26-28, 31, 34

Nosocomial Infections, 17, 19, 21

O

Obstetric Anesthesia, 103-104, 106

Output, 69-70, 75, 90, 135-136, 150, 152-153, 187-188, 197

P

Pentazocine, 62-67

Peribulbar Anaesthesia, 95, 101

Piroxicam, 62-68

Post-operative Pain Relief, 62, 64, 148

Postoperative, 1-6, 9-11, 29, 31-32, 37, 40, 42, 45, 55, 58, 62-64, 77, 81-83, 87, 89-95, 101, 108-112, 118, 124-141, 146-150, 153, 163, 173, 176, 179-181, 196-198, 200-201

R

Rectal, 67, 132-141

Refractory Trigeminal Neuralgia, 47, 53

Regional, 8-9, 11-12, 36, 42-43, 46, 52-53, 55, 57-59, 63, 66, 83, 87-89, 96, 101-103, 117, 123-126, 130-131, 135-136, 162, 164, 167, 169, 179, 181-182, 196, 200-201

Rocuronium, 70, 84, 95-96, 99-102

Ropivacaine, 40, 57, 83-84, 86-88, 94, 102, 130-131, 146-147, 181

Ruptured Intracranial Aneurysm, 26, 28

S

Sedation, 8, 18, 20, 26, 31, 40, 56, 62-65, 74-76, 89-95, 97-98, 100-101, 109, 112, 126, 134, 146-148, 163, 197, 201

Sevography, 22

Single Shut Spinal Block, 59

Spinal Anesthesia, 42-46, 58, 62-63, 100, 103-107, 117-118, 120-124, 134, 196-197, 200

Subarachnoid Haemorrhage, 26, 28, 34

Surgery, 1-6, 8-14, 23, 28-33, 35-37, 39-43, 46, 55-58, 62-64, 66-67, 69-72, 76, 82-85, 87-103, 108-114, 116, 130-141, 145-162, 164-169, 174, 179-181, 188, 192, 194, 196-201

Surgical Blood Transfusion, 1

T

Thoracic, 20, 36-37, 39-41, 67-68, 114, 135, 197, 200-201

Total Abdominal Hysterectomy, 146, 149, 201

Tramadol, 62-67, 71-73, 89-90, 92, 129, 198, 200

Transcriptome Analysis, 77-78, 80

Transesophageal Echocardiography, 142, 144-145

Transversus Abdominis Plain Block, 146

U

Unruptured Intracranial Aneurysms, 26, 30, 33-35

Urinary Retention, 44-45, 55, 57-58, 125, 134, 136, 139

V

Ventilator-associated Pneumonia, 17, 20-21

W

Web-based Education, 142

www.ingramcontent.com/pod-product-compliance
Lightning Source LLC
Chambersburg PA
CBHW080651200326

41458CB00013B/4811